D0312424

ALSO BY NATALIE ROBINS

Savage Grace (coauthored with Steven M. L. Aronson)

Alien Ink: The FBI's War on Freedom of Expression

*The Girl Who Died Twice: The Libby Zion Case
and the Hidden Hazards of Hospitals*

Living in the Lightning: A Cancer Journal

POETRY

Wild Lace

My Father Spoke of His Riches

The Peas Belong on the Eye Level

Eclipse

Copeland's Cure

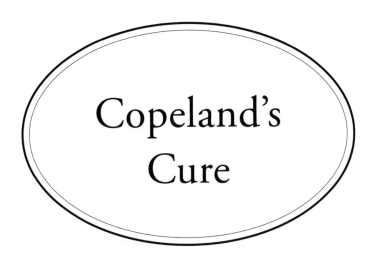

Copeland's Cure

*Homeopathy and the War
Between Conventional and
Alternative Medicine*

Natalie Robins

ALFRED A. KNOPF
New York / 2005

THIS IS A BORZOI BOOK
PUBLISHED BY ALFRED A. KNOPF

Copyright © 2005 by Natalie Robins
All rights reserved under International and Pan-American
Copyright Conventions. Published in the United States by
Alfred A. Knopf, a division of Random House, Inc., New York.
Distributed by Random House, Inc., New York.
www.aaknopf.com

Knopf, Borzoi Books, and the colophon are registered trademarks
of Random House, Inc.

Library of Congress Catalogue-in-Publication Data
Robins, Natalie S.
Copeland's cure : the war between conventional and alternative
medicine in America / Natalie Robins.
p.   cm.
Includes bibliographical references and index.
ISBN 0-375-41090-2 (alk. paper)
1. Copeland, Royal S. (Royal Samuel), 1868–1938. 2. Homeopathic
physicians—United States—Biography.   3. Homeopathy—United
States—History.   4. Alternative medicine—United
States—History.   5. Medicine—United States—History.   I. Title.
RX66.C67R63   2005
615.5'32'0973—dc22   2004048325

Manufactured in the United States of America
First Edition

For Greg Mears, MD,
and F. and R.

It is not enough to treat a disease by name, as is the practice of the dominant school, or to prescribe for a disease because of the peculiar manifestations which are common to all cases of the same disease. The remedy must be selected to fit the special symptoms presented by the individual patient. When so selected, the remedy fits the disease as the wing of a bird fits the air.

—ROYAL SAMUEL COPELAND, MD,
"What Is Homeopathy?"
1910

The facts are, the homeopathy of Hahnemann is as dead as a last year's bird nest.

—AMERICAN MEDICAL ASSOCIATION,
June 2, 1938

Contents

Illustrations

(Unless otherwise indicated, the source for the illustrations listed below is the Royal S. Copeland Papers, Bentley Historical Library, University of Michigan.)

Author's Note

I had never heard of Royal Copeland until his name turned up in some preliminary research I did after someone suggested to me that I look into the power struggle between conventional and alternative medicine in America. Eventually, I discovered that he was the person to use to tell the story I was uncovering, a war story that focused on homeopathy, the controversial alternative with definite rules of usage that had been developed in the West and used around the world for nearly two hundred years.

There has never been a biography of Copeland—a doctor, surgeon, homeopath, mayor, dean, commissioner, and senator—except for an unpublished PhD thesis completed in the late 1960s. This unusual man, who helped change medical culture in the states of Michigan and New York, and who championed his beliefs until they were written into a historically important federal law, deserves a full and comprehensive biography. This doesn't pretend to be that book; in fact, it is more a "biography" of homeopathy than of Royal Copeland. My intention from the beginning was to draw only upon the parts of his life that dramatized the life of conventional medicine (also frequently called "standard," "mainstream," "regular," or "traditional" medicine) and homeopathy.

Until I began this book, I'm not even sure I knew what homeopathy was. No doctor had ever suggested I use it, nor had anyone else I knew. But as often happens in such cases, soon after I decided to write about it, I started to hear neighbors and friends mention the sometimes odd, very dilute, remedies they often said "changed their lives." Their stories intrigued me. One neighbor, a newspaper reporter, told me that her two children, a daughter now twelve and a son sixteen, had never needed an antibiotic. She had always given them homeopathic remedies, especially one called Belladonna, made from the poisonous Deadly Nightshade plant, or "Devil's Herb," for ear infections. "It takes the pain right away, and my children have never had to get in the antibiotic and ear tube cycle," she explained. Another neighbor, a young lawyer with three daughters (ages six, nine, and twelve), first treated their ear infections with antibiotics, until she said, "I wised up." One remedy she gave for their colds was *Allium cepa,* made from a red onion. (She told me also that her husband's father was brought up by a mother who, at the onset of a cold, urged him to eat half an onion with hot water.) Both mothers said they wished they could convert the whole world to homeopathy.

How could an alternative often dismissed as the "no medicine medicine" still be in such favor? What does this say about science-based, conventional medicine? What does this mean in the twenty-first century? I decided to try to find out.

The method of action of most standard medications is often pretty much known, or understood on some cellular level, and they all have had extensive clinical studies performed on them, studies done not only at well-known research and medical centers, but studies that have been peer-reviewed, published in standard professional journals, and regulated by the Food and Drug Administration. But the method of action of homeopathic remedies is generally not known, very few of the remedies have gone through extensive clinical studies, and scientific proof is only a distant possibility. But this was changing, I discovered, because many modern homeopaths say they are performing clinical trials with the same discipline used by standard doctors.

In my writing (and life), I always want the two or more sides of every issue to be taken into account, counted, and accounted for. I want even-handed, balanced deliberations about all things, especially those that are considered controversial. I want to hear and analyze and understand the debates. Maybe I am asking the impossible. Maybe, as Wallace Sampson, MD, a leading skeptic of alternative medicine wrote me in an e-mail, there can be no "even-handed" approach to homeopathy, which, he said, "was not developed through rational, scientific channels." He went on to semi-mock me and say that "the equivalent [*of homeopathy*] in other fields would be Robbery in America or Embezzlement in America—even-handed, so we understand the mind of the embezzler—the rationale, the needs, the social justification, people who benefit from it. Analyze the pros and cons of laws against it from both sides—the dominant political authorities' hegemony over the embezzling communities, and the monopoly of the banking and business communities." He told me to "compare the businesses that run on laws and rules, ethics and professional standards as balanced as possible with the embezzling business. Explain the reasons for each's existence. Or better, one on alternative physics . . . free energy, zero energy devices such as energy from gravity and static magnets, perpetual motion machines, cold fusion devices. Those are the physical and economic equals of 'alternative' medicine.'"

Jennifer Jacobs, MD, one of the doctors featured in the last three chapters along with Michael Carlston, MD, writes that "homeopathy is essentially a method of applying drugs. These are drugs, however, that work with the body. These are medicines with eyes and ears." Carlston adds that "homeopathy's most unique capability is to alleviate chronic illness, because treatment of chronic illness is conventional medicine's greatest weakness."

Conventional vs. Alternative.

Here's what I hope is a fair-minded story about their battles.

Prologue

The knives that were once used by doctors to drain blood from the bodies of men, women, and children were folding, triple-bladed instruments with bone handles and highly polished sheaths. Or they were brass spring-loaded twelve-to-twenty-bladed tools that made quick punctures. Sometimes a wooden stick was tapped on the top of the blade handle to help push it into a vein. Always nearby was a shallow bowl—plain or ornate with delicate flowers or birds—to catch the cascading blood as it flowed from the diseased bodies. The pain of multiple incisions in the scalp, neck, wrists, ankles, back, penis, vagina, and forty other sites was invariably excruciating. Just as often the bites of leeches were used as an alternative to knives. Those who survived their bloodletting sometimes got better.

All across America in the eighteenth century and the early decades of the nineteenth, people believed that health was restored because the body's four "humors"—blood, phlegm, yellow bile, and black bile, first noted by the Greek physician Galen in 500 B.C.—were brought into proper balance by a medical therapy that actually dated back to the Stone Age. And if the removal of enough blood to cause the patient to lose consciousness—sometimes as much as 70 percent of the person's blood—didn't bring about a cure, there was always mercury, arsenic, or lead, which purged the body of its excesses if they didn't first poison the patient, or blistering, pulling teeth, sweating, ice, starvation, darkness, and silence. Illness was always dreaded; the popular treatments for it were hell on earth. Even babies were bled.

Royal Samuel Copeland had never been bled. His older sister, Cornelia Alice—"Nellie"—and their parents, Roscoe and Frances, had never been bled. No one in the Copeland family ever had to feel the sharp point of a knife pierce, over and over, the delicate veins of the body. No one had to endure, in the words of Royal Copeland, these "crude and disgusting ways of treating disease" either: "hearts of vipers, earthworms, green lizards, live frogs," or even, "the shavings of a man's skull that dy'd a violent death."

Copeland's Cure

ONE

"Like a Pleasant Dream"

T HE LAND near Dexter, Michigan, flat in some places, rolling in others, was, in the early 1800s, one of the healthiest-looking regions in America. Bordering the Huron River and Mill Creek, the territory was fertile and green. Crystal-clear lakes, rapids, streams, and marshes were surrounded by cottonwood trees, sugar maples, black walnuts, elms, and ashes. Meadows overflowed with wildflowers. Sunfish, perch, and bulletheads flourished in the waters. Red squirrels, grey foxes, turkeys, and wild pigeons roamed the thick woods.

Frances Holmes Copeland's ancestors had traveled from the Berkshires in Massachusetts to a region near Dexter in 1825, the very year it was founded by Judge Samuel William Dexter, who said he came to Michigan from New York "to get rid of the blue devil . . . which like a demon pursues those who have nothing to do." The town, in a county called Washtenaw, was laid out so that every house received sunlight. The early settlers lived in log cabins and grew corn and wheat, and later also barley, oats, clover, and apples. Sawmills soon abounded as lumber became an important business, and before long, the log cabins had sash windows, shingle roofs, and doors. The Potowatami and Mohican Indians lived nearby—first settling near the streams—and the people of Dexter eagerly exchanged liquor, tobacco, flour, or powder and lead for buckskins, beeswax, furs, and venison.

By 1847, when Roscoe Pulaski Copeland arrived in Michigan on a covered wagon with his parents, Joseph and Alice, and ten siblings, from Dexter, Maine (which had been founded by Judge Dexter's father), the

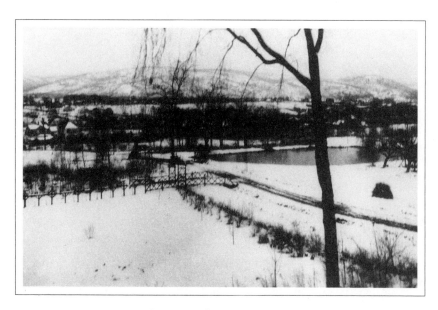

Dexter, Michigan, wintertime

area was thriving. They first rented a log house near Pontiac, in southeast Michigan, and then another log house near what was known as Webster Township, in Washtenaw County. When twelve-year-old Roscoe and his family finally settled in Dexter in the fall of 1850, it was, as he later wrote in a letter, "a busy little village." The family bought an 80-acre farm with an old white frame house and a small barn on Joy Road. Nearby were flour mills—"with farmers coming 20 to 40 miles with their wheat and other crops to sell"—a foundry, several dry-goods stores, a blacksmith shop, a wagon shop, four hotels (the biggest one was the Eagle, until it burned down) and four saloons. Cows, pigs, and chickens freely roamed the dirt roads. There was a small brick schoolhouse, where the children were taught that the world was flat, and four churches—Methodist, Baptist, Congregational, and Catholic. The Copelands were Methodists, and their church, built in 1841, had the only bell tower in the village. "The church was full every Sunday," Roscoe wrote, and "after a two-hour sermon, there was a one-hour recess so neighbors could visit and have lunch and then a two-hour service again."

The village had an apothecary housed in a two-story frame building on Main Street that also sold soaps, brushes, perfumes, paints, and varnishes. There was even a passenger train from Dexter to Detroit. Still, Roscoe wrote, "the first settlers had to go through many hardships . . .

dig out the stumps and stones—split rails to build fences and do all work with ox teams." He and his brothers slept in the unfinished upstairs of their house, and "the snow would blow in it and it was pretty cold for us boys the first winter."

In 1850, the apothecary carried a multitude of medicines—castor oil, camphor, syrups, digestives, salves, opiates, herbals, roots, and tonics of all kinds. Tonics made of licorice, saffron, berries, lime, iron, copper, mercury, arsenic, cyanide, opium, or cocaine, and bitters, which had an extraordinarily high alcohol content, were dispensed to aid the recovery of the men and women who made it through their bloodlettings. Sweet water and morphine was given to babies. Sometimes doctors made their own pills. When Roscoe Copeland and his siblings developed ague, or fever with chills, they were fortunate to be given mild Dr. John Sappington Anti-fever Pills, a well-known medicine made up of ½ grain of quinine and several other ingredients—usually bayberry, spearmint, ginger, yarrow, sassafras, garlic, or cayenne.

Ague was a peculiar illness. "Sometimes the whole family would be in bed," Roscoe explained. "The farm had a lake on the northwest and south. I had to go to school through the woods between two lakes, up a long hill to the school house. . . . I remember one week when school let out at noon I felt a chill coming on and I would start for home and before getting home the chill would be gone and the fever would be on. It would seem as if I would never get home, and Mother would hear me yelling. I would eat a good supper before I went to bed and the next morning feel as well as ever. Then I would go to school again the next day and be all right—but the second day I would have the chills and fever again." Roscoe Copeland said that two or three Sappington pills would break the chills. It was unusual that even one ingredient—in this case, quinine—was known; most patients didn't know what was in the pills they were taking. Secret nostrums, later called "patent medicines" (although there were no laws beyond protection from counterfeiters governing them), were becoming increasingly faddish, although many were of a questionable nature, mostly containing liquor or vegetable extracts. Some even contained dirt—plain, old-fashioned dirt from farmland.

Many residents of the area had heard that during the cholera epidemics of 1832 and 1849, a new kind of medical treatment had saved many lives. Even though the country was still close to twenty years away from the realization that germs caused disease, and over half a century away from the discovery of viruses, something new, or rather something old that had been made new, had been happening in various parts of America since 1827. This was a treatment that was kind to its users. It was called homeopathy, and it seemed to make people feel better than ever. It had helped during the cholera epidemic, if only because it replaced the chloroform given for spasms and cramps, and the purging and bleeding that made the victims of that miserable sickness even weaker.

Founded in 1796 by Christian Friedrich Samuel Hahnemann, a German doctor, literary scholar, translator, and uncompromising dreamer with a bad temper who was appalled by the harsh approaches to treating illness, homeopathy, a term he coined, expounded the principle of *Similia similibus curantur*—Like cures like. The doctor, known as Samuel Hahnemann, demonstrated on himself and many others in a series of what he called "provings" that certain substances had a curative effect if used in a special way. First, the substance had to resemble the very illness it was treating, and second, the substance had to be given in the smallest possible dose. These two "rules" were the exact opposite of the ones that other doctors followed. These doctors, or allopaths, as Hahnemann called them (*allos:* other), were also referred to as the "dominant" practitioners of the time, and they used large doses of substances that were very different from—in fact, the opposite of—the illnesses they were treating. Most doctors treated fever not only with bloodletting, but with great quantities of laxatives, such as jalap root, made into a powder, which also brought on strong bouts of nausea; emetics, such as toxic tartar crystals or powder, which also produced heavy sweating; large doses of lethal mercury (calomel)—sometimes 4 tablespoons or more a day—black pepper in whiskey, chloroform, zinc, iron, or cold baths and cold drinks. Blistering was a common treatment. Lethargy, weakness, or collapse was treated with quarts of whiskey or wine, rhubarb, massive doses of opiates such as opium, or even huge portions of roast beef. Those with toothaches often had their gums bled and blistered. Earaches were treated not only with purging, but with blistering of the ear lobes. Many doctors believed that specific organs had a separate existence from the body as a whole, or that most diseases were caused by impediments in the intestines, or that a poisonous fluid emanated from the hands. Some doctors believed that hair was a direct link to the body's entire nervous system.

The same year that homeopathy was founded, a smallpox vaccine had been discovered by the Englishman Edward Jenner. This vaccine was akin to homeopathic principles in that it used a small amount of cowpox disease to prevent smallpox. Hahnemann himself praised Jenner's discovery as an excellent example of the law of similars.

Hahnemann and his followers used small quantities of common herbs and minerals, various plants, mushrooms, barks, and insect, shellfish, or animal products. Wild hops, jasmine, tiger lilies, poison ivy, silver nitrate, lead, carbon, salt, onions, toadstools, sponges, oyster shells, spiders, human tears, extract of lice, gonorrhea discharge, and milk from female dogs. Most everything he and his followers used had been known for centuries—in ancient Egyptian, Greek, and Roman civilizations, in ancient Far, Mid, and Near East cultures, as well as in Native American tribes.

What was new was its method. Small doses. Like cures like. Because of its very special and distinctive methodology, homeopathy was a wholly Western invention, and it marked the beginning of the first worldwide, systematic option to bloodletting. Because of its painlessness, lack of side effects, and relative simplicity, homeopathy caught on like wildfire across America. It quickly swept aside another favored approach, something called Thomsonianism, a movement founded in New England which held that disease was caused by cold, and treatable by heat through the use of steam baths and certain pungent herbs that could clear the body's clogged systems. The John Sappington pills given to the Copeland boys were created by a Thomsonian doctor, who was also a savvy businessman. Dr. Sappington, always opposed to bloodletting, was later influenced by another botanical system called Eclecticism, a hodgepodge of allopathic, Thomsonian, and homeopathic theories that had come into existence in 1845.

Hahnemann had first discovered his theory of medication by ingesting large amounts of cinchona bark, or quinine, to see what would happen to his healthy body. He reported that "my feet, finger ends, etc., at first became cold. I grew languid and drowsy; then my heart began to palpitate and my pulse grew hard and small, intolerable anxiety; trembling, but without cold rigor. . . ." What happened was that he began to get the symptoms of malaria. He soon decided that if a large quantity of quinine could bring on the symptoms of malaria, then a small dose might be able to cure the disease. (Full-strength quinine had been in use for centuries as an antidote to malaria and fever, but it wasn't known why it seemed to help only sometimes. However, most allopathic doctors treated malaria not only with large doses of it—sometimes as much as

100 grains—but also with colonics and purgatives that left patients in a state of catastrophic exhaustion.) Hahnemann's experiments with small doses had successful results, even though Hahnemann still couldn't explain exactly why the bark was a cure for malaria, as well as for disease symptoms like nervous exhaustion, loss of body fluids, or certain types of headaches. But he saw that it worked. He believed in his provings. He also showed that lethal Belladonna, which brings on hallucinations and flushed skin—two symptoms of scarlet fever—could treat that disease if given in small doses. (The "dominant" doctors had long used large doses of it to treat spasms, and Indian tribes had used it for pain in general.) Pulsatilla, made from the windflower, a plant that can cause burning in the throat, was used by Hahnemann for coughs. (Roman doctors had used it for eye problems.) Nux Vomica, a toxic tree seed, from which strychnine poison is extracted, was given to aid digestion. (The dominant doctors often used it as a nerve stimulant.) Aconite, a poisonous plant once applied by hunters to their arrows, was used for severe pain and fever. Eventually, as homeopathy evolved, minute doses of opium were given to patients who had convulsions and a weak pulse (a symptom of an opium overdose). Bees were used to treat insect stings. Ambrosia, or ragweed, was used to help alleviate hay fever.

Hahnemann reported that he experimented with around one hundred different remedies. In every single case, he used small doses, and he came to believe that no substance was poisonous if taken in the proper quantity. In 1810, he published his discoveries in a book, *Organon of Homeopathic Medicine,* which had gone through six editions by 1842, the year before his death at the age of eighty-eight. "The highest ideal of cure is rapid, gentle, and permanent restoration of the health," he wrote in the Introduction. He also believed in prescribing one remedy at a time and concluded that only through a detailed evaluation of the patient would the correct remedy be discovered.

Hahnemann prepared most of his medicines by dissolving them in water or alcohol, which produced what he called the "mother tincture"; some of the materials he used were insoluble, so he first ground them into a powder. He eventually came up with the idea of the infinitesimal dilution after discovering that in many situations the body could best be healed with the highest possible dilution of the mother tincture. Dilutions, or what he called "spiritized medicinal fluids," of 1 part substance plus 9 parts water or alcohol, for a total of 10 drops, were designated by

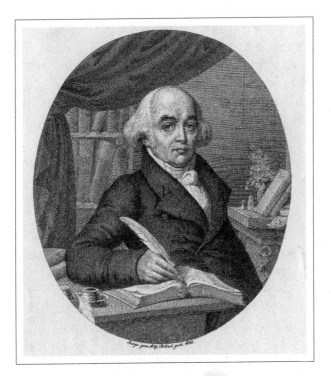

Samuel Hahnemann, MD

the Roman numeral X, and those of 1 to 100 (actually 1 part substance plus 99 parts water or alcohol, for a total of 100 drops) were designated by the Roman numeral C. Thus, 1X equaled and became known as 1:10, 2X equaled and became known as 1:100, and 3X equaled and became known as 1:1000, and 1C equaled and became known as 1:100, 2C equaled and became known as 1:10,000, and 3C equaled and became known as 1:1,000,000. He referred to the process of dilution not only as "potentization," but as "dynamization," and believed the medications must be shaken, rubbed, and banged upon forcefully because these steps, which he called "succussion," would make them even more potent. He said that the succussion developed "the latent, hitherto unperceived, as if slumbering hidden dynamic powers" of the raw material. (After succussion, a drop of 1C remedy, which is 1 part mother tincture and 99 parts water or alcohol, could then be mixed with 99 parts water or alcohol to become a 2C dilution.) Hahnemann wrote that "a well-dynamized medicine whose dose is properly small becomes all the more curative and

helpful, almost to the point of wonder," a sentiment that many homeopaths would come to believe meant that the more a substance is diluted,
the greater its overall power. Sometimes the end product was so much
more water or alcohol than remedy that, in fact, no molecules at all
remained of the original substance. The phenomenon defied the principle of what was called Avogadro's number, which set the point in the
process of dilution where a molecule of any given substance could theoretically no longer exist. (It was formulated in 1811, but not used much
until 1860.) But even if the dilution was so great that its usefulness
seemed to defy logic, it was thought that the solution "remembered"
what once had been in it. Homeopaths believed that the very shadow—
or memory—of the original substance was enough to effect healing. The
diluted substance, or "liquid potency," was generally added to and
absorbed by sugar tablets or pellets, which were then readily stored in
glass jars and easily administered to patients.

Dr. Hahnemann soon promulgated a theory that the body has a
"vital force," and that various substances, when used his way, restored
balance to this force, bringing about full recovery from illness. He further believed that long-term diseases were the result of "psora," an itch
that was the result of a negative spirit. This psora was connected to an
invisible "miasm," or weakness. The miasm contained a "sycosis," which
had its origins in the suppression of the venereal disease gonorrhea, and
a "syphilis," which had its origins in the suppression of the venereal disease syphilis. Later, other facets would be added to the miasm.

In one way, allopathic and homeopathic medicine were the same in
that both believed the body needed to get rid of its disease-causing elements. Many doctors of both persuasions also believed that the soul was
involved in disease, and that the body's very movements and motions—
walking, sitting, stretching, leaning—also had a bearing on illness. But
allopathic medicine got rid of disease primarily with bloodletting and
large doses of substances. Homeopathy got rid of disease with small, gentle doses of substances. Pain vs. Pleasure. This way of thinking soon won
the heart and soul of an America looking for relief beyond what the
Thomsonians or the eclectics could offer, and homeopathic practices,
periodicals, and journals began springing up across the nation like milk-
weed and clover.

In their Sunday sermons, ministers, who, along with members of
their congregation, sometimes received homeopathic tablets at no cost,

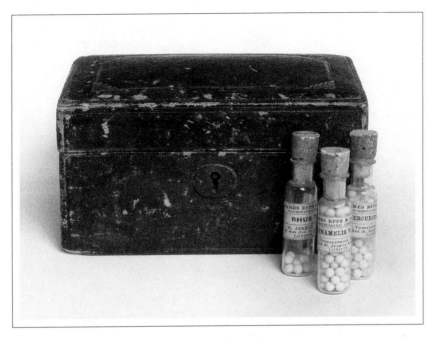

Homeopathic tablets and remedy carrying case

began preaching the benefits of the mild, comforting medicines. (They later even sold remedies.) Women, especially, became enthusiasts, particularly for their children. Invite in the "sugar doctors," the women urged, slowly winning over their more reluctant husbands. By the mid-1850s, homeopathy was being used by many of the 1,225 families in Dexter, and the apothecary, which had opened soon after the town's first doctor arrived from Vermont in 1826, now began to sell "Domestic Kits" filled with small blue-, green-, or clear-glass bottles of the remedies that could be used not only in the privacy of the home, but also over and over again, thus saving money on new medicines or further visits from a doctor. Still, after seeing rows and rows of many appealing jars and bottles with cork or glass stoppers lined up on the shelves—some of domestic origin, and others imported from Europe and the Far East—people sometimes were confused. Were they herbals, tonics, opiates, secret nostrums, or powders and pellets containing homeopathic remedies? At first, there seemed to be no way of knowing what was what, or what did what.

"After we went through those chills and fever for years, and found out

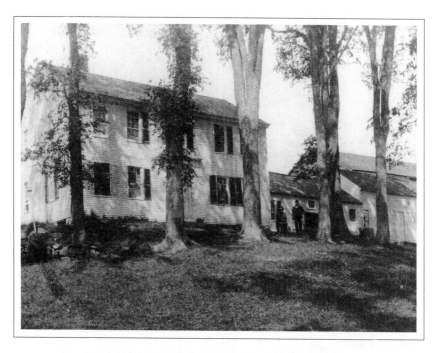

Royal Copeland's childhood home, in Dexter, Michigan, circa 1879

that quinine was the remedy," Roscoe Copeland wrote, "I heard Mother say that if she had known about the remedy she would have bought a ½ pound if they had to sell the last cow."

ONE SUNNY afternoon during the summer of 1879, eleven-year-old Royal Samuel Copeland, called Roy by his family, and his fifteen-year-old sister Cornelia, or "Nellie," stood by the open door of their parents' bedroom in the house on Huron Street in Dexter. Their father, Roscoe, age forty-one, lay in bed, deathly ill. From the side window they could see their mother's garden, full of yellow roses, white snapdragons, red carnations, and helitropes. Nearby, Roy had his own garden of white daisies, sweet williams, and wildflowers—butterfly weed, field thistles, buttonbushes, and showy sunflowers.

By 1879, many people in Michigan had embraced homeopathy with the fervor of religious fanatics. If they needed a doctor, they now wanted only a homeopathic one. Indeed, Dr. Edgar Frank Chase had recently opened his homeopathy practice in Dexter, and it was well known that he had received the same kind of medical training as a dominant doctor, except that he had the added bonus of learning about Hahnemann's therapeutics and remedies.

Roscoe Copeland was no longer a farmer, later telling his children that "farming began to get pretty hard work indoors and out," and so he began a lumber and building-materials business and moved to the center of town.

Roy watched as his petite mother, Frances, paced next to the bed. No one shooed him away from the door. As he watched with his sister, his thoughts drifted, he later said. He wondered if there would be a moon that evening. If there wasn't, he'd do his work as the village lamplighter, for which he was paid $8 a month. If there was a moon, well, he wouldn't have a job that night. The moon would light the evening.

Breaking into his reverie, his mother suddenly motioned him and Nellie into the kitchen. Two of his uncles were there. As Roy later wrote, "I sat in the wood box and listened to the lamentations of my relatives. Their fear gave me visions of a well-ordered country funeral, and I could almost hear the slow and measured tread of the mourners. The end of the world seemed near at hand. About that time the door burst open and in marched Grandmother. 'What is the matter?' she cried. Hearing that Roscoe was sick, she proceeded at once to the sickroom to examine the patient. Very shortly, she came forth with her diagnosis, 'lung fever.' "

Because Grandmother Alice Copeland saw the urgency of the situation, she didn't wait for Dr. Chase, who no doubt would have prescribed a tiny dose of two poisonous substances, Bryonia, or wild hops (often used for inflammation, headaches, coughs, and extreme pain) and Gelsemium, or yellow jasmine (often used for colds, headaches, and eye problems), or perhaps Belladonna. There was no time for that, and Dr. Chase probably would have agreed. So Grandmother Alice reached into her other domestic medicine chest. As Roy explained, "Grandmother ordered one member of the family to build a fire in the kitchen, another to fill the wash boiler and place it on the stove. Another member of the family was sent to the corncrib to get a dozen of the biggest and longest ears of corn that could be found. These were dumped into the wash boiler, while another member of the family tore up an old sheet in pieces eighteen inches square. By this time the fire was roaring and the water boiling. One by one, the ears of corn were wrapped in the linen, and I was on the run between the wash boiler and the sick bed, where Grandmother packed the steaming rolls around the patient. In an hour's time, he was in a pouring perspiration and red as a boiled lobster. Grandmother announced in triumphant tones, 'the fever is broke.' "

"As a very little boy I wanted to be a doctor," Roy Copeland said. His father's bout with "the onslaught of the angel of death," as he put it, would forever change his life, particularly when he saw the benefits of healing with "like cures like." His grandmother was following Thomsonian heat, or steam treatment, using heat to cure fever. It was not as brutal as allopathic treatments, especially the still-popular blue pills containing mercury, and Roy, observing carefully, would eventually follow a medical model—homeopathy—that he said was "like a pleasant dream."

"MY EARLIEST recollection is driving the old gray horse of our family physician," Roy recalled about Dexter's homeopathic physician. They had become pals right away, and the eleven-year-old revered Dr. Chase for his concerned eyes, his compassionate voice, and his ability to listen, to really listen to everything said to him. Young Roy also admired the country doctor's flair for business. He was one of the founders of the Dexter Savings Bank and was its first vice president for several decades.

As a child, Roy was a wanderer, and worried his mother to death, even when he was a toddler. He strayed all over the village on his own, crossing bridges, peeking into the mills and the wagon shop, looking in on the rug weaver, or watching leather shoes and boots being made. Roy, who had graciously curved slender fingers—doctor's hands—was once found by his Uncle Alpheus sitting on the top of a gatepost. "He commenced to climb when he was very young," his father said. Roscoe Copeland finally had to fence in the yard; it would be one of the few times Roy would let himself be restrained.

As he got older, he was given lots of chores to keep his active mind and body busy, and he spent a lot of time tending to his flower garden. Using his father's flintlock shotgun, he hunted for the rabbits, ducks, and wild pigeons that lived "by the millions," he said, in the nearby woods. And like his father, Roy, who also collected rocks and bugs, used to "watch birds to see where they built their nests and the kinds of eggs they laid." Later, he worked in a general store owned by his Uncle Samuel. While he was still in high school, he set type and wrote articles for the *Dexter Leader*, which was a natural development not only of an early gift for instructing, but also a happy consequence of his father's custom of reading aloud to the family—Charles Dickens was a favorite—every evening by the glow of the oil-burning light.

That Roy, as he wrote, once "drove Dr. Chase's gig over the end of a lumber pile," thus causing himself to be "projected from the carriage over the fence into the dooryard of a neighbor, which necessitated some hospital care," was not particularly traumatic for him, because, as he explained, "some of the happiest days I ever had were in a hospital, even as a patient."

This was true for most followers of homeopathy, "the disease-shortening, pain-alleviating method," as Roy would soon call it. But, surprisingly, as favored as homeopathy was when he was growing up in rural Michigan, where smallpox and malaria were the major causes of death, there weren't all that many carefree days for the "life-saving system"—far from it.

THE HOMEOPATHIC doctors had formed the first-ever national medical organization, the American Institute of Homeopathy (AIH), in 1844, twenty-eight years after the introduction of one of medicine's most fundamental diagnostic tools—the stethoscope—and just four years after the arrival of the anesthesias chloroform, nitrous oxide, and ether into general medicine (so pain was no longer a major deterrent to dominant treatments). Three years later, in 1847 (the year Roscoe Copeland and his parents and siblings arrived in Michigan), the dominant doctors formed their own national organization—the American Medical Association (AMA).

One of the first things the AMA did was to ban homeopaths from ever becoming members, even though their then two-year training was identical to that received by the dominant doctors. But the AMA wrote that homeopathy was an alien practice brought to America's shores by greedy, ignorant foreigners "who infest the land," a statement that seemingly ignored the fact that all the early allopaths had been trained in Europe. The AMA added that homeopathy was usually pressed upon innocent people not by physicians but by clergymen—"volunteer missionaries"—known to be antagonistic toward dominant medicine, clergymen, who, moreover, hawked the "evil" remedies to their parishioners. Homeopathy, much mentioned in newspapers, was making men good salaries, taking earnings that should have been allopathy's alone. "The newspaper press, powerful in the correction of many abuses, is too ready for the sake of lucre to aid and abet the enormities of quackery," the AMA announced at its first National Medical Convention in 1846, a year before the group was formally approved.

Most people didn't even know—or care, if they did know—that there were any differences between the two types of doctors. As Roy Copeland would later say, "Those who really practice medicine, who go about daily meeting the sick and the suffering, and trying to get them well are really brothers, no matter to what school they accidentally belong." In fact, the first American homeopaths graduated from the leading medical schools of the day—University of Pennsylvania, Harvard Medical College, College of Physicians and Surgeons of Columbia University in New York, Dartmouth Medical School—and only afterward became converts. Many received their post-medical-school training at the North American Academy of the Homeopathic Healing Art, which had been founded in 1834 by Constantine Hering, a devoted friend and follower of Samuel Hahnemann's, the first president of the AIH, and a man considered to be the father of homeopathy in America. Hering developed the economical "Domestic Kits." His two-volume book *Domestic Physician,* published in 1835 and 1838, helped spread the doctrine across the nation, and became a training manual for dominant doctors interested in learning about homeopathy (the book came with forty or so bottles of remedies). In 1848, Dr. Hering, who believed that people felt better emotionally before their physical symptoms went away, had created the first successful homeopathic college in America, the Homeopathic Medical College of Pennsylvania, in Philadelphia. Other such colleges followed, and by the end of the nineteenth century there were twenty-two of them.

Education was a serious matter to the homeopaths, and at the founding meeting of the AIH in 1844, two goals had been stated: "the reformation and augmentation of the materia medica," and "the restraining of physicians from pretending to be competent to practice homeopathy who have not studied it in a careful and skillful manner." The AIH resolved the following year to admit only members who had completed "a regular course of medical studies" and to require that they first pass an examination "before the censors of the Institute."

In Michigan (which had become a state of the Union in 1837), a dominant medical school was not organized until 1847. That same year, a bill was introduced into the state legislature making it a prison offense to practice homeopathy—this in a state where the doctrine was particularly widespread, and written about in the press. Indeed, the many friends of homeopathy managed to convince the lawmakers to defeat the bill. Four years later, in 1851, at the height of homeopathy's success in the United States, the Michigan state legislature received an unusual petition from influential homeopaths: a request to abolish the dominant medical school unless homeopathy was taught there. It took four more years, until 1855, for the homeopaths to achieve their goal, even though the students who took the homeopathic course were treated with great hostility. Yet a steady if uneasy alliance between the two schools of thought came into being in the state, including the eventual construction of a homeopathic hospital. Although the homeopathic will prevailed, it did not do so without many struggles over the years (it was "like trying to mix oil and water," Roy Copeland later said).

The struggle included even a few well-placed punches. One spring day in 1867, a professor of homeopathy, angry about the way his students were being ignored in the dominant medical classes, was strolling on the apple-blossom-strewn campus of the medical school in Ann Arbor. He saw a colleague, the dominant professor of surgery, coming his way. There was to be no handshake that day. Instead, the professor of homeopathy hauled off and hit his fellow professor on the chin. There were no words left to say. The professor of surgery punched his colleague right back, and soon they were engaged in a nasty fistfight on the campus path. They had literally come to blows over the place of homeopathy in American medical life.

Earlier that year, the Michigan legislature had passed a ruling providing for two chairs of homeopathy. The regents of the University of Michigan didn't want two chairs in the department of medicine—one was plenty—so they suggested there be a completely separate school of medicine for the homeopaths. It would take eight years for such a school to become a reality, and in the interim tempers became almost too hot to handle, even among venerable professors walking amid the bittersweet nightshade and common smartweeds of bucolic Ann Arbor.

The dean of the new homeopathic medical school said that "by closing your eyes you can easily imagine this is not Michigan, a sovereign state, but the land of Lilliput, and the question the great one of the Little Endians and the Big Endians." The dean would plead for peace: "Can't we bury all personal differences?" But the battle would go on, and include an attempt by the AMA that ultimately failed to ban as members graduates of the separate but equal homeopathic college. And in time, the dean would see what Roy Copeland saw: "The sunlight streaming through the vanishing smoke of battle, showing in each succeeding read-justment of medical thought, a closer approximation to homeopathic ideals."

Worldwide, too, the smoke of battle began to vanish. In Austria, where the first homeopathic journal had appeared in 1821, its practice had been forbidden until 1837. Although England and France at first rejected homeopathy, they later embraced it with a fervor more intense than that of any other countries in the world.

In 1847, the AMA called homeopathy "a delusion," and many of its 426 inaugural members (out of approximately 40,000 dominant doctors in America) went along with this, agreeing that the practice was illogical, inconsistent, and just plain absurd. "Its preparations were sometimes of a highly poetic and romantic nature," the AMA said. At the 1846 meeting that preceded the formalization of the AMA, homeopaths were called impostors who believed in miracles, and apothecaries were blamed for their contribution to the "deception." In time, the AMA ruled in a Code of Ethics that members would risk expulsion if they even consulted with a homeopath. One doctor who consulted with his wife who was studying to become a homeopath was ousted from his local medical society, and another was expelled simply for buying milk sugar at an apothecary. Homeopaths, which the AMA took to calling "irregulars," were consid-ered a sect, and sectarian medicine of any kind was not acceptable to the dominant, or "regular," doctors. The homeopaths were romantics, the dominant doctors realists. The homeopaths were spiritual, the dom-inant doctors logical. The homeopaths believed in "philosophic medi-cine," the AMA wrote in 1846. To counter this, the *Michigan Journal of Homeopathy* responded bitterly that the dominant doctors never ques-tioned any of their "accumulated wisdom of three thousand years."

As a further response, the AIH, which required that its members be graduates of one of the twenty-seven dominant medical schools in exis-tence in the mid-1840s, argued that the AMA, small and political, was jealous of the popularity and earnings of homeopathic doctors. This was true enough, many people agreed. But the AMA sidestepped such charges. It began looking at medical training and said that homeopaths weren't being taught proper science; by this it meant that homeopathy wasn't a legitimate science. At the time, the AIH did little to defend itself other than to say that acceptance of its theories would come in time—its truths would catch up to its popularity—and therefore patience was the best defense until that time when the dominant school accepted the superiority of homeopathy.

But the AMA and the dominant doctors could not accept Hahnemann's provings as scientific evidence because, they said, there wasn't a "well-directed series of observations," i.e., strictly dominant doctors who were doing the observing and documenting. The AMA called Hahnemann's provings "crude hypotheses" and an "entirely fabulous species of evidence," and said that homeopaths were simply "shrewd and designing men, ready and eager to take advantage" of the unfamiliarity of people with their native plants, both medicinal and nonmedicinal. The AMA also said that if homeopathy worked at all it was because of the power of suggestion, and the fact that "mischievous" homeopaths spent a lot of time talking to their patients, who probably would have gotten better on their own, especially since the doses were too insignificant to make a difference. At their 1846 meeting, the AMA described these doses as "often of known inertness or slight power." The AMA believed that the public was in rapture over homeopathy because of its gimmickry—"a straining after novelty for novelty's sake," it wrote, adding that "although it is not in the power of physicians to prevent, or always to arrest these delusions in their progress, yet it is incumbent on them, from their superior knowledge and better opportunities, as well as from their elevated vocation, steadily to refuse to extend them the slightest countenance, still less support." The AIH sat by, waiting with confidence and with the certainty that their Law of Cure would one day rule the land. The homeopaths waited for the validation that would almost certainly arrive in time. The dominant school, they said, was a group of "therapeutic skeptics." They'd see the error of their ways. They'd come to accept that homeopathy "carried with it all the elements of scientific permanency."

SOON AFTER excluding homeopaths in 1847, the AMA had created a committee "to study the indigenous medical botany" of the United States, "paying particular attention to such plants as are now, or may be hereafter during their term of service, found to possess valuable medicinal properties." It was an attempt to try to reconcile what was happening in medicine—people flocking to homeopaths, or using all sorts of botanics at home. It was also an attempt to slow down the flow of imported products from Europe and the Far East.

Most doctors considered the committee to be a sincere effort by the AMA to understand not only certain aspects of homeopathy, but also Thomsonian and eclectic botany, as well as Indian and other herbal medicinals in use at the time. The AMA acknowledged that America's "indigenous Materia Medica has received far too little attention from the profession," adding that many of the substances "have been imperfectly investigated," and only "partially understood."

The AMA also resolved in 1847 to study the possibility of establishing schools for the training of apothecary owners. The following year, in 1848, it further approved the recommendation of a law "to provide for the appointment of an inspector at each chief port of entry to examine all imported drugs and medicines." Two years earlier, in 1846, 7,000 pounds of imported rhubarb root headed for medicinal use as a laxative had been discovered to be worm-eaten and decayed. At the same time, imported opium, which the AMA said was "an article of priceless worth in the treatment of disease," was found to have two-thirds of its active medicinal properties removed and was adulterated by its exporter with licorice paste. One shipment was found "infested with living worms." There was also "imperfectly manufactured iodine put in the usual small bottles, very impure, black, and damp," which both dominant doctors and homeopaths used for problems ranging from weak muscles to coughs and bone pain. There was Castor, generally used as a laxative, of which the AMA said, "very little, if any, of the pure Russian castor finds its way to this country. An imitation compound of dried blood, gum ammoniac, and a little real castor, put up in artificial bags, is the article generally met with." Even "vastly important" blue mercury pills, the staple of dominant medicine, were found to be contaminated with clay and sand. Clearly, something had to be done about this situation. The homeopaths were less concerned about inexperienced apothecary owners, or adulteration by exporters, because they generally prepared their own remedies (unlike the dominant doctors who relied on apothecaries to make up the majority of their medicines). The homeopaths felt they were in a stronger position to control the purity of the small amount of ingredients they used, even the ones in the Domestic Kits. They didn't think the AMA's resolutions for inspectors at ports and training for apothecary owners were foolish, only unnecessary, especially since they believed homeopathy would soon become the predominant practice in American medicine.

There was one essential medicine, however, that straddled both camps—Peruvian bark, from which quinine was made. Of course, the dominant doctors used it in large quantities and the homeopaths used it in tiny amounts. (This was also true to a certain extent of the poison mercuric chloride, which dominant doctors used full-strength in the seventeenth and eighteenth centuries as a local antiseptic, and homeopaths diluted for eye, throat, mouth, and certain stomach problems, as *Merc. cor.,* or *Mercurius corrosivus.* Homeopaths also used dominant medicine's mercury, or calomel, as a remedy called *Merc. dulsis,* or *Mercurius dulcis,* for certain eye and ear problems. Digitalis, or foxglove, was also used by both dominant and homeopathic doctors to treat heart ailments.)

The AMA, calling Peruvian bark "an important article of medicine," said much of it was "entirely unfit" because it arrived in the United States "in a greatly deteriorated condition." Some of the imported quinine was mixed with plaster of Paris and chalk, and in such an "inactive" state that it had no value at all. Even though both dominant doctors and homeopaths were equally at risk in accepting adulterated or worthless shipments, only the AMA felt the problem needed to be addressed in a public way. The AIH still believed that homeopaths, with their training and experience, would be able to regulate and oversee quinine (and mercury and foxglove) on their own without assistance of any kind. It was a precarious position considering the AMA and its attacks, and it also risked negative public opinion. But the AIH held fast to its belief that its remedies were always safe. Judging from sales, most of the population in America agreed.

In 1849, the AMA decided to form a committee to study quack medications, "to enlighten the public in regard to the nature and dangerous tendencies of such remedies." (The word "quack" is derived from the Dutch *kwakzalver,* or quacksalver: "quack," from the gibberish or nonsensical sound of a duck, and "salver," a healer.)

Because of the confusion that existed over everything lining apothecary shelves, the AMA was on firm ground. The AIH, which continued not to see any problem with the raw materials its members used, imported or not, didn't look at the issue of quack medicine. It became easy for the AMA, for whatever reasons—economic, scientific, or philosophical—to start to include homeopathic remedies in its definition of "quack medicine." But the AIH pretended not to notice and held fast to its belief that the public would understand the difference.

Finally, the AMA decided that Congress should pass a law making it mandatory that all drugs and medicines be examined by "properly qualified" persons. In the meantime, while waiting for a fair and adequate bill to be passed, the AMA selected another option—"the wisest and safest course—condemnation, re-exportation, and destruction" of medicinals considered unsafe. In its mind, this tactic would settle things, if not once and for all, then for a very long time. And it did.

The homeopaths scarcely knew what hit them, nor, for that matter, did the public. But Roy Copeland knew, and eventually did something about it, something "militant and at the same time diplomatic," to make homeopathy truly acceptable in the nation.

"As Fixed as the Law of Gravitation"

A LOT HAD happened to medical care since Roy was a boy and had watched his father survive lung fever by the use of "like cures like." By the time he was a senior in high school, most dominant doctors had given up bloodletting and purging, and many had begun to reduce the size of their large doses of medications. Tiny doses were on the rise; Thomsonianism was on the decline, although it had been replaced in popularity by Eclecticism, which now offered its botanic remedies primarily in teas and/or in powder form. While eclectics were in as great demand as homeopaths for a long while—there were 10,000 of them in the 1880s—and even had their own schools, the approach lacked any exact systemic formula. Eclecticism didn't have the kind of structure or fixed principles that homeopathy did.

More than 90,000 Michigan men had served in the American Civil War from 1861 to 1865, though no battles took place in Michigan. As Roscoe Copeland wrote to his children, "When the war started, Joseph and son [his brother and nephew] enlisted, Joseph started as Colonel and Fred as Captain. Joseph organized a regiment afterwards and made General. He told me if I wanted to enlist I could start as Captain. If this happened before father had died I would have enlisted but as it was I could not leave my mother all alone."

The war dramatically altered people's views about illness. The formation of a United States Sanitary Commission had improved the terrible conditions in many of the battlefield hospitals, where filthy beds, dirty water, and inadequate meals had been the norm. The commission's goal was to create infirmaries that had plenty of fresh air, good food, and clean water. These were always Hahnemann's goals, too. Roy, who would learn to apply these ideas in both sickness and health, described conditions in 1875, when he was a seven-year-old boy: "When cold weather came, the windows were nailed shut and rags tucked around them to keep the air out of the home. The children were sewed into their clothing. Nobody took a bath until the ice went out of the river in the Spring. The result was they died young."

Other medical systems became known. Osteopathy ("bone-suffering") had been developed in America in 1874 (although the first school wasn't opened until 1892). This was an approach to healing that maintained that the human body required a proper alignment of its bones, muscles, and nerves. In 1875, a former homeopathic follower, Mary Baker Eddy, had created the Christian Science movement, which believed that God promoted healing and that medical care of any kind was really unnecessary. Eddy had formulated her beliefs in 1866, but it was not until 1875 that she published them in a book, *Science and Health*. The AMA considered all these practices "anti-medical." Most Americans did not.

Soon after graduating from Dexter High School on the balmy Friday evening of June 26, 1885, where he gave a class address titled "An Intelligent Purpose Is Necessary to Success," seventeen-year-old Roy taught for four months (his salary was $38 a month) in a one-room schoolhouse in nearby Sylvan Township. He was trying to earn enough money to one day attend medical school. He lived in a boardinghouse and had all his meals prepared by, as he wrote, "my good landlady . . . who often cooked spare ribs, boiled potatoes, pork gravy, and salicylic preserved strawberries." (Aspirin would soon be derived from salicylic acid.)

By the spring of 1886, Roy still didn't have enough money for medical school, but he had earned enough to attend some classes at the State Normal School, a training school for teachers in neighboring Ypsilanti. His mother (and later, his sister) studied there (such advanced schooling was very unusual for women from a country area), and his father, as part of his school board duties, "used to go down to the Normal School most every year to hire teachers." Roy majored in literature but was soon attracted to American history. This was not surprising, considering not only his sense of curiosity about his county, his country, and the world, but also his ancestry.

According to a family record, the name Copeland was first mentioned in 1248, in Scotland, where "Copeland castle stands on the north brink of the glen." The name Copeland also shows up early in Germany, where ancestors were called Kopffeldt, Kopf-landt, Coff-Landt, and Coplandt. In 1650, Lawrence Copeland came to America from England, landing at Plymouth; a year later he married Lydia Townsend in Boston. American Copelands fought not only in the Revolutionary War, but also in the War of 1812, and one of Roy's ancestors married the granddaughter of John Alden, who was immortalized by Henry Wadsworth Longfellow in his poem "The Courtship of Miles Standish," published in 1858.

In the mid-1800s, Longfellow, along with his Harvard colleague James Russell Lowell, the poet and critic, had been won over to homeopathy. Many other well-known people had also embraced it: Nathaniel Hawthorne, author of, among other books, *The Scarlet Letter,* in 1850; Daniel Webster, the statesman and orator; William Cullen Bryant, the poet and newspaper editor; and Harriet Beecher Stowe, best known for *Uncle Tom's Cabin,* published in 1852, which helped awaken the national conscience concerning slavery. (Coincidentally, Dexter, Michigan—specifically founder Samuel Dexter's house—was a stop on the Underground Railroad in the 1840s and 1850s.)

Homeopathy had been dealt a blow when, in 1842, it was attacked by the doctor and writer Oliver Wendell Holmes in a series of widely publicized lectures. Holmes, a colleague of Longfellow's and Lowell's at Harvard, and someone who had once trumpeted homeopathy, decided, after careful consideration, that Hahnemann's provings were the result of chance. Now calling the principles he had once endorsed not only "peculiar" but "improbable," he attempted to demolish Hahnemann's entire doctrine by using facts and ridicule. "When one man claims to have established three independent truths [like is cured by like, high dilutions, and the psora] which are about as remote from each other as the discovery of the law of gravitation, the invention of printing, and that of the mariner's compass, unless the facts are overwhelming and unanimous," he said, "the question naturally arises, Is not this man deceiving himself, or trying to deceive others?" He said that when some reputable dominant doctors had tried to reproduce some of Hahnemann's provings for Peruvian Bark, Aconite, and Arnica, among others, they could not, even though everything was done that was supposed to have been done. Holmes said that "in 1835, a public challenge was offered to the best-known homeopathic physician in Paris to select any ten substances asserted to produce the most striking effects; to prepare them himself; to choose one by lot without knowing which of them he had taken, and try it upon himself or an intelligent and devoted Homeopathist, and, waiting his own time, to come forward and tell what substances had been employed. The challenge was at first accepted, but the acceptance retracted before the time of trial arrived. . . . I think it is fair to conclude that the catalogues of symptoms attributed in Homeopathic works to the influence of various drugs upon healthy persons are not entitled to any confidence."

At the end of one of his lectures, Holmes asked how anyone "guilty of such pedantic folly" as Hahnemann was could possibly be considered as great as Sir Isaac Newton and his law of gravitation, or William Harvey, the English doctor who was the first to demonstrate the function of the human heart? But thousands of Americans—"the unprofessional public," Holmes called them—saw in Hahnemann a mind as great as any of the greats, and "a very extraordinary man," as Roy Copeland would later say, "one whose name will descend to posterity as the exclusive founder of an original system of medicine, as ingenious as many that preceded it."

Although his father always made a comfortable enough living as a businessman, especially considering his farming background, there was never money for extras. Roscoe Copeland, while steady and sure (he was president of the village for many years, as well as a member of its school board and head of the cemetery association), was a romantic. And as important as education was in the Copeland family, a major university was out of reach, even for a prospering rural family. While Roy was still in high school, where he took what was called the "Latin-Scientific course," his father bought part interest in a flour mill, which did quite well for a time until disaster struck. As Roscoe described it, "The farmers had commenced raising a new white wheat called the Clawsing. A good yielder and fine-looking, but when we came to mill it, it proved to be a very poor bread flour. After the bread makers had one try at it they did not want any more and all that good trade we had worked up was blotted out. The final result was it ruined all the mills on Huron River, and a good many of them never revived." Roscoe then went into the grain business, since he said he had received "such a good education" in it after his mill fiasco, and he remained in that business successfully for many years.

By 1885, a few dominant doctors across America had begun to ignore the AMA's ban on consultation with homeopaths, and some people were even hinting that perhaps the ban should be lifted completely. Many allopathic drug companies, a thriving industry since 1860, had started to wholesale homeopathic remedies, not only because they were so enormously favored by the public, but because their purity was still better guaranteed than that of some of the dominant medicines. This was good news for the AIH, which, of course, had never let go of its position that the high standards of its remedies would be acknowledged in time. And they were. In fact, with the purity issue partially sidelined, the dominant doctors went back (actually, they never left it) to the matter of tiny doses. How in the world could a tiny dose of anything—a tiny dose of nothing, really—cure a disease? Homeopaths, they said, even believed a remedy could be sniffed to elicit a healing effect. In 1855, the *Boston Medical and Surgical Journal* had published a report showing "no medicinal substance" whatsoever in the remedies. But despite the criticism, the public kept buying. The public was not going to be told what medicines to use.

After Roy's teaching stint (as well as his caretaking of the schoolhouse) was up—he earned a total of $152—the now nearly 6-foot-tall teenager decided to live at home while going to the State Normal School. He also decided to apprentice with his village doctor. Dr. Chase was thrilled to pass on his knowledge to his young protégé, who, like his mentor, took for granted that "the law upon which homeopathy is based is one of the great laws of nature, as fixed as the law of gravitation." By training with Dr. Chase, Roy was getting a foot solidly in the door, because he would be well versed by the time he became a medical student. "A very common school education" was all the preliminary training that many medical schools required for entrance at the time, although Michigan also called for a knowledge of Greek and Latin, and "evidence of good moral character." In this, in intelligence—as well as in looks—Roy was far ahead of the other sons of Washtenaw County.

Several significant milestones had been achieved by 1886 as Roy worked alongside Dr. Chase. Almost twenty-five years earlier, in 1861, the French chemist Louis Pasteur had completed his pioneering research on the germ theory of disease. Pasteur would revolutionize the preservation of certain foods, especially milk, with his process of pasteurization in 1864, as well as create a vaccine against rabies in 1885. The groundbreaking theories of the English surgeon Joseph Lister, who sterilized instruments with phenol to reduce infections during operations, had come to fruition in 1865. In 1876, a German doctor, Robert Koch, had established the definitive bacterial cause of anthrax disease (Pasteur would develop the vaccine), and later in the 1880s, Koch found the bacterial cause for wound infections, conjunctivitis, and tuberculosis. The work of these three major scientists proved that diseases did not arise spontaneously out of thin air—or ghostly presences.

It was against this compelling scientific background that homeopathy first began in the 1880s to question itself, barely more than fifty years after its arrival in America. Newspapers and journals started asking why dominant medicine was making such giant strides in terms of scientific discoveries, and homeopathy was not. Was that the way it was supposed to be? Since the remedies always worked, did it matter that homeopathy stayed the same? Wasn't this a good thing? Even so, shouldn't homeopathy try to evolve, too, to keep up with the latest findings? Was the miasm perhaps the same as germs? How did the germ theory relate to the "vital force"? Most homeopaths didn't think new discoveries were necessary, and would agree with a professor at the University of Berlin who said that "the bio-chemically-thinking" Pasteur's work "cannot be better characterized than by Hahnemann's word, 'Homeopathic.' " The world was beginning to catch up with what homeopathy always knew, so why did homeopathy need to change?

But some new ideas did appear. In 1877, *Repertory of the Homoeopathic Materia Medica,* by the American homeopath James Tyler Kent, a former eclectic, had been published abroad. This book introduced to homeopathy the concept of constitutional types and prescribing, and brought into being what came to be called classical homeopathy. Kent held that people with similar personalities and body types also had similar illnesses, and he said that the remedies should be prescribed according to the individual's physical appearance and emotions, as well as to his symptoms.

The majority of the members of the AIH began to challenge even the extreme dilutions and the number of necessary shakings, as well as the treatment of each symptom separately, which had always been a basic component. Some of these moderates, or revisionists, went along with the dominant custom of treating the disease and not the symptom. And so in 1880, the purists among the homeopaths, the doctors who wanted things to remain exactly the same (most of them did not believe that the germ theory had anything to do with medical treatment), dropped out of the AIH and created a new organization, the International Hahnemannian Association. Coincidentally, six years later, in 1886, the dominant doctors also split up, with some former AMA members starting what they believed would be a less political group, the Association of

American Physicians, which focused on the physician as an academic and a scientist.

In 1862, the speed of light had been measured and the earth's magnetic currents discovered. In 1876, Alexander Graham Bell invented the telephone, an instrument that forever altered the doctor-patient relationship by providing efficient communication and access (as would the automobile in the 1890s). In 1880, the development of the electric light would illuminate a doctor's work as no lantern ever could.

By the time Roy entered medical school in 1887, just two years after his high-school graduation, the profession of medicine in America was not only improving, but was also getting fairly complex and more than a little confounding. In addition to the split between revisionists and purists in homeopathy, and that between "political" doctors and "academic" doctors in dominant medicine, there was the matter of licensing. In the 1840s, most states had abolished it, saying that a diploma from medical school was license enough (with the exception of Michigan, New Jersey, Louisiana, and the District of Columbia, which never gave up the regulating of medical practice). In the 1870s and 1880s, most states began to reestablish licensing measures, and in this undertaking many dominant and homeopathic doctors cooperated. They worked to make things not only more professional, but safer for the public.

Roy became a student at the Homeopathic Medical School of the University of Michigan, which was one of approximately forty-four such schools in the United States. The Michigan Homeopathic Medical College and the Detroit Homeopathic College had been chartered in 1871 but had closed when homeopathy came to the University of Michigan.

He had managed to afford the tuition by talking his father into selling some land. Roscoe Copeland hadn't really needed much persuasion, because Roy was his prince (Roscoe and Frances's first son, Harry Lee, had died at birth the year before Roy was born). Royal (it was an old family name) was royal in every way, not only as a gifted student, but also as a son and brother—even his older sister, who worshiped him, always deferred to him. "No one knows the history of our country better than my brother," she gushed in letters to friends and relatives.

The Homeopathic Medical School was located in Ann Arbor, a village ten miles from Dexter that still looked like a frontier town, but one in an area full of bountiful forests, rivers, hills, and dozens of inland lakes. Telephone service had begun only six years earlier. By 1887, many of the original wooden buildings were slowly being replaced by brick ones, and electric lights were introduced, although gas streetlamps still existed and would not be replaced until 1894, when the Huron River was fully developed as a source of power.

Roy was one of fifty-eight students in his class. The majority of them were from Michigan, and the rest came from New York, Pennsylvania, Maryland, Iowa, Ohio, and Canada. Five women were classmates, an unusually high number at the time; in general, the homeopathic schools admitted more women than the dominant ones, which allowed very few to enter their ranks.

During the first year of training, where, as Roy explained, "the laboratory methods of science receive the same patronage and the same encouragement in the homeopathic school as elsewhere . . . in surgery, in gynecology, in ophthalmology, the same skill, the same methods are everywhere employed," his devoted father resolved to try to win his own fortune, once and for all. He contracted what he called "western fever." Roscoe and four friends decided to go to North Dakota to start a lumberyard "in some new town." But as it turned out, "it was just not the country we expected to find," he said, so he returned to Michigan and his grain business in Dexter. But the following year, Roscoe went away again, this time to Kansas to see about still another lumber business. That didn't work out either, so he "started back to Michigan, my Michigan." He told his children, "Michigan has been a pretty good stepping stone for you both. . . . We might have had a little more wealth, but there are many things superior to wealth."

His only son listened well. Roy always listened, as Dr. Chase had encouraged him to do, and then followed his own instincts, which included speaking often in a high nasal voice, sometimes incessantly, about what he had found out. His words were always accompanied by vigorous hand gestures. He said he was ready to "recognize his power so the world could be his," a world that now contained what he called "the priceless secret, the key to the shackles of disease, the relief from the bane of the ages."

The subjects that he studied were varied and rigorous. As Roy later summarized, "When I was a student, two courses of six months each (usually both alike) and three years in a doctor's office were all that was considered necessary to fit a young man for the most exacting of all the learned professions." These "two courses" actually comprised twenty different classes over a two-year period. All medical trainees at the time followed the same regime, and the only difference between the homeopathic and the dominant students was that the homeopathic ones additionally learned about Hahnemann's theories and remedies.

According to his brown leather class notebook, Roy studied the following subjects: general chemistry, qualitative chemistry, organic chemistry (Hahnemann considered homeopathy a principle of organic science), anatomy, practical anatomy—upper and lower, physical diagnosis, urine analysis, osteology (the study of the skeleton), histology (the microscopic study of tissues), microscopy, physiology (the science of the normal functions of the body), nervous disease, obstetrics, gynecology, ophthalmology (the study of the structure, function, and diseases of the eye), sanitary science (in another entry this is crossed out and replaced by "hygiene"), materia medica, and homeopathic therapeutics and practice. Later, he acknowledged how much he had learned from the eclectics, "who have given us some of our most valuable remedies."

All medical students attended four lectures a day and observed a clinical presentation on Saturday mornings. Although instruction was for six months, Roy said that "teaching used to 'let down' so to speak about the first of April. We did not do very much during April, and when the hot weather came upon us, we did still less. Little was required of the student after the Easter holidays." As it turned out, he was only an average student, receiving the just passing grade of 4.5, out of a possible 10. But very early on he began expressing his often outspoken views. His classmates respected him and began turning to him for leadership; these qualities had also been shown earlier through his active membership in the Methodist Young People's Society.

Roy and his fellow homeopaths didn't think of themselves as the "sectarians" or "cultists" the AMA accused them of being. As a student, Roy believed deeply that dominant medicine "is painstaking and honest and scientific" and said that homeopaths "cannot afford to let it pass." In fact, he often urged his future colleagues "to secure our share of the honey distilled by our brother doctors." From the very beginning of his medical career, Roy insisted that homeopathy was "but one of many methods of treating illness," and he said that "it does not replace surgery, hygiene, biological medicine, chemical antidote, or physical therapeutics." He always stressed that homeopaths must "not ignore the work of our friends of the other school," and he would repeat over and over to whoever would listen that homeopathy "is not all of medicine."

The words of one professor in particular, Wilbert Hinsdale, MD, led the budding homeopath to the specialty he would choose. Hinsdale,

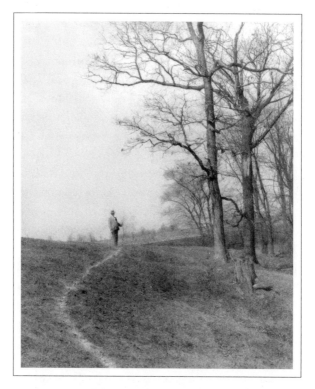

Professor Hinsdale walking "from Indian trail through the
woods to cowpath across the meadow" in Ann Arbor

who taught materia medica, told his students that the specialty of eyes,
ears, nose, and throat was becoming more appreciated and patronized by
the public, and he urged his class to consider this direction, even though
specialists were still rare at the time, and most students became general
practitioners. Hinsdale also lectured that "we look to the microscopist to
correct errors of diagnosis, to tell the surgeon when not to operate." As
always, Roy took it all in, and by the end of 1888, had found his calling.
He decided to become an eye specialist and surgeon who would offer his
patients homeopathic remedies. He had chosen a field that was not
crowded, where he could excel, and a field where he could combine the
best of homeopathic and dominant medical care. And it was a place that
Hahnemann himself would have approved, because his distrust of and
distaste for allopathic medicine had never included surgery. "There is
something appealing and fascinating in the thought of a brief surgical

operation and convalescence, with immediate escape from pain," Roy said; "why suffer the delay and ultimate disappointment of medical treatment, when the surgeon can so easily do both?" Thus, even as a student he began to understand that all medical treatment, even homeopathy, held the possibility of disappointing results, and that perhaps adding surgery to the mix offered the best chance for total recovery.

On Sunday, May 29, 1889, after two years of study, Roy S. Copeland, now sporting a mustache and a beard, was unanimously recommended as house surgeon and assistant to Dr. Henry Lorenz Obetz, the dean of the Homeopathic College and a professor of surgery, at a salary of $350 a year. Copeland was twenty-one years old.

THE AMA performed a sound function through its continued condemnation of impure and fraudulent medications. It never tested homeopathic remedies per se, although it recorded somewhat ambiguously in its House of Delegates minutes that it did so "in the few cases in which 'patent medicines' of the alleged homeopathic-type were being exploited." But the AMA's financial resources were not copious at the time, and in general its influence was not very broad.

With some dominant doctors now using homeopathic remedies, things seemed to be going smoothly, even though many homeopaths didn't appreciate this endorsement from rival allopaths, causing further division in their ranks. (In 1879, a homeopathic remedy, glonoin, or nitroglycerine, proved twenty years earlier by Constantine Hering, had first been used by a dominant doctor to treat angina, or cardiac pain. In 1867, the Swedish scientist Alfred Nobel had added an ingredient called kieselguhr to it, which gave birth to the explosive dynamite.)

The AIH met once a year to assess its own practices and "to present new thoughts in medicine and surgery." Within the AIH was a Bureau of Homeopathy that met more often. The bureau's role was "to discuss the scientific reasonableness "of homeopathy and to compare results with other practitioners. Arguments often occurred about the comparative qualities of homeopathic and allopathic care, and much enumerating of how many and how much of this and how many and how much of that each offered. But in the 1880s and 1890s, the AIH wasn't sufficiently organized or interested to launch a campaign to counteract some of the AMA's criticism, even though the Bureau of Homeopathy did consider "educational and propagandistic methods" that might advance the cause of homeopathy. But it was *their* cause, not the cause of medicine in general, that interested them. They just weren't going to get directly involved in the politics of quackery and the AMA's vested interest in it.

The AMA's attitude toward homeopathy remained disapproving. Its response to a patient asking about the effect of the remedies was that "it would, however, seem rather a waste of time for a practitioner to seek to compound his own remedies when the drug houses are in a much better position to furnish him the material he needs and have the facilities of their laboratories." In other words, go dominant, the AMA advised.

Yet homeopathy began more and more to be called the "new" school, and dominant medicine, the "old." Nothing substantial was done by the AIH beyond a modest recruiting strategy and the acceptance of dominant doctors as members. Copeland soon wanted more done, and urged that "a book or pamphlet be placed in the hands of some possible convert." He himself thought the issue of fraudulent medicine had to be confronted, but the majority of homeopaths disagreed.

In 1851, the American Pharmaceutical Association had been founded, and nearly twenty years later, in 1870, the AMA urged druggists (apothecaries were now called drugstores) "to organize themselves into societies." In 1872, the AMA formed a committee "on the relations between physicians and druggists," and by 1876, it accepted recommendations from the American Pharmaceutical Association for "dangerous, active medical preparations, noting their maximum doses." (The AMA and the APA would work together for years on behalf of doctors, hospitals, and patients.)

In 1879, the AMA had ruled that the advertising of drugs in medical journals was a violation of its code of ethics, and in 1884 it had denounced any doctors who endorsed drugs or the private mineral waters that were beginning to become all the rage. Four years later, in 1888, the AMA voted to disapprove of any member of the clergy or religious press who "recommended charlatans."

Copeland asked whether homeopaths, in addition to being considered sectarians and cultists, were also considered such charlatans. The short answer was yes. But the long answer was no, because the AMA and the homeopaths did live together, even if in confusion and with hostility. Despite a hint in the air during the 1880s and 1890s of some convergence between dominant and homeopathic medicine, the AMA kept using

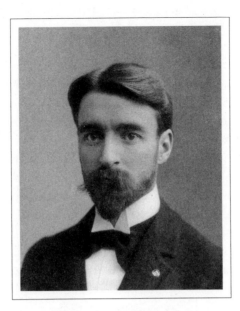

Roy S. Copeland, MD, 1889

negative words about homeopaths, and the homeopaths thrived as the underdogs.

As a new house surgeon, Copeland worked in the homeopathic hospital under the watchful eye of Dr. Obetz. Not all homeopathic surgeons were trained the same way. Some schools believed homeopathic remedies were "useless in all abdominal complaints," and instead preferred to use what they called "scientific surgery." (Obetz used both.) Some surgeons removed "the pelvic organs" in all cases of "troubles of women," as one report stated, and said homeopathic remedies did not work even as well as dominant treatments like Fenner's Epileptic Cure, whose ingredients were not listed.

One of the first complete homeopathic pharmacopeias had been published in America just seventeen years earlier, in 1872. It contained information on 1,021 remedies. Hahnemann wrote in his *Organon* (which Copeland would reread annually for decades) that the physician must discover all the "special details" of the patient's condition: "For example what was the character of his stools? How does he pass his water? How is it with his day and night sleep? What is the state of his disposition, his humor, his memory? How about the thirst? What sort of taste has he in his mouth? What kinds of food and drink are most relished? What are most repugnant to him?" Every detail was important, and every detail contributed to the discovery of the right remedy. Hahnemann stated that "the age of the patient, his mode of living and diet, his occupation, his domestic position, his social relation and so forth, must next be taken into consideration, in order to ascertain whether these things have tended to increase his malady, or in how far they may favor or hinder the treatment." Hahnemann further commented that "the old school physician . . . would not listen to any minute detail of all the circumstances of his case by the patient; indeed, he frequently cut him short in his relation of his sufferings, in order that he might not be delayed in the rapid writing of his prescription, composed of a variety of ingredients unknown to him in their true effect." And so it became known to patients everywhere that in addition to the mild medicine offered, the homeopath listened, and had to listen well in order to find the proper cure.

The University of Michigan Medical School was the first medical school in the country to have its very own hospital, built in 1869, although a homeopathic hospital was not founded there until ten years later. Until the late nineteenth century, most sick people were treated at home, and the hospitals that did exist were not particularly agreeable places to be housed. Early on, the homeopaths had decided to try to develop their own hospitals and mental asylums, and in time most patients preferred these institutions. Pleasant medicine brought pleasant hospital treatment, and by 1892, homeopaths supervised over a hundred hospitals across the nation.

Young Copeland's first operation with Obetz, on October 1, 1889, had nothing to do with his chosen specialty, but was performed to treat an enlarged testicle. There was more bleeding than expected, Copeland wrote in his casebook, where he kept detailed notes, and the two surgeons put in a drainage tube, but the patient, Copeland wrote, "did not do well, kept bleeding more or less. Not a bit of fun." The man remained in the hospital for a month. Two weeks later, on October 15, Copeland, with Obetz's help again, operated on his first cancer patient, a man with a rectal malignancy. The two men removed a two-inch tumor, and the new surgeon noted in his casebook that his patient "recovered from shock in 8 hours. Complete Recovery." He also assisted Obetz in castrating a patient "because the patient kept bleeding." There is no further explanation in his notes.

Copeland always used homeopathic remedies on his patients—both the surgical and nonsurgical ones. His 1890 patient's book indicates that he gave a woman with sciatica, or pain in the lower back, *Arsenicum album,* made from a compound of the poison arsenic. This remedy, which smells like garlic, was usually given to people with severe pain, fear, and/or digestive problems, but the complete list of its uses and symptoms, as well as that of most other remedies in the *Homeopathic Pharmacopeia,* is extremely long. The list for *Arsen. alb.* is minutely detailed, even more so after the "Arsenicum personality profile" came into being—along with profiles of most other remedies. This was why Copeland later said that "every garment [remedy] is made to order and is fitted only after careful consideration of many patterns." His casebook mentions that his sciatica patient didn't get any better, so the remedy was changed to *Citrullus colocynthis,* made from a fruit called bitter cucumber or bitter apple (although it resembled a pumpkin); it has roots that burrow deep into the earth, and the remedy, which dominant doctors had often used full-strength as a purgative, was made from the dried fruit without the seeds. Homeopaths gave it for digestive upsets, certain kinds of headaches, and nerve pain. (Deep pain—deep roots.) Copeland's sciatica patient was also given *Rhus toxicodendron* (*Rhus tox.*), the mother tincture of which is made from poison ivy leaves. Its main uses are for joint and muscle pain; burning, itchy, and swollen skin problems; and digestive problems. The dilution given was 3X, or 1 part poison ivy tincture to 1,000 parts water or alcohol, and is the only dilution recorded by Copeland in this casebook. Tiny milk sugar pellets were impregnated with the solution, which patients then dissolved on their tongues. (Hahnemann wrote that sometimes if the pellet was dissolved in water first, and stirred well, it "will produce a far more powerful medicine for the use of several days.") Copeland's notes go on to say that "a local exam found slight laceration on the cervix" of his sciatica patient, and that "Dr. Obetz operated. Improvement of sciatica at once." Glycerinum, or glycerine, and *Carbolicum acidum,* or carbolic acid—a powerful irritant and anesthetic (not always considered homeopathic)—were prescribed on a tampon as a salve. A man "with nightly emissions but no history of depravity" was given *Aurum metallicum* 3X—gold, ground into a fine powder. This was often prescribed for depression, congestion of blood in various organs, liver problems, undescended testicles, and emotional oversensitivity. (Dominant doctors used gold for tuberculosis.) In general, sexual complaints of any kind were treated as very serious ailments that required punishing treatments. Encasement of the penis in plaster, leather, or rubber devices, and circumcision were sometimes used to prevent masturbation in young men. Full-strength carbolic acid was sometimes placed on the clitorises of young women. In later years a mother begged Copeland to find a solution other than reform school for her teenage son who masturbated daily.

For rheumatism—pain, swelling, and stiffness in muscles and joints—Copeland gave a patient three remedies (it was very unusual in America to give three at one time, although it was customary to do so in Europe), but he was clearly experimenting with his prescriptions. The first remedy he chose for his patient was *Bryonia alba,* or Bryonia, 3X (1 part wild hops root with 1,000 parts water or alcohol). Homeopaths used Bryonia for headaches, constipation, and pain; its full-strength root is bitter and poisonous and can kill a person in an hour or two. The second remedy he chose was *Rhus tox.,* in the same quantity he used for his patient with sciatica pain. The final remedy was *Arnica montana,* also known as leopard's bane, mountain tobacco, or sneezewort (because the flowers cause sneezing). Its main use was for shock and pain. He prescribed *Cocculus indicus,* or indian cockle, and Belladonna, which he called "the wonderful medicine," to a woman with heavy menstrual periods. In a proving by Copeland's own Professor Hinsdale, *Cocculus indicus* was found to "affect the cerebrum, but will not cure convulsive seizures proceeding from the spinal cord." It was said to especially help "light-haired females" with "profuse dark menses." Belladonna was often used for infections and inflammations, as well as labor pains and toothaches. Copeland later wrote in a seven-page article that Belladonna affects every part of the nervous system.

Copeland finally got to operate on a woman with an eye infection—acute conjunctivitis. All patients undergoing eye surgery received ether, which had been in use since 1846, or the newer cocaine eye drops, which had been developed in 1884. It is not recorded in his casebook exactly why an operation was needed for conjunctivitis, or pinkeye, nor what type of operation was performed, although Copeland later observed that "most of the eye conditions which can be considered strictly emergent are largely surgical." Copeland does note in his casebook that his conjunctivitis patient "had to be on cocaine to relieve pain because the procedure was tried too often by students," meaning that this patient was being used as a teaching case—over and over—and suffering because of it. Boric acid, a chemical with mild antiseptic qualities, was used as an eyewash on the patient, as well. Some homeopaths (but not Copeland) were taught to treat eye problems with "simple means," not ever with an operation, or even homeopathic remedies. One doctor wrote in a journal that "nothing is so harmful to healthy eye action as only one bowel movement a day, and with conjunctivitis ('pink eye') we must have three corresponding to the meals."

As the year went on, Copeland saw more and more patients with eye problems. He gave a patient with a detached retina *Kali iodatum,* made from iodine and potassium iodide. (Dominant doctors once used this remedy full-strength for syphilis.) He also prescribed the same remedy in a 2X dilution to a patient with "Arteria-sclerosis with a hemorrhage at the base of the brain." For a patient with eyestrain, he prescribed Bryonia, which he had given to his patient with rheumatism. He also gave this patient Belladonna 3X, plus Nux Vomica, derived from the same seed that produces strychnine poison, which Hahnemann had proved for digestive problems, and which was now also used for insomnia, colds, menstrual complaints, and suppressed anger. Dr. William Boericke, an American homeopath who graduated from the Hahnemann Medical College in Philadelphia in 1880, and who was the cofounder in 1881 of the Pacific Homoeopathic [*sic*] Medical College of San Francisco as well as of Hahnemann Hospital (later part of the University of California), wrote in his Homoeopathic [*sic*] *Materia Medica* that Nux Vomica "is frequently the first remedy, indicated after much dosing, establishing a sort of equilibrium of forces and counteracting chronic effects." Copeland heard Professor Hinsdale lecture on this remedy, a favorite of his, in class the previous year. Hinsdale told his students Nux Vomica had been known as a drug since 1540, and that strychnine "acts very rapidly, the effects being felt in 5–30 minutes, and death usually occurring in one hour if the dose is fatal." After hearing such words, it was not hard for the homeopathic students to grasp quickly the concept of the infinitesimal dose. Hinsdale also described for his students the "temperament" of the Nux Vomica patient: "While Nux is adapted to all people, it is especially indicated in thin, spare, shriveled patients, rather than in those who are corpulent. The characteristic Nux patient is dark and sallow, of nervous, irascible temperament, quick and active in all his motions." He reminded the soon-to-be doctors that Nux Vomica "is perhaps used more than any other drug on our materia medica because its pathogenesis covers a class of ailments most commonly met with in practice."

Equipped with Hinsdale's difficult but skillful lectures, as well as those of his other teachers, his year with his village doctor, and his assistantship with Obetz, Copeland was ready to open his own medical office.

Before he left Ann Arbor, he wrote his sister, who was now a high-school teacher in a nearby district, that he had promised to lead a Sunday afternoon prayer service at the homeopathic hospital. The subject was "brotherly love," and he told Nellie to "please look the matter up and give me some pointers at once. Look over the papers, etc., and give me a good send off." He stressed to her that "I must make a good speech for the first one you know," reminding her that "I cease to be an infant now and begin life as a man tomorrow."

THREE

"We Shall Deserve to Win and We Will Win"

Royal Samuel Copeland, MD, ophthalmologist, surgeon, and homeopath, opened his first private practice in the bustling town of Bay City, Michigan, approximately one hundred miles north of Dexter. The twenty-two-year-old, with one year of internship—"the probationary period," he described it—heard opportunity call and he took notice, for Bay City, situated close to the mouth of the Saginaw River, which fed into Saginaw Bay, Lake Huron, and the Great Lakes waterway, was not only the major distribution point for shipping on the Great Lakes, but was also home to more than fifty lumber mills and 25,000 residents. There were a lot of potential patients in this fast-growing town— "a pioneer town," the new doctor called it—huddled in the midst of a rich white pine forest. Copeland quickly found himself a comfortable office in a sturdy wooden building at 303 Chilson Street, which was two blocks south of the main street, Winona, where he could hear the continual clacking of the horse-drawn trolley that brought shoppers—and patients—to the area. He rented a room at the nearby Rouech House and was ready to begin life in a town one of its founders described as "a little hamlet on the bank of a broad, beautiful river." For recreation— when time allowed—there was plenty of bird-watching, since large flocks of Great Egrets, two hundred kinds of songbirds, and waterfowl visited the nearby shores. There were also particularly large mosquitoes to dodge. He became a member of the local YMCA, where he could exercise and socialize (Hahnemann had been a proponent of exercise as part of the total homeopathic healing process). He also joined the Bay

City branch of the Epworth League, a national young people's group founded in 1889, named after the boyhood home of John Wesley, the founder of the Methodist movement. Religion was never far from his thoughts; in fact, he read the Bible several hours a day.

On New Year's Day of 1891, three months after he had settled in, he married Mary DePriest Ryan, who lived in Adrian, Michigan, a farming community forty miles south of Dexter. Mary, whose father was a Methodist minister, had met her groom at an Epworth maple-syrup-and-biscuit supper. After their marriage, Copeland left his boarding-house, and the newlyweds rented a house at 319 North Madison Avenue, close to his office on Chilson Street.

By 1891, there were close to 14,000 practicing homeopaths in the United States (and more than 80,000 practicing dominant doctors). Copeland became determined to do his part to change the balance of those numbers, and he took an active part in the Homeopathic Medical Society of Michigan, whose motto was You Need It, and It Needs You. He became a member of the Saginaw Valley Homeopathic Society and soon was elected its president. "We must clothe ourselves in the panoply of war and go forth to more aggressive battle than has yet been recorded in all our splendid history," he would command his fellow homeopaths right at the beginning of his leadership.

The year before, Mark Twain had published a positive article about homeopathy in *Harper's Magazine*. He wrote that homeopathy "forced the old school doctor to stir around and learn something of a rational nature about his business," and that everyone should "feel grateful that homeopathy survived the attempts of allopathists to destroy it." That same year, Robert Koch developed tuberculin, which was made from the tuberculosis bacillus and was used to test for the disease. Even though it was not an antitoxin, a dominant professor at Harvard Medical School commented that "the use of Tuberculin is a form of vaccination which illustrates better than any example known to me the approval of homeo-pathic principles by our school."

Not only was Bay City booming, but so was Copeland's specialty, just as Hinsdale had predicted it would. With surgery now painless and mostly infection-free, patients were no longer as afraid of the knife. Copeland's skills soon became well known around town. He described a particularly nasty operation performed under messy conditions at a local bar on Water Street: the removal of an eyeball. "The memory of the saw-dust and filth through which I passed to see the suffering bartender in the loft above, conjure up thoughts which are indeed nightmarish. In that filthy place, and with no better one available, the operation was performed in the light of a smoking kerosene lantern." He reported in his casebook that his patient made "a happy recovery," also noting that "later he turned from his evil ways and became a pillar of the church." Such an observation was natural for Copeland, who liked to say that he was "one of those old-fashioned persons believing that medicine is a calling . . . just as much as the ministry is." Many people in Dexter once thought he might become a minister, but now his medical practice was like a ministry. He called doctors "the shepherds," and patients "the flocks," and said that "if homeopathy were not of God, that is, if it were not in harmony with the laws of nature, it would have come to naught." He was particularly proud of a letter he owned that Hahnemann had written to one of his patients, in which he mentioned, Copeland said, "his dependence upon the God of Hosts, and his reliance upon divine guidance in the practice of his profession."

The "wild and wooly westerner," as he teasingly called himself in a letter to his parents, continued to use a variety of homeopathic remedies on his patients. "I had been but a few months in Bay City, and was a candidate for all the business I could get," he said. "My bank account demanded that it should come mighty fast. An old gentleman, the father of the congressman of the district and proprietor of a great ship building plant, presented himself in my office. I was nearly terror stricken when I learned of the prominence of the patient. . . . He had a chronic corneal ulcer which had persisted in spite of, and I am frank to say, probably by reason of the long continued treatment he had had from the allopathic oculist. The family was a homeopathic one, and learning that a homeopathic oculist had come to town, I was consulted." Copeland prescribed *Mercurius corrosivus* (*Merc. cor.*), in a 6X dilution (1 part remedy and 1 million parts water) and reported that his famous patient had "an early cure." (The remedy is derived from mercuric chloride salt, a poison used as an antiseptic in the seventeenth and eighteenth centuries.) For a patient with a pain in his side and back, he prescribed Pulsatilla 2X and Colocynthis 2X, telling his patient to alternate the remedies every half hour, which was a new approach for Copeland. He tried that experiment again on a woman with "profuse menstrual bleeding and pain," prescribing Colocynthis 2X and Belladonna 2X every half hour. The patient told him that "complete relief followed." In another experiment, he told a patient with a chronic cough of "several years" to take *Calcarea carbonica*

(*Calc. carb.*) 3X every three hours, and even though the patient told him he was feeling better, he increased the dilution to 5X, and added Pulsatilla 2X for a newly developed stomachache. He believed that eyestrain contributed to many stomach problems.

He had learned in medical school how Hahnemann believed that "the dynamic force of minerals, magnets, electricity, and galvanism act no less powerfully upon [the] life principle and they are no less homeopathic" than the customary remedies. Hahnemann also said that "baths of pure water prove themselves partly palliative, partly as homeopathic serviceable aids in restoring health in acute diseases." Copeland decided to try something else that was novel for him. For a patient with "gastric distress," he prescribed a common substance full of "the dynamic force of minerals," a substance that, though ordinary, would nonetheless get him into a lot of trouble later in his career, especially with the AMA. "Rx H2O," he began writing often in his patient casebook—for sore throats, headaches, and stomach ailments. Water, prescribed four times a day. A cool drink of water.

Copeland was beginning to be aware that although his cures were as sought after as ever, and that as well as "the people who agree with us and the people who oppose our views," there was now a third group, "deserving no thought whatsoever—those who hold no fixed views on any given subject." Still, despite not wanting to think about such unworldly persons, he hoped one day to reach even them. He wasn't sure how, yet while still a young doctor, he knew that after first attacking the problems in his profession, he wanted to be an aggressive advocate for maybe even more than just homeopathy. Meanwhile, he recognized that "we would be blind indeed, however, if we were to imagine for one moment that the homeopathic profession is universally united." He was referring to the continuing conflict between the purists and the revisionists, or moderates, who slowly but surely were beginning to disagree about everything under the sun. Copeland always followed a saying found on the flyleaf of most homeopathic journals: "In essentials: harmony / In non-essentials: liberty / In all, charity." He believed that Hahnemann's basic principle of "like cures like" was the essential doctrine, and that "the size of the dose prescribed and the repetition of the remedy have little to do with homeopathy" and could be considered nonessential factors.

"I suppose I could go on indefinitely in pointing out the reasons why the doctor has an important place in public life," he would soon write, adding that "the medical man is so devoted to his profession that he hesitates to leave it to take on the larger work of helping to heal the ills of a nation." So the desire to help his country came first in a small way. In 1892, just a year after opening his practice, Copeland, who had worked hard for the Bay City Democrats to help elect Grover Cleveland president, asked his congressman for support in getting a place on the local Board of Pension Examiners, which handled disability cases. "My every vote since legally qualified has been for and in support of the Democrats," he told Congressman Thomas Weadock, whose father he had cured of a corneal ulcer. "I am sure our country would be better if more men of the medical profession entered the field of politics." He easily won a place on the board.

His activism continued, and the following year, 1893, when he was just twenty-five years old, he helped form the Christian Union, a group opposing the fanatical American Protective Association, which was attacking Catholics in Bay City. Copeland called the APA "the most unkind, unjust, un-Christian and un-godly movement of its generation," and in time, and after speeches by many people, the APA left the area. That same year, he was elected secretary of the Homeopathic Medical Society of Michigan, which now had 1,400 members. His lifelong balancing of medicine and politics began in earnest. It involved not only civic duties, where he would learn to handle a Republican and Democratic seesaw, but complex medical issues, which he would referee with deft, often stunning, conciliatory powers. His views were never the expected, and sometimes they clashed with the very side he seemed to be on. Nowhere was this truer than in a new fight at his alma mater that began in 1893.

Dr. Obetz, with whom Copeland had worked side by side as a surgical trainee, wanted to ride the wave of the allopathic-homeopathic alliance that had been slowly advancing. Obetz believed that it was now time for the two separate medical schools to merge into one. The majority of homeopaths were irate, and even wanted Obetz to resign (he eventually did), and most allopaths, as expected, wanted no part of any homeopathic college. They had never really left the warpath. Newspapers mostly favored the homeopaths, and one article reported that "the professional representatives of the regular school often overlook the fact that there are large numbers of people in the state who prefer homeopathy and employ homeopathic doctors. Nearly all of them are voters, many of them taxpayers, and heavy ones at that." But at least one article called the plan for consolidation "a most encouraging and refreshing sign of advancement in the science of medicine." Copeland got drawn into the fray because his state homeopathic society opposed a merger of the two schools. Some members even wanted the homeopathic college to leave Ann Arbor and move to another city altogether, possibly Detroit, forty miles to the east, where it could be completely independent and out of harm's way. Copeland wanted things to remain as they were—no merging and no transfer, although he somehow managed to convey to one of his close colleagues that he was actually in favor of moving the college to Detroit. Spoken—or unspoken—like the true politician he was in the process of becoming.

Meanwhile, resistance and resignations reigned at the University of Michigan, and when in the end the homeopathic college stayed in place and his former professor Wilbert Hinsdale became the new dean, Copeland was asked to become part of the faculty. He was invited to become a professor of ophthalmology and otology, replacing the friend who had been in favor of moving the school out of Ann Arbor. And so, in 1895, Roy and Mary left Bay City so he could return to what he called "one of the fairest towns in all this land." Ann Arbor now had an electric streetcar, though most residents still rode bicycles, and a sanitary sewer system. It was stepping up, as was Copeland, who was also stepping over, and in just six years he would become its mayor.

THE STUDENTS at both the homeopathic and the dominant—the new and the old—medical schools now attended classes for nine months, spread over a four-year period. They were required also to have at least two years of high school. The catalogue for the dominant medical school said "that the rapid development of medical science has necessitated the introduction of many new subjects," and while the homeopathic college tried to follow suit and evolve, it didn't attract as many students as the dominant school did, even though both schools stressed laboratory instruction, and both schools were officially recognized.

In 1895 and 1896, medicine continued to progress. Submicroscopic viruses, or infectious agents, were first observed in 1895, and this remarkable discovery would eventually refine and help track certain diagnoses. X-rays were developed that year, another diagnostic tool that would be of inestimable value in the treatment of illness and injury. In 1896, the magnetic detection of electrical waves was discovered, and the following year, the actual electron particle, which carries a unit charge of negative electricity, was first observed.

In 1895, Sigmund Freud had formulated his theory of hysterical neurosis that led to psychoanalysis and psychotherapy, or the "talking cure." Symptoms could disappear just by talking about them. A mind-set could be altered. Behavior could change. Patients could improve without medication. Homeopaths, with their lengthy interviews, had always used and believed in what was to them an age-old technique. Copeland had always held that the "mind and brain are so interlocked that when the mind is aroused, the brain sends its message to every part of the body, including the heart." He said that the average allopathic doctor, unlike the homeopath, "pays little attention to the moods and mental condition of his patient." Paying attention was a critical tool in discovering the correct remedy. Most homeopaths spent hours figuring out a single case, causing many dominant doctors to decide that this facet alone brought about relief from illness, and the actual remedies played a smaller role or even none.

Copeland would tell his students to "study the modern ideas of disease and morbid processes as they are now understood, delve into physical chemistry as it is taught in every university of the world, listen to the forensic eloquence of the physicist, the chemist, the physiologist and the pathologist; then take from the shelf the '*Organon of the Art of Healing.*'" Hahnemann's voice, he lectured, remained attuned to all medical advances "in perfect sweetness" and "in one symphony of perfect harmony."

In addition to his prestigious new teaching position, Copeland opened a practice on the busy corner of State Street, where all the stores were located, and North University Avenue, across from the campus. The office was, he said, "eight or ten" blocks from the train depot, so patients could come for homeopathic care from neighboring towns. He and Mary lived nearby at the Cutting Flats.

"I have been rushed, working like a slave since I returned," he wrote a friend in Bay City. Whatever his growing political aspirations, he was first and foremost a doctor, and performed more and more elaborate surgeries. A new five-story granite and grey pressed-brick homeopathic hospital, with five acres of lawn, had been built in 1892. It looked more like a large manor house than an institution and had been constructed without square corners or angles inside that could attract dirt and germs. Spreading oaks surrounded the hospital, and an apple orchard lay in the back, leading Copeland to quip that the unripe fruit would "doubtless furnish many cases of acute illness for the benefit of future doctors."

He was asked to operate on the eyes of a blind Civil War veteran, and when the time came for the bandages to be removed, he said that he "took them off and asked: 'What do you see, Mr. Webster?' His voice quivering with emotion, the old man answered: 'You, the handsomest man I ever saw.' Copeland said that his chest swelled justifiably, but collapsed a moment later when his patient added: 'But where did you get that awful big nose?' "

Belladonna, Bryonia (wild hops), and Nux Vomica became his most frequently used remedies now, and by 1895, most of his dilutions were 3X, or 1 part remedy to 1,000 parts water or alcohol. Most of his colleagues used this dilution. Occasionally, he went lower, as he once did with a patient with a brain hemorrhage, when he prescribed *Kali iodatum* 2X. (*Kali iodatum,* derived from iodine and potassium hydroxide, was generally used for swollen glands and diffuse pain.) He continued his experimenting, and sometimes tried slightly higher dilutions, as he had with his corneal ulcer patient, offering *Merc. cor.* in a dose of 6X. He also tried this remedy on a patient with a retinal hemorrhage, and wrote in his casebook that he had "seen marked improvement." This success encouraged him over the years to use even higher dilutions. (Still, 2X, 3X, and 6X were considered low potencies by most homeopaths, 30X to 200X were considered medium potencies, and anything above the 200th was considered high.) The split that had begun in the 1880s between the purists, who strictly followed a dictum that the higher the dilution the stronger the curative powers, and the moderates, like Copeland, who didn't believe the dilution was as important as the right remedy, persisted well into the 1890s and beyond. "In the true sense," Copeland told his somewhat bewildered students at the University of Michigan, "the dose is not the amount given at one time; it is the total amount administered. If this be true, one cannot state positively that the 6th, the 30th, or the 200th is indicated."

He greatly enjoyed trying out new techniques, and described in detail his treatment for a thirty-year-old woman "who has all her life suffered from violent headaches." He had hoped that "the adjustment of proper glasses might be of benefit" and recorded in his casebook that he "made a careful examination. The ophthalmoscope, retinascope, and other instruments of precision were employed and the error of refraction carefully measured. Astigmia and slight muscle imbalance were found for both," of which, he said, he made "the usual corrections." But, he also recorded, "absolutely no relief followed." He reviewed the case and came up with the same prescription for glasses. Finally, he advised using some homeopathic remedies, and he and the patient discussed her symptoms for two hours. "The patient complained of having a 'hard ache' [*sic*] in the top and back of the head and in the temples. Every jar was painful and she said that the smallest drink of wine, or exposure to sunshine, brought on the headache. For two days before the appearance of the menses, she would have the blues and, for days at a time, intense melancholia. There were occasional periods of blindness when she could not distinguish form . . . the pain was as if there were a hot iron against her eye, the head seemed full of blood with occasional nose-bleed." He decided to try *Calc. carb.* 12X, which was 1 part ground oyster shells and 1 trillion parts water or alcohol. There were probably no molecules left of the original powder after such a dilution, yet two months after the patient tried this remedy, she reported that she felt "marvelously better," and Copeland recorded that "on the strength of the improvement, I discontinued the glasses entirely." Two weeks later, the patient said that she had had "one slight headache," so he gave her another dose of *Calc. carb.,* this time in a higher dilution of 30X. He reported that three months later the patient's husband told him that the patient "was well and happy, had had no return of the symptoms and was in better general health than in the years before."

Copeland said that he had one patient—an inmate at the Michigan State Prison—who "was seized with an acute inflammatory form of glaucoma in both eyes" and was paroled to his clinic at the governor's request. "The pain of this disease seems unbearable almost," Copeland wrote in his casebook. "It radiates from the eye into the temple, the brow, and, indeed, to every part of the head." He explained that "since the prison was at that time under old-school control, it was probable the victim had had opiates without limit." Copeland, an acquaintance of the governor, thought about "puncturing" the eyeballs, but decided to "wait until the acute symptoms subsided." The prisoner told him that "his eyes seemed as if on fire," and Copeland saw not only that "the lids were swollen," but that "the man was sweating and restless, and had a great thirst and fear of cold." He decided to prescribe *Arsenicum album* (*Arsen. alb.*), 6X, a remedy he had tried as a student doctor on a patient with back pain. He reported that "in all my experience I never saw a remedy act more quickly. Had it been a narcotic, the effect could not have been more magical." But he believed that the body's reaction to the correct remedy was a chemical reaction that was definite and positive. The "old" doctors forced the body to accept medicines that didn't work properly, and doing this was, he said, "like forcing upon the body a lazy and unproductive spouse."

At homeopathic meetings, members continued to bicker. Young Copeland always tried to reason with them: "My friends, is there not a middle ground? Can we not bury our theoretical differences, and meet on the common ground of expediency, if one must use so cold a word?" Homeopaths had to stop their infighting, because, he told them, "we have a common cause and a common enemy." The common enemy was the old-school doctor who wouldn't accept homeopathy as a legitimate science. The AMA, for its part, didn't care anymore whether the dilutions were infinitesimal or large. It was simply homeopathy's "means of selection," the chosen remedies themselves, full of nothing, that angered, baffled, or threatened them, and while it would never stop calling homeopathy "popular," it never called it scientific.

Copeland urged others to "show that homeopathy has the numerical strength, the capability of united organization, and the intellectual ability to impress its theories upon the whole known world. When we do that we shall deserve to win and we will win," he said, wearing the bright smile he wore every day. He was a happy man in Ann Arbor.

In 1896, the American Naturopathic Organization was founded. Naturopathy was the treatment of disease by heat, light, cold enemas, hot and cold (even air) baths, massage, and diet. It incorporated some of homeopathy's beliefs about the importance of diet and fresh air, but used no medicine, and its practitioners were generally not medical-school graduates. The public became enthralled with its nonchemical, down-to-earth, gentle, hands-on doctrines.

The AMA became frustrated with this new player, which it considered not only fake, but dangerous. Three years later, in 1899, it would include chiropractic, the spinal manipulation therapy invented in the United States, in the same light. Both naturopathy and chiropractic claimed to use the body's energy as part of their cure, a facet that particularly infuriated the dominant doctors. The AMA wrote of naturopathy that not only was it "unscientific," but "the cult seems to have no basic idea but to be rather a nature-cure hodgepodge with a decided antipathy to drugs. In fact naturopathy has developed in part as an effort to broaden the scope of chiropractics [sic]." The AMA was particularly incensed when it learned that a naturopathic doctor had a patient send him a sample of her saliva on a blotter. This doctor then diagnosed the woman's illness (although the AMA was not told what it was), and the patient was prescribed 18 cups of cabbage broth daily and a tea made out of peach tree leaves.

Most naturopaths believed that the germ theory of disease was wrong, and that, in fact, it was the disease that caused the germ. So did, of course, most purist homeopaths. In 1889, at a meeting of the IHA, the International Hahnemannian Association, a doctor announced that the germ theory involved dominant medicine's "haste and want of reason." Another doctor replied, "If the germ theory, or the causation of disease by germs be true, of course our therapeutics are no longer of any use."

Under the right conditions, Copeland said that he "had no objection to certain forms of drugless healing." He particularly favored "air baths," saying that they toned up the texture of the skin. Still, for him, the right conditions included one big one: that the healer have a full-fledged medical degree. He said that his "criticism of the drugless healer is not that he depends upon unusual methods and scorns to give medicine. My sole objection to him is because the average drugless healer is ignorant of the fundamentals of medical knowledge." As one of the few homeopaths willing to talk about quackery, he said he was against "pseudo-medicine," acquired in "so-called studies that lasted from one week to six months." He stressed that "no person is qualified to set himself up as a healer of disease, nor is he justified in taking charge of a sick person, unless he is fully informed regarding the physiology, anatomy, and histology of the human body, and unless he is so well founded in pathology as to be able to differentiate between the serious disease and a trifling one, between a dangerous contagious disease and a harmless one, between a curable condition and a fatal malady." In this, Copeland and the dominant doctors saw eye-to-eye.

But his true feelings about "drugless healing" were reflected in one change he made in a draft of a speech about the new therapies. He first referred to chiropractic as a "faith cure," and then later crossed out those words and wrote in the term "drugless healing." That change, more than any of the words he actually spoke, showed that he believed drugless healing, unlike homeopathy, "was not of god."

On January 20, 1896, the faculty of the homeopathic medical school met at the Hotel American in Ann Arbor for their weekly meeting. Copeland, now the new secretary of the faculty, wrote that it was "moved that Dr. Hinsdale ask the Board of Regents to establish a training school for nurses" at the homeopathic hospital. (A nursing school had been in existence since 1891 at the dominant hospital, and in fact, the actual profession didn't exist at all until after 1870.) Eleven days later, at the next meeting, held at the Copelands' house, he wrote that it was "moved that Dr. Copeland be appointed to head a committee on the training school, to prepare the course of study, arrange the faculty, etc." In other words, Copeland, not busy enough with his activism, teaching, and medical practice, would take charge of creating a nursing school. "There is nothing in the atmosphere in Ann Arbor which encourages softness and self-indulgence," the industrious doctor later remarked to a colleague.

On February 14, he was officially appointed dean of the nursing school. It was agreed that a three-story stone house would be built as a residence for the first class of twenty nurses. The requirements for admission were a high-school education, "good health and temper, and a love of the proposed profession." The training consisted of "three years of text book and clinical work" to prepare them for a twelve-hour day.

"From earliest times, the homeopathic profession made much of the natural methods," Copeland lectured. "So much indeed did our forebears depend upon hygiene and bedside attention that our early rivals said we were not doctors, but clever nurses." He said that Hahnemann himself called attention to the value of "the ministrations of the nurse." It is "a noble art," and a "blessing," Copeland said, adding that "I have the feeling that a nurse to truly succeed must be conscious of her high calling." He would become a strong advocate of nursing care, forever believing that the roles of both doctors and nurses were equally played out with "a devout spirit," "in a sacred place." He would also become an advocate for women doctors, saying that only homeopathy offered them a special "reign." After all, he noted, hadn't his class in medical school, unlike the old-school class, boasted a Miss Peck, a Miss Backhouse, a Miss Carey, a Miss Wheelock, and a Miss Hill?

IN 1891, the AMA had tabled a resolution that a chemist be appointed to analyze all secret nostrums, although that same year it approved a recommendation that the U.S. government publish a report identifying and analyzing these drugs. Adulterated, worthless, and fraudulent products on the market continued to be a serious problem throughout the century, but the AMA wanted someone else to do the examining. Three years later, it found that someone else in its old friend the American Pharmaceutical Association, which, in 1894, began contributing reports to the AMA on all secret nostrums.

The homeopaths still maintained that they could regulate the raw ingredients of their remedies, and, in fact, homeopathic remedies were not actually singled out by the AMA at this time, although most dominant doctors, when they weren't giving them to their patients, still considered them quackery. But the AMA's focus was mostly on such fakes as "a native herb from South Africa" called "Umckaloabo," which contained glycerine and alcohol, or Dr. Charles' Flesh Food ("The Great Beautifier"), which was composed only of starch and suet.

In 1895, the AMA's House of Delegates adopted several resolutions submitted to them by the American Pharmaceutical Association. These resolutions "condemned 'the prescribing and dispensing of proprietary medicines,' protested 'against any system of protection which permits one manufacturer to retain the exclusive control of a pharmaceutic product indefinitely,' and recommended that 'the working formula of every pharmaceutic preparation should be published and a technically correct scientific name given to it,' and recommended the use of the U.S. Pharmacopeia and the National Formulary." A pharmacopeia was, of course, an official list of drugs and their preparations recognized by the medical profession. The *U.S. Pharmacopeia* was first published in the 1820s (although a version was published in 1778 for use by the army only). The AMA's 1895 resolutions left the homeopaths out in the cold, which was precisely where the organization preferred them to be. There was no mention of a homeopathic pharmacopeia, although the homeopaths didn't expect or want at that time any mention by a group that had banned them. (Two years later, the Committee on Pharmacy of the AIH published an official, comprehensive *Homeopathic Pharmacopeia,* which the AMA ignored.)

Still, it was considered a small triumph to some homeopaths that even though most dominant doctors scorned the use of their remedies, at least publicly, they did give homeopaths credit for introducing the concept of "sugar-coating" to medications. Copeland and his colleagues resented such credit. "Sugar-coated pills are pleasant to take which may add to their danger," he said, explaining that "that is the reason they are coated with sugar. They are less drastic," but also "habit-forming because they appeal to the taste."

Copeland, unlike many of his colleagues who objected to any

attempt to be friendly with the AMA, said he "had no quarrel with the AMA as a scientific group." Indeed, he would always try to maintain cordial relations with the organization and didn't fear any of its "modern ideas."

In 1898, an AMA Committee on Scientific Research was established to provide grants for medical research. The following year, when the world heard the first magnetic recording of sound, Dr. George H. Simmons, a former homeopath from Lincoln, Nebraska, became the editor of the *Journal of the American Medical Association* (*JAMA*). He would bring new medical, political, and financial energy to the group. Simmons, who graduated from both the Hahnemann Medical College of Chicago (a homeopathic institution) and later the Rush Medical College of Chicago (a dominant institution), opposed antagonizing homeopaths. He favored a more balanced approach, although by no means a conciliatory one. At some point, homeopaths would have to go, or would go, because nature would phase them out. He agreed with the dean of Rush Medical College, who argued that "we cannot have a homeopathic science of medicine; we cannot have an eclectic science of medicine, and we cannot have an osteopathic science of medicine." There can be, the dean said, "but one science of medicine." Copeland would counter this reasoning by saying, "The truth is—why dodge it?—medicine, as it is commonly practiced, is but the expression of the individual art of the individual doctor." Dominant doctors "have not looked squarely and without bias" at the "facts and results" of homeopathy, and, he argued surprisingly, it was not from "ill will" but from "inertia"! Copeland said that dominant doctors (now also called "orthodox" doctors) had "an implanted and nurtured skepticism, naturally enough, because in their early years their colleges mocked and vilified us, and ever since they have fed upon a blinding literature of prejudice and injustice." These were fighting words.

By the beginning of the twentieth century, "the whole known world," which Copeland often lectured about to his students, knew about alpha and beta rays in radioactive atoms, knew about the quantum theory of energy, matter, and motion, and had heard human speech transmitted by radio waves. The world also learned about the fever-reducing and pain-relieving qualities of aspirin powder, a non-narcotic derivative of salicylic acid, from the bark of willows—which was formulated by a German company, Friedrich Bayer & Co. Orthodox doctors prescribed it regularly to their patients. Homeopaths stayed far away from it.

Copeland, taking an even more forceful role, now asked, "Will it not be well for us to take a glimpse at the present state of homeopathy, and the conditions necessary to perpetuate its practice? Unless we, ourselves, recognize the limitations of homeopathy, on the one side, and its unbounded possibilities, on the other, and unless we devise plans to properly present its scientific claims, it bids fair to be overlooked in the crowded highway of the world's progress." He concluded, "with Christian Science, Osteopathy, Chiro-practice, the many cults based on psychological or physical theory, the biological teachings, and the multitude of 'isms'—with each of these making insistent demands for recognition, it behooves homeopathy to inventory its possessions." These were bold words (especially his use of the word "cult") from a doctor who "conscientiously believed that the superiority of the homeopathic practice has been proven in every disease, in every climate, in every season."

FOUR

"Much Missionary Labor Yet to Perform"

In 1898, when he was thirty, and past middle age (life expectancy at that time for males was 47.9 years), Copeland, dapper in his dark pin-striped suits, high-collared crisp white shirts, and colorful silk ties, with his wavy hair parted on the side, brushed dramatically across his forehead, and covering his thick eyebrows, added a brand-new distinction to his career. He published his first professional paper, an up-to-date primer for medical students on measuring vision: "Refraction," about the deflection of light as it enters the eyes. The ambitious homeopath, who would himself begin to wear glasses—or spectacles, as they were still called—when he was forty, was determined to keep up with the best of the ophthalmologists in the country and to teach the newer ones what he already knew. In fact, because he saw no real distinction between his ways and those of allopathic doctors, each new twist and turn he learned or understood better than before involving his specialty of the eyes made him a better homeopath as well.

Eye surgery was becoming easier because of the use of cocaine drops that made the operations not only painless but less subject to complications from general anesthesia. This was particularly true for cataract surgery, in which cloudy lenses that caused blurred vision were removed. Still, the operation was not simple, infection was still a real possibility, and recovery was not quick. In the past, bloodletting and full-strength mercury were used to try to dissolve cataracts, and doctors (without anesthesia) pushed the lens to the base of the eye with a sharp knife, a procedure that more often than not caused inflammation, infection,

Copeland's first book soon became "important."

and eventual blindness. In the eighteenth century, doctors removed the entire lens and capsule, also without anesthesia, and by the time in the late nineteenth century when Copeland learned the operation, it involved removing only the lens. He got so good at it that by 1902, when he had been teaching at the University of Michigan for seven years, and had also become, two years earlier, the head of the eye and ear section of the American Institute of Homeopathy, he decided to write a paper on the operation. He had by that time seen "thousands of cases of cataract," he said.

He emphasized that "the chances of success or failure" in cataract extraction had to do entirely with the elasticity or inelasticity of the cornea, the transparent tissue that shields the front of the eye. He said that an indication of the cornea's structure could be discovered by pinching and releasing the skin on the back of the hand. If the skin was flabby and inelastic, he believed that the wound in the eye would not only not heal properly, but infection would probably occur as well. With respect to infection, he said that it was important that "the night before the patient is given a bath and shampoo, with thorough scrubbing of the eyebrows, forehead, nose, and cheeks." In addition, the patient's eye was to be irrigated with a boric acid lotion and then covered with a "thick pad of gauze" dipped in bichloride of mercury solution. He had first used *Merc. cor.* (mercuric chloride) successfully in Bay City on his congressman's father. He also used it to treat certain stomach problems.

For twenty-one pages, Copeland detailed the operation, stressing skill and cleanliness as its most important components. He also said it was better if the patient could be in an airy and sun-filled room, even though his account of his only failure (from infection) contradicted this advice. In a report that was a perfect example of what set him apart from his allopathic colleagues, he told of a patient who "was a 'roustabout' in a livery stable . . . careless regarding personal cleanliness, wore two suits of woolen underwear, summer and winter, slept in his clothes in the hay loft, and would seem to be immune to exposure of any sort." Before the operation the patient was given a bath, a thin nightshirt, and a clean bed. But this pre-op routine proved "too much," Copeland decided: "A few hours after the operation, he had a chill, followed by a high fever, and pus appeared in the wound on the second day. I honestly believe, that had this patient been left in his normal dirty condition and sent to the barn after the operation, he would have made a nice recovery." He concluded that in this case the "the radical departure from the accustomed habits" of his patient caused an "acute systemic disturbance," or infection. In other words, an imbalance in his "vital force" made the recovery somehow go wrong. Hahnemann would have agreed.

Before beginning cataract surgery, Copeland sometimes first used a homeopathic remedy called *Calcarea fluorica,* or calcium fluorite, made from a dark grey mineral stone found in parts of North and South America and western Europe. *Calc. fluor.* was used to keep tissues flexible, and was one of twelve "tissue salts" identified in the mid-1800s by Wilhelm Schussler, a German homeopathic doctor who maintained that some diseases were partially caused by mineral deficiencies. He claimed that patients could be helped if they received the missing minerals (*Calc. fluor.* exists naturally in tooth enamel, in skin and blood cells, and in connective tissue). Other Schussler's "tissue salts" included Magnesium Phosphate (*Mag. phos.*), used for cramps and spasms; Potassium Chloride (*Kali mur.*), used for inflammation; Sodium Phosphate (*Nat. phos.*), used for indigestion or gout; Calcium Phosphate (*Calc. phos.*), used for anemia or cramps; Calcium Sulfate (*Calc. sulf.*), used for boils; Iron Phosphate (*Ferrum phos.*), used for inflammation; Potassium Phosphate (*Kali phos.*), used for nervousness; Potassium Sulfate (*Kali sulf.*), used for skin ailments; Sodium Chloride (salt; *Nat. mur.*), often used for colds and anxiety; Sodium Sulfate (*Nat. sulf.*), used for liver and gall bladder disease; and Silicea, used for boils or night sweats. Most tissue (or cell) salts had multiple uses.

Copeland said that he saw improvement in only one or two cases of cataracts when he used *Calcarea fluorica,* admitting that "this remedy could not be expected to do much." For all his talent and studiousness, Copeland didn't think his prescribing skills were as good as his surgical skills. In a rare moment of modesty, he admitted that when it came to prescribing he was not a "master."

Still, he described a successful case of using a remedy to cure a severe optic-nerve problem that usually led to blindness. He wrote in his casebook that "on the 22nd of March, 1898, Mrs. M.H.R, aged 49, visited my clinic in Ann Arbor, complaining of . . . failing vision." Her optic nerve showed atrophy, or degeneration, causing a loss of functioning, and Copeland said that this type of problem offered "an unfavorable prognosis." He also reported that Mrs. M.H.R. complained of "an obstinate stomach trouble, great distension with frequent belching." This additional symptom was what led him to try *Argent. nit.* (silver nitrate) on his patient, a remedy that he had learned could be used for anxiety and digestive complaints, as well as for inflammation of the eyes. (In Bay City, he had used it on a patient with diabetes.) He gave the remedy (the dilution is not mentioned) to Mrs. M.H.R. for nine months; he said that he saw her only "occasionally" during this time. On December 30, 1898, he recorded in his casebook that her vision "was practically normal in each eye, and every ophthalmoscopic evidence of atrophy had disappeared." In a lecture on this case, Copeland said, "contrary to the almost universal testimony of the authorities and in spite of the natural course of the disease . . . I am perfectly satisfied that the homeopathic remedy has cured at least one patient of optic nerve atrophy. I doubt exceedingly if nature, unassisted, could have ended the case so happily."

SIR WILLIAM OSLER, the leading orthodox doctor of the day— Copeland called him "one of the greatest medical authorities in the world"—was quoted in a newspaper on January 27, 1901, as saying, "No one will deny that as many patients recover under homeopathic treatment as recover under any form of treatment." Homeopaths who read these words either shrugged in a finally-he's-come-to-his-senses sort of way or simply shrugged it off because they were too busy listening to and sometimes trying to shut out the noisy arguments within their own ranks. Even so, as unusual as Dr. Osler's statement was, he was not so much endorsing homeopathic remedies as he was his belief that the less medication given, the better off the patient.

Some local orthodox medical societies began slowly reaching out to homeopaths to become members as long as they severed their relations with sectarian organizations, i.e., the American Institute of Homeopathy, which now had a membership of over 2,000, although there were an estimated 10,000 homeopaths in practice. The International Hahnemannian Association had 1,300 members in 1892. The AMA had 8,000 members in 1901, out of an estimated 104,000 orthodox doctors.

This courting was an attempt to get homeopaths to acknowledge that there was but "one science of medicine," something most of them would never go along with; they saw the wooing as a bid to control them, and eventually to dissolve them. The orthodox doctors had even suggested the removal of the word "homeopath" from titles and said they would accept them as true equals if they became part of the mainstream. The trouble was, homeopaths believed that *they* were the mainstream. Copeland's response to the courting was curious. He said the attitude of allopathy brought "a new danger to homeopathy," because it "is not accustomed to an environment of friendliness." Homeopathy, he said, "must now face new conditions." Yet he was sure that with the "divine guidance" he believed in, homeopaths would be able to face the future.

On May 21, 1901, four months after Dr. Osler's observation about homeopathy, the new president of the Homeopathic Medical Society of Michigan gave an address called "Homeopathy in the Twentieth Century." The president was Copeland. It was no wonder that his marriage to Mary was beginning to crumble; with no children and her husband's heavy schedule, Mrs. Copeland was often alone and adrift. She had few friends. The year before, Copeland had spent time away from home at a lengthy Methodist Church conference, and he had also decided to become president of the Michigan chapter of the Epworth League.

In his presidential address to his fellow homeopaths, Copeland reminded his audience that "homeopathy was born, it grew up and conquered a large share at least, of the English-speaking world during the Nineteenth Century." In his by now typical style of weaving history and religion into his speeches and class lectures, he said that homeopathy "need not weep, like Alexander, for more worlds to conquer, because it has much missionary labor yet to perform." Also, this speech would have warmed the heart of the new president of the AMA, George Simmons, because of its acceptance and praise of allopathy. Yet for all of Copeland's trust in "the revelations of the laboratory," "chemical and microscopical tests," and "bacteriological examinations," he didn't want to see homeopathy subsumed by orthodox medicine. He felt that the new laboratory methods increased the possibility of discovering a more exact homeopathic diagnosis. He told the audience that he was sure that Hahnemann would have come to the same conclusion. He remarked also that his family had "a standing order" that in the event of an illness so severe that it left him unable to speak, they were to call in a homeopathic doctor, "no matter how despised and hated of men, in preference to the most popular and clever prescriber of the other school."

Copeland was particularly enthusiastic about "the most recent laboratory advances" of "blood examinations" and the new light they cast on "some obscure diseases, such as leukemia." He then spoke of a case by a fellow homeopath: "A middle-aged woman of rather strong build, mother of two children, of good personal and family history, began to suffer pain in the left side under the short ribs. The pain was aggravated by deep breathing and overexertion. Sometimes she was annoyed by nausea and vomiting. She consulted a physician, who diagnosed pleurisy and treated her case as such. As her strength persistently failed to return, other physicians were called from time to time. An enlargement in the left hypochrondrium [upper region of the abdomen] finally became noticeable, and an addition was made to the diagnosis—'with empyema [pus] bulging down into the abdomen.' The bulging area was aspirated a number of times with no evidence of the presence of pus or other fluid."

Bryonia was prescribed but didn't help. Eventually the blood was examined, and as a result leukemia was diagnosed. Copeland added that the blood exam "did more than to determine a brilliant diagnosis," it also "proved at once that Bryonia could not cure, because it is never indicated in such conditions. It called to mind Arsenicum, Phosphorus, the mineral acids and snake poisons. It made possible a prescription, the early carrying out of which would prolong the life and comfort of the patient and widen the reputation of homeopathy as a system of medicine." The laboratory was homeopathy's new ally.

Arsenicum, or *Arsenicum iodatum,* considered a minor remedy, was made from metallic arsenic and iodine, and was given for tuberculosis and lymphatic cancer. It was never used by orthodox doctors in any form. Phosphorus is a nonmetallic mineral that glows in the dark; first discovered in urine, it is found naturally in teeth, bones, and bodily fluids. Orthodox doctors prescribed it for malaria, pneumonia, rheumatism, headaches, and epilepsy, while homeopaths prescribed it for nervousness, heavy bleeding, and digestive problems. Copeland's reference to mineral acids was probably Schussler's tissue salts. Snake venom was used for vascular and circulatory problems, and the remedy was made from bushmaster snakes (the American homeopath Constantine Hering first proved this venom in the mid-1800s), adders, cobras, rattlesnakes, or yellow pit vipers.

Copeland went on to lecture that "our materia medica teems with symptoms which sound ridiculous to the lay mind and are scoffed at by our rivals of the other school. Under 'Alumina,' for instance, is this startling symptom: 'Desire for [to eat] clean white rags.' This symptom is an indication, merely, of a perverted appetite." Then in his presidential speech, he asked one of the most important questions, one that was on the minds of many orthodox doctors in America: "Is it possible to find a scientific explanation for a symptom which seems so absurd?" His answer was yes, and he called for every single homeopathic proving to be revised "in the light of modern science." He asked that this be done under the direction of "expert diagnosticians, expert chemists, and expert pathologists." Homeopaths would show that every symptom had a scientific basis.

One month later, in June, Copeland was the graduation speaker for the Class of 1901 at his alma mater. His speech echoed many of the themes in his lecture on homeopathy in the twentieth century, and even extended some of them. He now called for the establishment of "a great laboratory of drug pathology." He reminded the medical-school graduates that "the successful consummation of this scheme will involve much labor. It will be every day and every hour kind of business." He then announced that the American Institute of Homeopathy would act on this recommendation, and a laboratory would be created, although he gave no timetable for what he said would be the " 'magnum opus' of the present century."

That fall, Copeland began to understand that he had to do even more than he had already accomplished in his thirty-three years. He had a feeling now that a position beyond his norm might hold the secret to some future promises for homeopathy, and he would soon begin a pattern of reaching outside medicine to achieve certain medical goals.

WHEN ROY and Mary Copeland returned from a much-needed vacation in California to try to pull their marriage together, it became clear what the new position would be. Copeland said that his work with the faculty of the Homeopathic Medical College "brought him into more or less intimate relations with the political powers of the state and particularly of the immediate locality." He went on to confide that Ann Arbor was "a boss-ridden community" and that "the leading political party was sadly divided." Sophisticate that he was becoming, he even made a reference to the corrupt politics of New York City, saying that certain things in Ann Arbor "flavor too much of Tammany tactics." He was the man to change things. He was asked by some influential friends to became "a compromise candidate for Mayor." In no time at all, the former Democrat became the Republican candidate, marking the first of several party changes and political upsets that continued throughout his life. He wrote a friend in Bay City that "the fact is I couldn't stand William Jennings Bryan and left the Democratic party."

A magazine article about Copeland later characterized what happened: "The mayoralty of Ann Arbor shanghaied him when he was out of town. . . . Why is the public so ravenous for Dr. Copeland? Two explanations have been offered. One, furnished by relatives and friends in Ann Arbor, is that he is a man of destiny. There may be something to this. . . . The other theory, recently worked out, has less superstition in it. This theory is that Dr. Copeland had not been the plaything of chance, but has bossed his own destiny with great intelligence and pertinacity."

Whatever the reason, in 1901 Copeland became Mayor Copeland of Ann Arbor, Michigan. It was a close election, which he won by only 232 votes out of the 2,618 that were cast. Plaything of chance or master of his destiny, he was in charge of a city of 14,400 residents at a salary of one gold dollar a year.

His inaugural address, according to the *Detroit Free Press,* "struck a popular chord." An editorial said his message "reveals the fact that he is an optimist. He has faith in the public, faith in the city council, and faith in himself. With good health and plenty of enthusiasm he may go

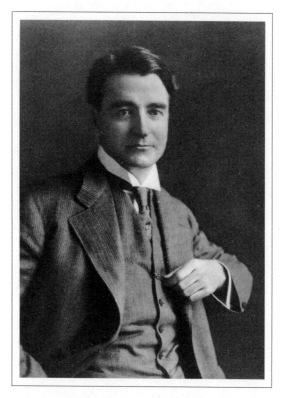

Mayor Copeland, 1901

through his term of office without coming to believe that the public is unappreciative and the city council dishonest." The local Ann Arbor paper, the *Argus,* described the morning he took his oath of office: "He was asked if he had made up his mind as to the appointments and a look of pain shot over his face as if he was just having a molar pulled out with a monkey wrench. 'No, I have not,' he answered, 'but I hope to before the end of the week. It seems as if every man who voted for me represents a different class that must be represented in the appointments. One thing is certain and that is I will not have any trouble in finding men who are willing to sacrifice themselves for the city's service. I have not been obliged to go out into the highways and byways to find men who would accept the appointment.' The appointments that Mayor Copeland will make will be scanned very closely. . . . Dr. Copeland is an eye specialist. Can he see anything green in the eye of an anti [those who opposed him]?" He must have, because two weeks later the *Argus* wrote that he had "reconsidered his announcement that he would this week acquaint the public with the men upon whom he would call into a self-sacrificing devotion to the interests of the city. . . . 'Do you want to save yourself any further annoyance' he was asked by The Argus. 'No, I'm getting used to it. In fact I would hate to become lonesome after such a strenuous training of two weeks.' 'Will you announce your appointments now?' 'No, I cannot for the reason that they had not yet been decided upon.' " He later said there had been "the most unseemly scramble for patronage."

But eventually the appointments were decided upon, and so was a lot more. He didn't take any of his duties lightly. He ordered more sidewalks to be built. (The first ones had been built five years earlier, in 1896.) He sought a plan for the general sprinkling of the streets, noting mischievously that "aside from the heat, which is not excessive in our shaded streets, and upon our fresh and fragrant lawns, the dusty driveways and dirt-impregnated atmosphere are the chief causes of discomfort in the summer season. Personally I do not object to this condition of things, because it promotes and aggravates diseases of certain organs which afford me a living." He requested more garbage collection and complained of "foul-smelling dump heaps" in parts of Ann Arbor, which now counted piano-building and furniture- and rug-making among its milling, brewing, and gas-fixtures industries. Copeland wanted better snow removal. He created park improvements, and in fact created a park system where none had existed before. He sided with labor in all disputes. He announced that he favored "a raising of wages in the case of teams to $3.50 a week." He fought the water power interests, and was taken to court in an effort to defeat his requests for lower rates. According to the *Argus,* "One day the Mayor's telephone bell rang. 'President of the Water Company speaking,' said the voice. 'If you don't withdraw your ordinances for lower rates, we'll take the case to the Supreme Court of the United States. We'll give you just two hours to decide.' 'Wait a minute, wait a minute, don't hang up,' said Dr. Copeland, 'I don't need two hours—I'll tell you now. You take the case to the Supreme Court or take it to hell—I'll never quit!' That is his style. But what happened in this case? 'All right,' said the Water Company President, 'we will accept your ordinance.' It was the last bluff of a blustering official who had never been defeated before. Dr. Copeland won his fight. In this same war it took him a year and a court decision to win his right to appoint his own corporate counsel, a man true to the people's interests. But he won.

He is interested in the human side of government." He even protected the old-line telephone company from prospective competition.

But later the *Argus* charged that he won all these battles by being secretive and by costing the city large sums of money. In an article headlined "As Mum as an Oyster," the paper now wrote satirically about a waterworks meeting: "After the mayor and the committee assembled all the doors were locked and the windows shut so that nothing could escape. Key holes were stopped up with blank votes and the transoms closed. . . . Secrecy breeds suspicion." Yet the paper also believed that "had it not been for his efforts to bond the city, for which undoubtedly others were more to blame than he was, he would have gone out of office as one of the most popular men that have held it." Still, in the end Copeland got what he asked for, all except reelection in 1903.

In 1899, the AMA encouraged passage of a law for compulsory smallpox vaccinations, an action that pleased those homeopaths who saw the resemblance of vaccines to homeopathic dilutions. But most homeopaths saw vaccines as interfering with the body's own immune system, creating a barrier to healing and cure. (Chiropractors saw little value in vaccinations, and naturopaths, none.) By the turn of the century, there were also antitoxins for rabies, typhoid, tetanus, and diphtheria, and by 1907 there would be one for cholera.

Even though Hahnemann had lauded Jenner's smallpox discovery in 1796, many doctors, both homeopaths and allopaths, didn't see much of a resemblance because the active ingredient in the vaccine was not only larger than that found in a remedy, but could actually be measured, unlike that in a highly diluted remedy. In addition, a vaccine was given to large groups of people and was not individualized according to special symptoms. Still, Copeland told an audience of homeopaths that the use of vaccines "is a remarkable instance of 'the old school' stumbling toward the light." His friend and colleague at the University of Michigan, W. A. Dewey, MD, speculated that "it is not improbable that homeopathic remedies act as toxins, and by dynamization cause to be developed in the human economy antibodies or antitoxins which effect the cure." Between 1885 and 1890, a remedy called Tuberculinum had been proved. It was made from the lung tissue of tuberculosis victims, and was used not as a vaccine but as an aid for all respiratory illnesses.

In 1907, members of the AIH heard a lecture about the use of "a splendid piece of homeopathic practice," a smallpox vaccine called Variolinum, which was made "from the contents of the ripened pustule of smallpox . . . not the virus of cowpox," and was given by mouth, not inoculation. Multiple provings had shown that "in exceptional instances, smallpox will occur in spite of the fact the Variolinum had been used." But the report went on to say that the same is true of the inoculation method, and that, in fact, smallpox occurs "with much greater frequency" with this method, the one orthodox doctors used.

Under the careful eye of George Simmons, the AMA continued to cultivate its more level approach toward homeopaths. In fact, in 1903, the Code of Ethics that had excluded them was slightly revised, not with any outright approval of their membership, but more with benign neglect. They were not mentioned at all. It was by that time well known that orthodox medical societies wanted to bring homeopaths into their fold, under their supervision. They wanted to bring them into the twentieth century. After all, they believed, what doctor—homeopath, eclectic, or orthodox—could resist the exquisite advances that were being made in medical science?

In 1900, the study of genetics, first discussed in 1858, became a separate area of scientific inquiry, although it was not until two years later that the term "gene" was originated. In 1901, the hormone adrenaline, which controls metabolism, the chemistry of body fluids, and secondary sexual characteristics, was discovered, and the following year secretin, which controls pancreas function, was first seen. These discoveries of the body's chemical messengers were not only advances for orthodox medicine, but regarded by most homeopaths as advancing their cause as well, and not just because of Copeland's belief that each new medical breakthrough helped homeopaths find a more precise diagnosis and remedy. Many homeopaths saw the revelation of microscopic-sized hormones as good news because the dilutions depended on microscopic-sized ingredients, and if there was acceptance by orthodox doctors that hormones existed, why not acceptance that highly diluted remedies had real qualities, too?

That same year, the body's blood groups (A, B, AB, and O) were identified, which meant there could now be safer blood transfusions, particularly during surgery. It was also determined in 1901 that yellow fever was carried by mosquitoes. An entry on homeopathy two years later in *Scientific American*'s encyclopedia, *The Americana,* said that when the cause of an illness cannot be ascertained, homeopaths attribute it to "the occult." It also said that homeopathy "does not cure directly," emphasizing in italics that "*the homeopathic medicine is a specific-restoration-stimulant, only and always.*" This was a brand-new public definition, at least brand-new in an encyclopedia with the reputation of a journal like *Scientific American.* It had been written by one of Copeland's acquaintances, a well-known homeopath by the name of Pemberton Dudley, of the Hahnemann Medical College in Philadelphia. The purists wondered if this entry had been devised by a bunch of revisionists in order to keep in step with modern science.

In 1903, the ultramicroscope was invented by two German scientists. This device allowed doctors to look at objects smaller than those observed under a regular microscope. Objects as small as 5 millimicrometers in diameter could now be seen. (One millimicrometer equals $\frac{1}{25,000,000}$ of an inch.) That same year, the first practical electrocardiograph, a machine that records the electrical activity of the heart, was developed. It transformed cardiac care because of its specific interpretations of the actions of the heart. Yet with all these gains, it would still be years before orthodox drugs would match such diagnostic triumphs. Copeland told a group of nurses that "a prominent allopathic neurologist in one of the large cities of the continent" said to him, "I am an honest man trying to help my patients, and there is nothing, absolutely nothing in our materia medica to give a ray of hope to the afflicted." He concluded, "I am helpless as a babe in the presence of disease, and feel myself to be a useless barnacle on the hull of society." Aside from aspirin, orthodox doctors still offered such staples as Dover's Powder, a combination of opium and ipecac, a plant that induces vomiting; bismuth, a by-product of lead; chloroform; and morphine. The homeopaths knew, as always, that the best path toward relief and cure was their mild "therapeutic procedure." Dr. Dudley had written in his entry in *Scientific American's* encyclopedia that the "specifically curative power" of this procedure "resides not in [the drug's] physical, nor yet in its chemical properties, but in its capacity to produce change in the functions of the organism." How could any newer medicine top that kind of action, Copeland and his Michigan associates asked.

Orthodox doctors who were opposed to any concession to homeopaths still complained that there had been no advances in the field. None at all. Homeopaths were stuck in another century, although the public was not grumbling. Copeland, of course, wanted his colleagues to look toward the twentieth century, become part of it, and even change with it. This didn't mean that he was disillusioned with homeopathic remedies. Far from it. He was still hoping that the AIH would create what he had called "a great laboratory of drug pathology," but so far this had not happened. Meanwhile, homeopaths were earning a lot of money dispensing their remedies, and the orthodox doctors were not happy about that either.

Pleasant medicine was no longer a novelty to Americans, nor was it always what it seemed it be. In December 1901, Copeland's Professor Hinsdale wrote in a homeopathic medical journal about his combined use of homeopathic, eclectic, naturopathic, and allopathic measures in a case of mercuric chloride poisoning.

Hinsdale wrote that he was "called at two in the afternoon to see a young woman who was vomiting profusely," and whose complexion was "a pronounced blue color." He reported that "without further delay, a stomach tube was passed, and three gallons of water turned into the stomach, a quart at a time, and siphoned out." He added that "immediately after the stomach washing, raw eggs were turned into the stomach through the tube and allowed to remain." The young woman, who had swallowed an undetermined number of poison tablets, was then taken to the homeopathic hospital in Ann Arbor, where she was treated for the next fifteen days, showing signs, Hinsdale said, of "great depression and anguish."

The first day in the hospital, she was given an enema of hot milk and brandy, which, Hinsdale, recorded, she "did not retain." This was followed by an eighth of an ounce of whiskey that "was injected into each leg." She then received the Schüssler tissue salt *Kali phosphoricum,* or *Kali phos.,* which contains potassium. This remedy is generally used for physical and mental exhaustion. She was also given "the whites of two dozen eggs in water," and "gum-arabic mucilage as a drink," an herbal remedy that had a soothing effect on inflamed mucous tissues. The next day, she was given two dozen more eggs, as well as "some milk." Hinsdale reported that she "complained of great pain in her throat, stomach, and bladder," but whether it was from the poison, her medical treatment, or something else, he does not say. That evening, the patient received "an infusion of Digatalis," and the following day she was given "a hypodermic of an eighth of a grain of Pilocarpin," or jaborandi, a shrub with grey bark and leathery leaves. This remedy, used to increase secretions, was injected into the young woman's left breast. The patient was also offered a mouthwash made of Calendula, from the *Calendula officinalis* marigold plant, which was often used by homeopaths, eclectics, and allopaths as an antiseptic. Over the next few days most of these procedures were repeated, with the addition one night of ⅛ of an ounce of Apocynum (Canadian hemp or dogbane), a toxic herb used for fever, for "irritable and congested uterus," and as an accompaniment to Digitalis. (People often used its stems to make rope.) Other extras in this patient's care included an occasional steam bath; a rubdown with hot, wet blankets; a dry, hot air bath; and flax-tea, salt, and turpentine enemas. Hinsdale even force-fed her 35 ounces of buttermilk. He also tried some other homeopathic remedies: Nitric Acid, or *Nitric ac.,* often used to burn off warts; Calcium Sulfide, or *Hepar sulf.,* which Hahnemann prescribed as an antidote for mercury side effects; Phosphorus, or *Phos.;* Lachesis, or venom from the bushmaster snake; *Crotalus horridus,* or venom from a rattlesnake; and finally, *Strychnia sulphuricum* 2X (one of the few times a specific dilution is mentioned). Strychnia Sulphuricum is a rare remedy made from corrosive sulfuric acid and the alkaloid of either Nux Vomica or Ignatia amara.

The patient died three hours after receiving the Strychnia, yet an autopsy revealed that she did not die of any kind of poisoning, nor from the assault of medicinals given to her. She died from acute nephritis, a kidney disease for which there was no cure. Hinsdale reported that had this disease not been present, his patient "would have undoubtedly recovered." Still, he also asked, "How much were the conditions modified by the drugs and antidotes given?" This question would be asked often in other medical circumstances.

EVEN THOUGH former Mayor Copeland had said that he didn't want a second term, some people in Ann Arbor thought this wasn't true. What was true was that he missed the authority and attention that public office gave him. In 1903, he decided to become a Republican candidate for the United States Congress. While many people were not pleased with this decision, those in his hometown of Dexter definitely were. He would be forever their special son. Copeland, who more and more, especially in print and in lectures, began to use his full name of Royal, was determined to keep his name visible, especially after he failed to win his party's nomination. But the following year, when he and Mary finally separated (she left him), he became the parks commissioner of Ann Arbor, a trustee of the Board of Education, and a member of the Michigan Tuberculosis

Board of Trustees, as well as president of the American Homeopathic Ophthalmological, Otological, and Laryngological Society. One way or another, he would keep working to remain noticed and to make a difference.

Two years earlier, in 1902, while he was still mayor of Ann Arbor, Copeland had learned about "artificial stone." The following year he had invested in a factory with two neighbors, and they had formed the Ann Arbor Brick Company. The bricks were made in a secret process out of marl—clay and calcium carbonate—from Bass Lake. An engineer reported to the owners that the raw material covered an area of "two million three hundred and seventy thousand square feet, with an average depth of three and two tenth feet." Such unusual business dealings would become a regular offshoot of Copeland's future vocations—and avocations—and some of them would become controversial, leading his opponents to agree with the AMA's later wisecrack, "Royal seldom overlooks a good thing!"

FIVE

"The Sacred Fire of a Wise Ambition"

Copeland and his cronies met often for lunch at the Cutting Café in downtown Ann Arbor. A bachelor once again (although he and Mary would not divorce until 1907), he looked forward to these get-togethers. When he wasn't involved in board meetings, teaching, and lecturing, he continued to see private patients. Now and then, politics humorously entered his diagnoses. He wrote to a patient, "I judge from what you say regarding your eyes that you are in proper condition for an operation at any time. With your faith in republicanism, the GOP, and Theodore Roosevelt, I judge that you will come out all right."

The situations that he now encountered in his practice became more complex, and his solutions more original. He wrote an optical company in Detroit about a patient who required "a very small artificial eye," and suggested "one such as used by taxidermists for the owl." He said that "if such eyes are not made for human use," it should be a simple matter to take the owl's eye and "angle it so the edges would be smooth."

He also began stressing psychology as part of his treatment. He told a woman whose cataract he had removed successfully but who was complaining about her glasses that "I wish you would not worry over your condition. It does you no good and so depresses you that your eye, as well as the rest of your body, is unfavorably affected." He continued, "Once in awhile you get the blues. I have read somewhere that when you get the blues, you should not think about the troubles you have, but about the good times you have had. Now just take for granted that you are going to be all right, as I firmly believe you are going to be, and you will find yourself in better spirits, and as a result your eye itself will be better. . . . Keep this letter on file and when you get the blues take it out and read it. . . . I have not permitted your depression to affect me."

He began to experiment with electric light. For a patient with a detached retina, he prescribed the remedy Bryonia, as well as "an ordinary electric light bulb, except of high candle power," to be "hung from a cord" so it can "swing back and forth across the face." He prescribed this treatment for ten minutes three times a week, for its "stimulating effect." He also encouraged the use of electrical current for generating heat in the body, cautioning that only "an expert" should perform this therapy. He did not say if he had actually used it himself.

All sorts of electrical treatments were in fashion, and vivid advertisements about them appeared in magazines and newspapers. Many people believed that electricity contained a magical dimension. There was an electrical device said to cure tuberculosis, hernias, prostate problems, and uterine problems. There was an electric hairbrush said to cure headaches and constipation. There were electric belts, corsets, rings, braces, throat protectors, and even spectacles, said to cure a multitude of ailments, including paralysis. People were willing to try them all. While Hahnemann believed that electricity had curative powers that worked "on the life principle," he also said that its use "still lies too much in the dark" to make homeopathic use of it. But manufacturers and distributors took full advantage of the rage for things electric.

As an influential official in homeopathic circles, Copeland was fully aware of the squabbles within his "flock." What he had to say was now being heard and read about all over the country, not just in Michigan. For several years, he had asked for a truce, in a voice that one newspaper described as "melodious, breaking into a sobbing vibrato or a bark of defiance." His current message that the orthodox doctors, specifically the AMA, actually had little to do with any problems in homeopathy was falling on deaf ears most of the time. Still, he did not let up on his "bark of defiance."

He loved to talk, and people loved to listen. He scolded that "it is not to be expected that any party or organization can long survive a condition of absolute noncohesion. We have learned from a study of physics that cohesion is a force strong in solids, weak in liquids, and probably absent in gasses. I fear our present condition is at least semi-gaseous." A magazine article depicted his face as having "the severe lines necessary to oratorical impressiveness," and said that these lines "soften into curves, dimples, and tiny wrinkles, expressing sympathy, sincerity, humanness and comradeship." It went on to note that "his laughter comes in quick explosions. His head flies back with a sudden recoil like the kick of a shotgun." He would help bring homeopathy into the twentieth century even if he had to do it with most everyone kicking and screaming.

A new problem had to be addressed. For reasons homeopaths across America didn't yet fully comprehend, enrollment in their twenty-two medical schools was falling, even though the popularity of homeopathy was still high. Part of the problem was the ongoing differences between the moderates and the purists, which focused more and more on single remedies—that is, whether to give one remedy at a time or multiple remedies. (Hahnemann had called homeopaths who gave more than one remedy at a time—which the moderates sometimes did—"pseudo-homeopaths.") The homeopaths also debated whether to use sedatives, narcotics, or palliatives in their practices, and argued about the place of chiropractic and osteopathy in their work. They questioned the use of "electrical" and "psychic" therapeutics. Could they use these and still be called homeopaths? (The AMA said all such therapeutics were ludicrous.)

But the most crucial problem concerned the new directions that medicine in general was taking because of its new diagnostic tools. Copeland asked himself if this could be a factor in the low enrollment in homeopathic schools. Some homeopaths considered the tools a detriment. Since the purists didn't believe that the pathology of disease had anything to do with selecting the correct remedy, they continued to say that the only thing that mattered was the symptom. They believed, as one homeopath wrote, that "the cause of disease cannot be often known, and if known, can aid but little in the healing of the sick."

Copeland, eager to remain a peacemaker, argued that "the most radical opponent of homeopathy would not say that in the choice of a drug, the presence or absence of the germ would influence his selection of a curative remedy. It would simply decide the question of climate or the general disposition of the patient," and like the purists—like all homeopaths, really—he would agree that "the chief cause of illness lies within us. It is a predisposition."

The American Institute of Homeopathy remained sympathetic to the moderates, as the International Hahnemannian Association did to the purists. The homeopathic medical schools were caught in between and struggled to keep the disagreements and rivalries from affecting their basic teaching of the materia medica, but over time the curriculum entered the fray. It was inevitable. What was taught and how it was taught were not necessarily the same anymore, even though most of the twenty-two colleges were controlled by moderates. The quality of the teaching varied from school to school. In addition, the converts from orthodox medical schools were fewer, mostly because these students were so exhilarated by the advances in orthodox medicine that they wanted to stay where they were, and not "go back" to homeopathy. Of course, most homeopaths saw their profession as being forward-looking, not backward, and a great many also believed that an allopathic-homeopathic alliance would settle the matter for good, anyway. The best of the two worlds would merge to create a force to be reckoned with in American medicine. Still, some graduates of homeopathic medical schools ended up not using homeopathic medicines at all, and others, even if they offered them, did so without using the word "homeopathic," following the suggestion of the orthodox doctors. A newspaper article at the time commented that "the potency of homeopathic medicine has been gradually augmented until the theory of that school now is along the line of 'assisting nature.'" Cure was not necessarily the expected payoff anymore, just as *Scientific American*'s encyclopedia entry had said.

Copeland had told the graduates of his medical school in 1901 not to let orthodox medicine pass them by and to "acknowledge your dependence upon others," but at the same time "to learn to separate the kernel of truth from the mass of chaff of doubtful theories and absolute falsehood." And he intoned, "With your soul filled with the sacred fire of a wise ambition you will be drawn forward by an irresistible force." That irresistible force was homeopathy. Orthodox graduates, on the other hand, often wondered why homeopaths like Copeland always needed to sound so self-important and blustery. They could show a little restraint. As early as 1846, the AMA had criticized their "figurative language." Medicine wasn't a sideshow or a religious revival. Not anymore.

IN 1902, the AMA had created a committee on medical education, and two years later it turned this committee into a more formal Council on Medical Education, with the goal of making high standards the only standard at all 155 medical schools in the country. These schools included homeopathic, eclectic, and orthodox (now also called "conventional," "regular," or "standard") institutions. The council recommended that all potential medical students must complete four years of high school before entering medical school and that the medical-school course should be four years, which had been the case, anyway, in most schools since 1895.

The AMA also began to look into the state licensing records of medical-school graduates. It reported that from 1900 to 1905 the failure rate on these exams was 16 percent for standard graduates and only 9 percent for homeopathic graduates—welcome news, of course, for the homeopaths when they heard about it. Additionally, the AMA began its own informal evaluation of medical schools, using such criteria as the general condition and ambiance of the school, including its curriculum, teaching equipment, laboratory facilities, libraries, and museums. It considered the school's hospital affiliations, whether or not its faculty was full- or part-time, and whether or not its faculty was engaged in useful research. It assessed entrance requirements and whether the school was interested primarily in profits. The homeopaths, when they learned about this evaluation process, didn't want to be included in it, however informal it seemed to be at the time. Just as they believed that their remedies should be exempt from AMA-influenced oversight of any kind, and just as they didn't want to get involved with the question of quack medications, or patent medicines, they believed that their schools should be evaluated only by other homeopaths. In fact, most homeopaths, Copeland included, believed that the standard doctors were simply too "materialistic in their views" and thus could not properly evaluate what did or didn't go on in a homeopathic school.

In 1903, Copeland and his friend W. A. Dewey represented Michigan at a meeting of the AIH's Inter-Collegiate Committee. Twenty doctors from across the country assembled to discuss medical-school issues, and several important questions were raised: Has Christian Science exerted an influence in decreasing the number of students? What influence has osteopathy exerted upon attendance at our medical schools? Are homeopathic practitioners to any extent sending their sons to old-school colleges? "Is medical practice less remunerative than formerly, and therefore less attractive to the American student? What percentage of students leave homeopathic schools for the purpose of entering some old-school college? What would you suggest as a remedy for the alleged decrease in the number of students? Such questions would be discussed for years, and there would be no easy answers. According to the minutes of the

1903 meetings, it was urged that faculty members be encouraged "to listen to criticism no matter how brutally frank." Conditions were called "discouraging," and it was noted that "it is a fact that it be [*sic*] impossible to produce any material change for the better at once." Eventually the Inter-Collegiate Committee would develop into the College Alliance of the AIH, for the express purpose of "maintaining and defending the vested rights" of homeopathic colleges and their graduates.

In the address Copeland had given to the graduating class of 1901, he had touched on some of the concerns, urging Michigan to require the equivalent of a high-school education before permitting a student "to take even an entrance examination to a school of medicine." In other lectures, he talked about chiropractic and osteopathy and how they must be practiced "under proper restrictions." He saw them as he always had, not as a threat to homeopathy, but as another "specialty in medicine." Yet he once told a cautionary tale: "I have in mind a man who came to me as a patient, suffering with a peculiar sore throat and inability to swallow. When I sent this patient to a colleague for an X-ray examination, he found that two vertebrae of the neck had been broken by the application of cruel force, which he said was applied by a chiropractor." Copeland never wavered from his stand that "four or five years of technical study following a first-class preliminary education, are necessary to prepare one for the practice of any form of medicine."

Osteopaths, who had founded a national organization, the American Osteopathic Association (AOA) in 1897, took a two-year course (later expanded to three, then four) that included anatomy, physics, toxicology, and clinical demonstrations. Chiropractors had far less detailed training, with the focus on spinal adjustment techniques. Most of their schools had but a single room containing a few tables.

Copeland said that he "respected" Christian Science, and in fact once conceded that it had "beaten to a frazzle" homeopathy in terms of "organization, means of publicity, and popular success." He acknowledged that Christian Science, osteopathy, and chiropractic were making "insistent demands for recognition" but maintained that all homeopathy had to do to compete was "cast out its stock worn goods, freshen its shelves, and adapt itself to modern requirements."

He never gave up his "bark of defiance." In discussing the statement made by the dean of Chicago's Rush Medical College that there can be "but one science of medicine," he had called this standard doctor not only "absurd" (the very word standard doctors used about homeopaths) but "narrow and bigoted." Yet he wouldn't cut himself off completely from standard medicine or its organizations.

On June 23, 1904, Copeland gave an address on the potency of remedies at a meeting of the AIH held in Niagara Falls, New York. In addition to all his other responsibilities, he was now the chairman of the AIH's Bureau of Homeopathy and a corresponding member of the British Homeopathic Society.

In his AIH speech, which he considered one of the most important so far in his career, he said that "modern" science had now shown that certain chemicals had a "selective" affinity for certain bodily tissues. In other words, these chemicals didn't affect every single organ of the body, but instead were attracted only to particular ones. He lectured that, for instance, carbon is found in the connective tissue of the joints and lungs, but not in the kidneys; or silver, "taken into the system," is found only in the lining of the base of the brain and in no other linings of the body. He speculated that this is "probably" due to "specialized metabolism." This idea was important to homeopaths because it demonstrated that a drug, no matter how small, is used by a particular part of the body because the cells of the body are "demanding" it, he said. The substance is drawn to the cells because these cells need it—so the amount of the substance is not as important as the fundamental need of the cells for the substance.

He spoke of "the new very interesting development of physical chemistry," that chemicals, or electrolytes, dissociate into tiny particles called ions when dissolved in certain mixtures. The more dilute the solution, the greater the dissociation and the more numerous the ions. Thus, Copeland reasoned, "complete ionization is possible only in infinitesimal doses." Homeopathy works! Homeopathy is "not only true in theory, but the research of the chemist seems to prove it." And he said loud and clear that "homeopathy, at least the infinitesimal dose, is as reasonable, as explainable, as scientifically sensible as is any other of the natural sciences." He confessed, however, that he rarely prescribed "above thirtieth decimal dilution," because he doubted that much of the original remedy remained in anything more diluted. He maintained that if it was now understood that remedies acted chemically, then a given drug, "high or low, in dilution or crude form, will thread its way through the blood stream and a sufficient quantity be appropriated by the disturbed cell to satisfy and correct its chemical equilibrium." The body will use only what it needs, so, as he had been maintaining for years, the dilution was not as important as finding the correct remedy. Yet in an apparent paradox, he also affirmed that Hahnemann's advice was still pertinent: "Too large a dose of medicine, though homeopathic to the case, will be injurious." Too large a dose was, still, too "standard" a dose.

He discussed what he called the new "popular" theory of immunity—"the ways by which the human system protects itself against the invasion of ever vigilant disease." He spoke of how "blood serum" can protect a person because it "overcomes the effects of infection" and "destroys the bacteria" by "counteracting the toxins developed." He called this "hypothesis" "extremely complicated," and said it would have future importance to homeopaths because "the protective action of the blood may be interfered with, then, by drug effect upon the cell." In other words, the right remedy might cause the body to create a natural immunity against certain diseases (just as Dr. Dewey had speculated), yet Copeland also thought that too much of a remedy or the wrong remedy could interfere with the body's own "protective forces." But most important, he was announcing that a vaccine might keep a remedy from doing its work, a new observation for him.

Copeland stepped out even further into new territory. He said that there was no reason for homeopaths to need the "vital force," because now "all the bodily processes can be explained in chemical terms." Disease was a disturbance of chemical equilibrium. It was "unnecessary to fall back upon a mysterious 'dynamus' or 'psora.'" There were no evil spirits. There was science. Among homeopaths, this was a controversial—and perplexing—statement. Most homeopaths would be loath to give up the actuality or even the symbolism of the "vital force" and all it had come to stand for. (Dewey had lectured that homeopathy's opponents ridiculed the "psora," calling it "the itch doctrine.") And what about the body's "predisposition" to illness? But Copeland held that "every feature of the homeopathic doctrine" fits into every modern idea of disease, and that Hahnemann, who knew nothing of the "modern laboratory idea," nonetheless formulated a system "in perfect harmony" with the "whole temple of science." (In 1897, the International Hahnemannian Association acknowledged modernity by publishing a proving of X-ray—alcohol exposed to an X-ray machine and "brought up to a 6C potency"—that showed "its penetration into that invisible interior of the human body which is under the dominion of the life-force." Another

X-ray proving, however, reported that old symptoms were resurrected, "some unheard of for as much as thirty years.")

As for the law of similars, Copeland now said that although some homeopaths "can demonstrate the law by showing experiments to verify it," they might not always be able to explain it "sensibly or convincingly." He said that "the theologian has the same difficulty with the immaculate conception," and even maintained that "the chemist can hardly account for some of the chemical affinities familiar as working truths." He reasoned that "thus it may be excused the Homeopathist, perhaps, if he fails to scientifically account for the theory of similars." Even so, he still insisted that this most basic belief of homeopathy was a hypothesis that could be explained by the very fact that, well, it worked, and therefore could be considered a law.

The purists were not happy with Copeland, who was sounding more and more like a standard doctor to them, even though in another speech given shortly after his one in Niagara Falls, he fully backed the single-remedy theory, which gratified them. "It must be admitted," he said, "that in the ideal prescription, there is demanded one, and but one, remedy. There can be no other to truly fill the needs and satisfy the cravings of the crying cell. The single remedy, therefore, is an expression of the highest type of scientific prescribing."

He pressed the scientific point of view over and over in everything he now talked about, in informal gatherings and before large audiences. "Chemical reactions are definite and positive," he said. He had to make his colleagues realize that they had the backing of chemistry and biology in their diagnoses and prescribing, and they had to make sure that their colleges were teaching the science of the new century. He himself was preparing a paper titled "Blood Pressure as a Factor in Eye Disease." Many of his colleagues, not understanding at all where he stood, suspected that he was leading them to an unhealthy alliance with allopathy. But he wanted homeopathy to remain "a distinct school of thought." He was enjoying his influence; everyone seemed to be listening to him, even if they disagreed with him. At one AIH meeting, he was described by a colleague as "a spirit like the roaring of the wind and filling the place where they were sitting." Copeland had almost forgotten Ann Arbor politics.

Across the country, opiates were still a favored treatment, especially for pain. Many people were addicted to them, and it was a matter that the AMA would soon rigorously address. A great many patent medicines contained opiates and liquor, especially sweetened whiskey, unbeknownst to patients. Copeland said repeatedly that homeopaths rarely resorted to strictly palliative methods of treatment, and stressed that as a doctor he "rarely employs the hypodermic syringe" and rarely gave opiates to his patients. He said "victims of induced habits are seldom found in homeopathic families" and that this absence of addiction was one of the reasons for homeopathy's continuing acceptance in America. Another was that many homeopaths promoted physical fitness and exercise along with the remedies. "Enthusiasm will do the same thing" as exercise, Copeland sometimes lectured his students; "earnest interest in one's daily tasks has exactly the same effect as exercise. It stimulates the heart." He recommended that a patient with serious retinal and optic-nerve problems be "sent to Florida for the winter" for a healing "out-of-door life." He said that "with improved health and strength," and "perfect peace of mind," his patient would show "improvement in her nervous system" as well as in her eye condition.

A common belief at the time was still that the illnesses of most women were caused either by their ovaries, uteruses, and vaginas, or by some mental disorder. Rest cures were commonplace. Newspapers ran features and advertisements on how "nervousness and female weaknesses ruin many lives." One article described eleven symptoms, including irregularity, bearing down, and/or a bad taste in the mouth, as being the result of female delicacies. Copeland wrote his sister that their mother's herpes "is looked upon as a neurosis, and a change of climate is frequently recommended by physicians in this disease." He also believed, as many doctors did, that "the verdict of incurable is often a home-made decision." But, for him, a homeopath on the scene could always change that verdict.

As BUSY as he was with his medical affairs, the nursing school, and teaching, Copeland found the time to keep up with his Ann Arbor political associates. He usually had an ulterior motive. On October 3, 1904, he wrote an official running for office a long letter about the homeopathic school. It was not exactly a threatening letter, but pretty close. "At the request of eighteen prominent and influential republicans, I submit to you three questions upon the answers to which will depend their attitude towards you in the coming election," he began. "For myself," he added, "I feel no need of a statement of your present position. Your attitude in the past regarding these matters makes me certain your future career will be entirely satisfactory." Copeland wanted to make sure that the school's autonomy would not be violated. "Will you protect the interests of the Homeopathic College the same as you would the university as a whole . . . ?" he asked. "If you hear of any measure, bill, 'rider,' or other scheme or movement threatening or seeming to embarrass the college, will you immediately inform its friends and lend your assistance promptly and persistently to defeat any measure the same as you would any other attack against any of the fixed institutions of Washtenaw County?" His letter was as clear as it was blunt. "It is possible," he went on, "that some one not in sympathy with the college or the ideas for which it stands may attempt to revive former schemes for removal, annihilation, amalgamation." Copeland was going to do his best to use his widening circle of friends to help not only his own career, but homeopathy's as well. He asked a friend of the governor's if a homeopathic doctor at the state penitentiary could be made the superintendent of a home for the feebleminded, saying "he and a large circle of friends will be greatly disappointed" if the appointment does not occur.

He would also always try to help his father. On August 23, 1906, he asked the head of the Michigan Central Railroad to do him a favor, which "when the time comes, I will be glad to reciprocate." He said that "for many years my father has purchased grain at Dexter," using the railroad's elevator. "It seems," he explained, "that the bridge leading up to the elevator is not considered as safe as it should be, and is in the need of repairs." He asked for intervention, and said he "would consider it a personal favor, indeed more than a personal favor, because you and I take more interest in the welfare of our respective fathers than we do in our own welfare, of course."

He was continuing to focus on ways to bring the old-school doctors around. He began to use grimmer language, now calling their skepticism "almost nihilism." He suggested that the AIH appoint a committee to write a statement "as would induce a fair-minded Old School man to make a trial of homeopathy." He thought that what was written "could not go elaborately into case taking." It would have to be "brief" on the subject of symptoms, as well as the method of choosing a remedy. He thought it best to "recommend the lower doses" and cover "but a dozen remedies" so the doctors would not feel overwhelmed. He recognized that doing it this way would "entail possible criticism on the part of the sticklers for Hahnemannian exactness." But he didn't care. He suggested that perhaps twelve remedies could be selected and "each of our homeopathic pharmacies be invited to prepare a medicine case. . . . A price should be placed upon this outfit, so very low as obviously to exclude the possible criticism that the whole thing was a drug advertising scheme." He hoped to see "scores of conversions" and many new members of the AIH. "Joy shall be in heaven over one sinner that repenteth more than over ninety and nine just persons, which need no repentance," Copeland sermonized.

"What else can we do as a profession to assist the cause of homeopathy?" he asked. He urged his fellow members to search their communities for "young men and women who would make excellent physicians." He said that high schools were graduating students who "might easily be induced to take homeopathy. Somebody has said: 'boys are like watermelons; so many get ripe every year.' We ought to be gathering our share of the luscious fruit." He did not prefer one homeopathic college over another, he said. He just wanted more and more "disciples for homeopathy." The age of doctors' offices sending students their way was over. "Whatever work is done today in the way of influencing young people to study homeopathy or any other kind of medicine must be done in the home."

The home. It was the place that mattered most to Copeland, despite the long intervals he had been away from his, and despite the breakup of his thirteen-year marriage to Mary. But he was determined to re-create his happy Dexter days in his adult life, to marry again, and to affirm a notion he had that "the schools teach everything except how to live." A close friend would later say that "to him home was the sweetest word in the lexicon of worthwhile things."

IN 1904, the AMA, which now had 44,362 members out of a total physician population of 128,950, veered away from new attacks on "the little pill doctors," another of its pejorative terms for homeopaths, and focused again on drug purity. It strongly supported a federal bill for preventing the adulteration and misbranding of foods or drugs. The AMA had long dreamed of legislation that would regulate the traffic of hundreds of fraudulent products, and it finally had enough financial resources to become involved in lobbying efforts. There had to be government regulations, and Congress had to pass such a bill now. The AMA said that the average person "believes, unfortunately, that any disease can be cured by taking something out of a bottle. . . . On this fallacy is built up a vast superstructure of fraud." The group also said that "it is an axiom that false and misleading advertisements are the life-blood of the 'patent medicine' business . . . blatant lies characterized nostrum advertising." (It wasn't until 1901 that the AMA itself restricted advertisements for nostrums and other secret preparations from the pages of its journal.)

The AMA's ire was less fixed on homeopathic remedies and more on such products as "Hoff's Consumption Cure," which, when analyzed by government chemists, was found to contain morphine, arsenic, potassium, and cinnamon. None of these ingredients was listed on the package. A cough medicine was found to contain alcohol, codeine, and chloroform, also not mentioned on the label. A nostrum called "Mother's Friend," for pregnant women, was found to contain only oil and soap. Other products contained unmarked plant ash, weeds, turpentine, camphor, beef fat, pebbles, and sand. The AMA also reported that "it has been frequently pointed out that most nostrums contain well-known products as their essential constituents. These are often disguised under fanciful names and sold under extravagant claims and at exorbitant prices. . . . Cane sugar for curing tuberculosis. Milk sugar for hay fever." In the production of food, "shady processors adulterated fertilizers, deodorized rotten eggs, revived rancid butter, substituted glucose for honey." Health hazards lurked everywhere. In 1905, the AMA established its own Council on Pharmacy and Chemistry to set standards for drug manufacturing and advertising. It was going to join the battle one way or another, with or without the government's help. It also reprinted and distributed a series of well-received articles about quackery that had run in Collier's magazine.

In the late 1890s, several private groups had signed up for the crusade against nostrums: the National Temperance Society, the National Pure Food and Drug Congress, the General Federation of Women's Clubs, and the American Public Health Association. Muckraking journalists added their voices. Meanwhile, by 1902, in Washington, D.C., the Bureau of Chemistry in the Department of Agriculture (a precursor to the Food and Drug Administration) had gone to work under the direction of Harvey Wiley, MD, the chief chemist and chief crusader, producing masses of documentation concerning fraud. This bureau had existed in various forms since 1862 and under Wiley's leadership since 1882. Also in 1902, the Biologics Control Act was passed, a bill that ensured the safety and purity of vaccines and serums. By 1904, there was talk of trying to create a law to fight quackery. Such talk was not exactly new. Since the late 1880s more than one hundred food and drug bills had been introduced to Congress. All had been defeated.

Finally, in 1905, the 59th Congress prepared a pure food and drug bill that would require drugs to meet a certain standard of strength and purity. They had to be labeled a certain way, and had to abide by the standards set in *The United States Pharmacopeia* and *The National Formulary* (both prepared by pharmacists and standard doctors). Adulterated and impure medications could still be marketed, but if the government could prove they were fraudulent and not bona fide, they could then be removed from the market. It wasn't much of a law because the burden of proof was not on the manufacturer, but it gave the public "some measure of protection," and the AMA recommended "early consideration" of the bill, which would be passed on June 30, 1906. It was not perfect, and it had many enemies (the liquor industry and various food processors, among others), but it was a start. Not a bad start, everyone agreed, even though some companies began using the labeling requirements as part of their advertising campaign, printing "approved by the Pure Food and Drug Act of 1906" directly on their labels.

The homeopaths did not fasten onto the new law in any particular way because they prepared their remedies according to the standards of their own pharmacopeia, and had continued confidence in their methods. They saw no need to conform to the law requiring them to label their remedies with their alcohol content, and even Copeland seemed to agree with this antigovernment position. He said that "the physician himself becomes responsible for the purity and the accurate preparation of the remedy." He added that the standard doctors "suffer defeat in the struggle with disease" because of problems that homeopaths never have. Homeopaths do not have to worry that "incompetent" pharmacists will substitute one ingredient for another, or carelessly prepare the medicine. Homeopaths, unlike allopaths, did not have to worry about "the presence of alien matter" in their remedies. Homeopaths had an "advantage," Copeland boasted, making his associates proud. He emphasized that "many mistakes and many failures in medical practice have resulted from the indirect methods of the pharmacist and the brief, unsatisfactory directions written on the label of the medicines." Homeopaths had an advantage economically because of "savings in drug bills," since the remedy "is made on the spot, and the directions regarding its use made clear by explanations of the physician himself." It wasn't exactly a kick in the pants to the AMA, or the Pure Food and Drug Act, but almost.

A year later, the AIH's Committee on the Pharmacopeia sent Copeland a letter asking him to "rally around" the "acknowledged standard in the Homeopathic Pharmacopeia of the U.S." The letter, sent to all officials of state societies, went on, "The New Pure Food Law passed by the present congress and which went into effect on the first of January 1907, makes the United States Pharmacopeia the standard of strength of all preparations sold. . . . [I]t is therefore a question of great importance that the homeopathic fraternity shall endorse its own standard that we may not suffer from discrimination in the enforcement of this law which requires that the alcoholic strength shall be given upon the labels of all our tinctures and dilutions."

Copeland would mull over that letter for the next thirty years, wondering what to do about it. As always, he would figure something out, a way to "rally around" homeopathy.

EVEN THOUGH the AMA still regarded homeopaths as "irregulars," it no longer confronted them as directly as it had in the past. But it also believed that if homeopaths wouldn't cooperate with the new FDA law, they must be hiding something "irregular." At the same time the AMA was criticizing homeopathic secrecy, it was still offering them membership if they would stop calling themselves "homeopaths." The times were tense, and most homeopaths still declined the AMA's invitation. As always, they tried to avoid medical politics and simply wanted to practice the medicine they believed in. "Homeopathy is healing for the nations— and homeopathy must go on confident in the conviction of cures impossible by other means," Copeland continued to say.

He now pleaded that the AIH "do one great thing every year." He asked again that his organization at least "carry a practical knowledge of homeopathy into the offices of five or ten thousand Old School doctors!" He said "this plan might result in scores of conversions," and, in fact, "the institute, a year hence," might be able to vote into membership "many long time practitioners of old school medicine." But the "old school," with the Pure Food and Drug Law passed, had other things on its mind. Not membership, not medicines. The standard doctors, specifically the

AMA, had inspection in mind; its Council on Medical Education now planned to visit every medical school in the country. It would even grade them A for acceptable, B for doubtful, and C for unacceptable. Copeland, who had found that the nursing-school deanship took up too much of his time and resigned his position there (he also resigned as secretary of the homeopathic-school faculty, saying "many of the functions of the office were disagreeable"), went along with his colleagues, who said that the AMA had no authority to investigate homeopathic schools.

The AMA's initial inspection, for the most part kept secret and never published—although it became known that only 82 out of the total of 155 schools were fully approved—was highly criticized by standard schools as well as homeopathic and eclectic ones and did not at first carry much weight. Copeland commented somewhat stiffly that "the well-known success of the homeopathic surgeons and their high professional standing, not only by the rating of the Homeopathic School of The University of Michigan, but also when measured by the standards of all other systems of practice, places the homeopathic operation above criticism." His surgical clinic had clearly received an A. He didn't remark on any other aspect of the rating except to worry whether the curriculum was "encumbered with a useless collection of time-consuming courses," as well as to suggest that "the junior and senior years of the medical curriculum are crowded with hours devoted to specialties quite beyond the possibility of practical value or safe application." Although he was implying that the AMA was pushing for better courses, the AMA, in fact, wanted fewer schools so there could be better quality.

Most doctors—of all persuasions—believed that confidential investigations resulted in "abuses." All doctors were concerned about the "lack of uniformity." As Copeland would explain, "In a given state, for instance, with private control there will, of necessity, be as many standards of admission and graduation as there are private corporations." He said that "some schools are essentially scientific; they are really research institutions. Others are emphatically clinical. Comparisons are odious." Homeopathic and allopathic schools must be judged separately. Some institutions have "different ideals, different features, and employ different methods of instruction." So, he asked, "how are standards to be established? Where is the authority for this or that level?" They were questions homeopaths would ponder for the next few years as they worried about "bureaucracy, politics, narrow-mindedness and sectarian bias."

In a speech before his fellow professors, Copeland repeated that their arguments were a great "stumbling block responsible for much trouble in our own ranks and undoubtedly one of the important factors in the small enrollment of our colleges." And he once again tried to get "the high potency wing" to cooperate so there could not only be larger attendance at the homeopathic schools, but also better and more consistent teaching. "One of our greatest weaknesses, in my opinion," he said, "is that we have no platform of accepted ideas." The dissension had to end. His "wise ambition" was getting restless.

In the fall of 1907, Copeland was elected to a one-year term as president of the AIH. His influence would be even more direct—and public—now. "I am going to win in this fight," he confided to an old friend, "if it takes every minute of my time. . . . even if I do not earn a cent in my private practice."

SIX

"Eventually Those Who Came to Scoff
Will Remain to Learn"

O N DECEMBER 7, 1907, a frustrated Copeland spoke before the Northwestern Ohio Homeopathic Society, in Toledo. He was replying to Henry Beates, Jr., the president of the Pennsylvania State Board of Medical Examiners, a standard doctor who had recently written that homeopaths belonged in—actually, he said they should be "securely placed in"—insane asylums. Beates thought this even though at the same time he acknowledged that their training was equal to that of his own doctors.

The affable new president of the AIH, who had recently added to his honors an honorary degree from Lawrence University in Appleton, Wisconsin, was sick and tired of the allopathic obsession with an area of medicine that was causing no harm, had never caused any harm, and, most important, was thriving. How could doctors, or anyone, still believe that homeopathy was a delusion? After all, most homeopaths, while not in favor of a full-fledged reconciliation, were utilizing the many advances of general medicine. "The sputum examination, for instance, in the diagnosis of throat and lung disease, is given the same importance in the homeopathic world that it receives elsewhere," President Copeland pointed out. But the "proof of the pudding is in the eating," he liked to say. He had seen "glaucoma, acute infections of the eye, and other definite and unmistakable disease disappear" with the correct homeopathic remedy. "Homeopathy is the method by which the facts of the sciences of pathology and pharmacology are brought into correspondence for the purpose of cure when cure is possible," he now lectured endlessly.

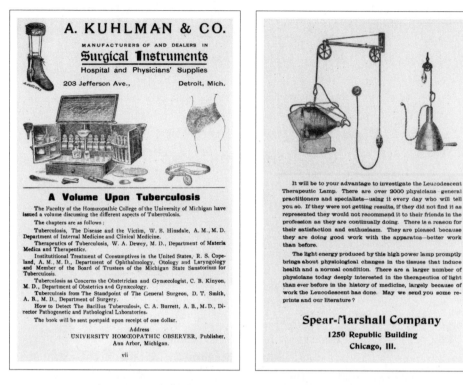

Surgical instruments and therapeutic lamp advertisements from *The University Homeopathic Observer.* Dr. Hinsdale was a supervising editor, and Copeland was one of four associate editors. Both standard and homeopathic doctors used these products.

Many of his colleagues continued to charge that the antagonism with standard medicine, now reaching into their medical-school enrollment, was because they *were* still thriving, and getting a big share of a market that standard doctors wanted for themselves. This was by now an old suspicion. Copeland wanted to try merely to eliminate the antagonism, and it didn't help (but he couldn't help himself) that he joined in the name-calling. He not only called the newest attack by Dr. Beates confused and distorted, but he called the doctor himself "a narrow-minded bigot," and a "poor, innocent, ignorant ass" who was the one who belonged in an asylum. Why couldn't this "joker" see the science underlying homeopathic principles, and see that they are not "at variance with the facts"? And why couldn't he see homeopathy not as a system of medicine and surgery, but as "the therapeutic specialty, which it is"?

Copeland had now touched on an area that would cause even more divisiveness (although it wasn't his intent to do so) than the other disagreements. If homeopathy was a "specialty," why shouldn't it then be taught as an option at allopathic medical schools, as the University of Michigan had once wanted, and some other schools still wanted and were beginning to plan? Paradoxically, Copeland and the majority of homeopaths continued to favor separate-but-equal schools, and the standard doctors, as the years rolled by, sought to end both separate and equal. Even though homeopathy might be a specialty, Copeland also said that "the aim of the medical colleges"—and he meant both homeopathic and allopathic schools—"is to develop a well-grounded, well-rounded, substantial and sensible general practitioner." He was against what he called "a composite product, the blurred image of a dozen specialists." He wanted clarity and excellence in the medical profession. He also said that the AIH had to recognize "the limitations of homeopathy on the one side, and its unbounded possibilities on the other." Homeopathy worked in some circumstances, but not in all, he now said, also veering away from calling Hahnemann a genius, saying only that he was "the chief scientist of his time." Even though a political slant was always close by, such pronouncements contributed to a misunderstanding of his intentions for American homeopathy.

At one meeting of the AIH, Copeland announced that the group had to encourage "plans to properly present the scientific claims of homeopathy" so it would not be overlooked "in the crowded highway of the world's progress." He proposed a World Homeopathic League. He wanted the AIH to think big, and then think even bigger. The standard doctors wondered anew if perhaps homeopathy was not only too missionary in its pursuits, but getting too cocky for its own good.

In a letter to a colleague in Connecticut, Copeland wrote that although "socially" the homeopaths and the standard doctors were on "the best of terms," this was so only because the homeopaths were "content to be in the minority." He conceded that "whenever we suggest an enterprise involving equal representation, the Old School is just as aggressive as it ever was." When, in his capacity as chairman of the Board of Control of the Michigan Homeopathic Society, Copeland had suggested that homeopaths "should be given equal representation on the Board of Registration," he said that an allopathic doctor "jumped from his chair," purple-faced and angry, and "denounced" the suggestion "as the purest nonsense" and "unworthy of consideration." At that time, Copeland started to understand as he never before had that if homeopathy was ever going to extend its borders, as he put it, it would need to do so with the same "aggressive and concerted work" he felt standard doctors used to keep it in its place.

First he decided to extend his own borders. He would move to New York City and accept a job as the dean of the New York Homeopathic Medical College. His colleagues in Michigan were stunned when they heard the news. Copeland said that New York Homeopathic had "more privileges, more opportunities to master practical medicine, a broader and more comprehensive education than can be found in any other college, allopathic or homeopathic, on this continent." It was also a school that he more humbly described as "in more or less poverty-stricken condition." It did not receive state money the way the homeopathic college in Michigan did, but it ranked first in the state in terms of graduates who passed the licensing exams. It was a college waiting for Copeland's imprint, and he would be going to live in the world's second-largest city, after London. New York was a city of opportunity and dreams for immigrants from abroad and from within the United States. (In the early 1830s, Hans Burch Gram, a European-trained surgeon born in Boston, had almost single-handedly turned New York into a homeopathic center.)

Some of Copeland's associates didn't believe he was leaving, because he had neither resigned his position nor asked for a leave of absence. Some didn't believe it even after the campus newspaper, the *Michigan Daily*, reported that "Dr. Copeland's action mystifies authorities and has placed the university in a peculiar and embarrassing position." But on September 7, 1908, just as the new semester was beginning, he wrote the baffled president and Board of Regents the following letter: "It is with genuine sorrow that I feel obliged to resign my long time connection with the university. As student, instructor and professor, I have spent seventeen years in this institution, a longer period of time than I spent in my father's house. During these years, I have come to have the same feeling for the University that one has for his own dear home. Naturally, then it is hard to say that the happy relationship must be dissolved." Copeland, who was soon to turn forty, used all the power of his charisma to lessen the impact of his sudden resignation, especially in his explanation that "the call to the New York Homeopathic Medical College has been made to appear the call of duty. Were I to consult my real preference, I should decline, but under the circumstances I am constrained to accept."

The offer had come fairly casually over the summer when he was in New York delivering a speech, and he immediately saw it as the promo-

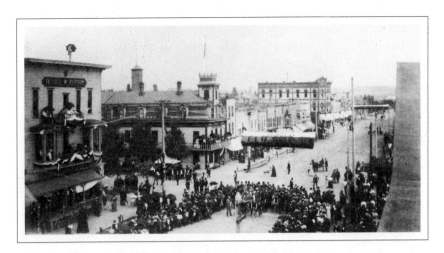

Mitchell Street, Cadillac, Michigan, July 4, 1896

tion he needed to take himself and homeopathy to a new level. It was also a way to begin a new life with a new love in his life. Frances Ellen Spalding, a graduate of Northwestern University, where she majored in music, had been born and reared in Cadillac, Michigan, 192 miles north of Ann Arbor. Cadillac, next to Lake Mitchell and Lake Cadillac, was in white pine country, and her father was a wealthy lumberman. She was self-sufficient and creative, not unlike his mother. Royal and Frances were married in Dexter on July 15, 1908.

An old friend from Bay City, now a member of the Michigan Board of Registration in Medicine, expressed the sting felt by so many of Copeland's associates in Ann Arbor: "I have probably reached the limit of my usefulness to you." This friend also conceded that "I think you are going to win in this game. First because you always go into such a game as this with the determination to win. And, second, because as I look back over the years you spent at Ann Arbor, I can not help but feel that this is going to be an easier job than that, even if it is larger in its scope."

On the train from Ann Arbor to New York with his new bride, who was decked out in a wide-brimmed feathered hat that enveloped her round face, and a long, lightweight cloak, Copeland wrote a note to himself with the newfangled fountain pen he had received as a gift from his parents. He scribbled on the back of the homeopathic journal he was reading: "No back step." There would be none of those for Dexter's golden son.

The new job would, in fact, be easier in at least one respect. As Copeland said in a speech in New York shortly after his arrival, "The one word that spells success in the up building [*sic*] of the present medical school is c-a-s-h! We are facing the Napoleonic doctrine that 'God is behind the biggest guns!' Show me the medical school with the richest endowment, and provided there be honesty, squareness, and intelligence in administration, I'll show you the most successful medical school. This is true in allopathy and it's equally true in homeopathy." In another speech, he made a more sweeping statement and said he was "convinced that the future of organized homeopathy is purely a matter of dollars and cents." Everyone would eventually agree, since most homeopathic colleges, especially the smaller ones, had nothing more to lean on than the tuition they charged. They rarely had any other source of income.

But Copeland had some big ideas. He told the audience honoring his appointment as dean, "It is significant that this year of grace, 1908, has been marked by activity in the progress of our cause," pointing out that "from Massachusetts to California, there is an awakening and a previously unheard of enthusiasm," and that "thousands of dollars have been contributed." He immediately appealed for additions to the college library and asked for "our own electric light plant, refrigeration system, and vacuum cleaner." He said that "above all else, the college building demands extensions," that it was crowded, that "every corner is in use, and important laboratories are tucked into unsuitable quarters."

Calling himself a New Yorker for the first time, he asked to be considered "simply as one of the New York physicians." He didn't want any honors or prominence. (He had declined the New York State Board of Regents offer to admit him to practice in the state "on the grounds of conceded eminence and authority in the profession," and, instead, took the licensing exam, receiving "an average of 95%.") He asked the audience to forget that he came to the college "under unusual circumstances," a reference to the swiftness and secrecy of his appointment and the fact that he was an out-of-towner—"a rural professor"—picked as much for his expertise at making demanding changes as for his teaching and doctoring skills.

He plunged into his new job with confidence and diligence. He replied to every interested applicant as if he were the last one. He told them all, "As a means to a livelihood, a young man makes a serious mistake to enter the old school. . . . There are many, many cities of the country, and literally hundreds of small towns where there is a crying demand for homeopathic graduates." His aggressiveness worked, and he soon had a freshman class larger than that of previous years. The faculty felt energized by his focus, and the alumni bulletin wrote that they were "undertaking their work with renewed zest."

Just a month after his tenure began, he wrote a rich doctor in Connecticut, who had wanted to give a substantial gift in the form of a prize to a graduate, that it might be better just to donate the money to the college. Copeland, as practical as he was visionary, suggested that it be used to buy "two dozen comfortable chairs" for the library, or for "improvements of the dispensary . . . the gateway to the clinic." This dispensary, located in a converted five-story house, was where medicines were given out five hours a day; it needed new floors and better lighting, and needed to be painted. Copeland said that these improvements would bring new patients and "increase the clinical material available for our students." He wrote his parents and sister in Dexter that he had "stayed awake more nights worrying over the finances of the hospital" than he ever did over his own finances.

No detail was too small for his attention. The windows in the hospital's kitchens needed screens. The laundry needed a better drain. The patients' clothing had to be stored in a better place than the employees' dining room. He asked a friend in Ann Arbor to send the formula for the black paint that had been used on the laboratory tabletops there, so he could use the same paint in New York.

Royal and Frances Copeland bought a wood and stone cottage at 72 Liberty Street in the small rural town of New Rochelle, which was twenty miles north of New York City in Westchester County. "The Queen City of the Sound," as the town was called, had a nine-mile waterfront and was halfway between New York City and Connecticut. The area was not unlike parts of Michigan. Copeland called Westchester "the most beautiful residential county in the United States."

He soon noticed that "every country road throughout Westchester was treated with crude petroleum" to keep its surfaces "hard, dry, and absolutely dustless," and he found the time to ask the mayor of Ann Arbor to consider using the same system on Michigan roads. The mayor, pleased that Copeland was "keeping in touch with the dear old town," said he would oil West Huron and Packard streets in a trial run. Copeland also wrote a letter of recommendation for a Republican candidate to the Michigan Board of Regents. He would not forget his former colleagues.

The enthusiastic new dean raised the money to buy two motorized ambulances to add to the three horse-and-buggy ones owned by Flower Hospital, the teaching hospital connected to the medical school. He hoped that these new "machines," as he referred to them, would bring patients to the hospital faster and more efficiently; the crews were made up of orderlies and interns from Flower. A year later, in 1909, Copeland said that approximately 130 cases a week were being brought to the hospital, "representing almost every variety of injury and disease," so that the students and interns had "an excellent opportunity to see a great variety of cases, both medical and surgical."

Copeland also raised the money to buy and remodel a nearby tenement as a residence for up to twenty nurses. When he first arrived in New York, he had noticed that the nurses lived in "inconvenient quarters." He told the Board of Trustees that "it is not to be expected that a young woman just out of her teens will submit herself to the self-sacrificing duties of a three years training to the exclusion of all social privileges. . . . A home for the nurses should be a home in the real sense. There should be provision for dancing, a study room and a library, a place where a young woman may receive a friend, and where she may talk with her parents or others without running the gauntlet of all the rest of the school."

Copeland also saw a need to improve what he called the "scandalous" housing of the hospital's domestic staff. He needed to find the money to install an elevator in the surgical building, too. As proficient as he was at such fund-raising, after only a short while he began to find it a distraction, and he admitted to the board that although he would continue to assist in any way, nonetheless he could not constantly "lasso the prospective giver," which seemed more and more a requirement of his job. He had other things to do now that he had settled into the job.

In 1907, the AMA's House of Delegates had applauded the defeat of a bill that would have licensed osteopaths in the District of Columbia. Benign neglect of them was one thing—acceptance, another. Osteopathy was still considered a cult, and the standard doctors for years to come would urge the states "to limit the practice as it sees fit." Like homeopathy, eclectics, chiropractic, and naturopathy, the AMA said, osteopathy was peopled with "freaks." They were all "a motley collection of pseudo-scientists."

That year, *JAMA* had published a series of articles on vaccine therapy. The journal authors protested the use of "mixed" vaccines, as they called the combining of several, and urged "the precise vaccine suited to the individual patient." The AMA said "many failures arise from the use of the wrong vaccine." Copeland seized on these statements as illustrative of, at the very least, a convergence of thinking between the AIH and the AMA on the matter of "definite and precise methods of medication," which, of course, was done in all homeopathic cases.

Precision and scientific proof were always on Copeland's mind. He spoke a year later, in 1908, to a group of students about the high-potency experiments of a Spanish scientist he identified only as "M. Cahis of Barcelona." Copeland told the group that "if these demonstrations are to be depended upon and if they can be reproduced by other experimenters, the homeopathist need no longer be without unanswerable argument regarding the truth of his hypothesis," adding that he himself "cannot personally vouch for the reliability of these wonderful results," although scientists at the New York College lab are in the process of trying to "substantiate or to disprove" the claims. Cahis's experiments were performed on rabbits, and Copeland said he "received private advices from Europe confirming the truth" of them.

Cahis gave strychnine poison "in a minimum mortal dose" to the animals, followed by "tetanotoxine" [*sic*] as an antidote because of its "toxicological resemblance" to the poison. He first used the tetanotoxine in 30X, and then gradually increased the dilution until he reached the dilution of 4,500C, in which the antidote was diluted trillions and trillions of times. At this otherworldly dilution, the animal survived! Copeland quoted Cahis as saying that "according to the studies of modern physical chemists there are no atoms in our lowest centesimal solutions, but as in these experiments it is demonstrated to an absolute certainty that there is something in our high dilutions which acts pharmaco-dynamically, it will be necessary that the learned men agree on this apparent contradiction and if necessary, invent a new science." Most homeopaths now accepted that above 24X (or 12C, Avogadro's number) no molecules of the original substance remained in the mixture. The experiments of Cahis were not successfully duplicated, but Copeland was optimistic that they would be one day and said, "Eventually those who came to scoff will remain to learn."

As dean, he continued to read the journals and follow any research work being done. In 1906, the American Homeopathic Ophthalmological, Otological, and Laryngological Society had performed what was considered a successful re-proving of Belladonna. The tests were done on fifteen patients in eleven cities across the nation. Copeland lectured about an English scientist who had recently written a book on radioactive waves, and a French doctor who did experiments on gold, silver, and platinum, and discovered "that almost infinitesimal doses are endowed with very great activity." The English scientist experimented with radium bromide, which he heated until gas evolved. The amount of gas "would not exceed a pin's head," yet when mixed "with a million millions times its own volumes of air," it was found to have "all the properties of pure radium." Copeland said that "the consensus of opinion today and the teachings of every laboratory in the world is that the finer the division of a chemical substance, the more active it is, and its activities are not fixed qualities except in infinite dilution. Samuel Hahnemann knew this a century ago."

"The sea of science, like the ocean itself," Copeland told his students, "is a restless, agitated, rarely quiet body." It was important to listen and learn, and to make practical use of "the new biological truths." The program of a homeopathic convention in New York clearly illustrated the dean's point—there were lectures on the tonsils, fractures of the hip, hyperthyroidism, and appendicitis. It was hard to distinguish these seminars from those a standard doctor might attend, and it was one of the reasons the AMA had been encouraging homeopaths to leave their own groups once and for all and join "the regulars."

THE DAILY commute by locomotive from New Rochelle to Grand Central Depot in Manhattan (a train shed that at the time held only twelve tracks), and then by trolley or electric taxicab to Flower Hospital, between 63rd and 64th Streets on Eastern Boulevard (later renamed York Avenue), proved to be too much for Copeland. It proved to be too much for his bride, too, who was left home alone a lot, just as Mary had been. "The poor girl is not well," Copeland confided to a doctor in Ann Arbor who had once treated Frances Copeland for "nerves." A month after their arrival in the East, Copeland gave his wife a remedy for nervous symptoms she was having. He prescribed *Argent. nit.,* the compound of silver nitrate, often used for agitation and stomach problems. (He had once prescribed it for a patient with diabetes.) Standard doctors had used it for epilepsy, eye infections, and the cauterization of wounds. Copeland gave his wife a 12X dilution, or one part remedy and one trillion parts water. The remedy helped her feel better, he said.

After a year—"a long year," as Copeland described it—the couple moved to a large ground-floor apartment at 58 Central Park West, on the corner of 68th Street, in New York City. Mrs. Copeland, now less isolated, and thus less distressed, began a tradition of pinning a red carnation—her husband's favorite flower, she said—on his lapel before he left for the hospital in the morning. She also decided to become a hostess. She was ready to adapt and move ahead with her enterprising spouse. As a young girl in Cadillac, she had learned well at her church's weekly chicken-pie suppers the importance of a strong social life. Very early on she understood, as she put it, that one was "either in or out of society, so to speak." She became determined to remain in society, and by the time she met her husband, she had grown into a fun-loving, stylish, and adventurous young woman who would one day host a dinner for one hundred guests on a railway car in Grand Central Terminal and have a thousand carnations on display at another big party.

NEW YORK Homeopathic Medical College had been founded in 1860, and its first president was William Cullen Bryant, who was, of course, an early advocate of homeopathy. The college's first class had fifty-nine students, many of whom were graduates of Columbia University (which New York Homeopathic's first faculty of eight professors also had attended). Seven years later, in 1867, the New York Ophthalmic Hospital came under its supervision, so, like Copeland, the medical students had a chance to learn about the eyes in detail. In 1889, New York Homeopathic Medical College built its own hospital—first called the Flower Free Surgical Hospital—a large brick building close to the East River. Its name didn't come from any homage to a remedy, but rather from Roswell P. Flower, a New York congressman and, later, New York governor, who helped finance the hospital.

Flower Hospital was next to crowded tenements and factories, and the squalid view from its windows mirrored the lives of many of the destitute patients inside. Copeland had chosen to further the cause of homeopathy smack in the middle of New York's biggest slum. Instead of flowers at Flower, he saw rows and rows of clothes drying on lines strung

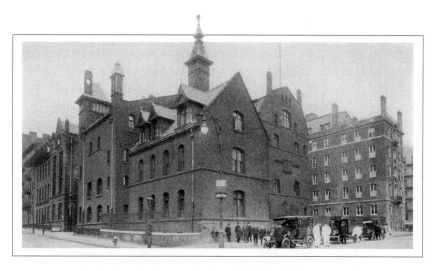

New York Homeopathic Medical College and Flower Hospital, 1917

between the dank buildings, and the blinking electric sign of a neighboring brewery. Misery and disease were prevalent in the area. "I can take you to thousands of families where twelve persons live in three rooms," he would write, "where four sleep in the kitchen every night. In hundreds of so-called homes they live inside rooms without light or ventilation."

Flower's motto was In This Hospital the Interests of the Patient Shall Be Paramount, and Copeland often reiterated that "this epigram became the law of the institution, and no patient is refused admission if there is a bed in which to place him." He reminded his interns that the patients "are mostly foreigners, and are apprehensive and distrustful, and afraid to go to the hospital. They go there not to see special doctors, as do private patients, but because they must."

At the time of its founding, New York Homeopathic Medical College had three laboratories—anatomy, qualitative chemistry, and histology (the microscopic study of tissues). By the time Copeland became its dean in 1908, it had more than two hundred students, and the classes and laboratories included bacteriology, dermatology, pathology, physiology (the functions of the normal body), physiological chemistry, embryology, ophthalmology, pharmacology, clinical medicine, physics, and biology. Copeland told a high-school graduate from Asbury Park, New Jersey, "You get everything you would get in an allopathic school and besides that, you get Homeopathy."

According to the catalogue, "homeopathic therapeutics will be given special prominence," and courses were also offered in hydrotherapy and electrotherapy. Students were told they would greatly benefit from the connection to Flower, and there would be "2 hours daily of operative work in surgery and gynecology (these clinics will be devoted to simple operations, to major operations, to orthopedic surgery, to fractures, and to dislocations)." The medical staff consisted of nineteen consulting and thirty-three attending physicians and surgeons. (Copeland later admitted that "the average number of Attendings daily could not be ascertained as no record of the physician's attendance is kept.")

Proving a maxim that the busier the person, the more time for other things, the new dean, whose one-year term as president of the AIH was over, opened a private practice in eye, ear, nose, and throat diseases. He saw patients for three hours a day in an office in his apartment and performed some surgery there, too. He often ordered small crystals of cocaine from a New York pharmaceutical company, telling them it was "for use in my practice." The company sent the cocaine to Central Park West without receiving the signed order required by state law, so as not to cause him "any inconvenience." But it sometimes took two letters to remind him to mail in the document.

He continued to see patients at Flower—not only for eye problems but for fractures and other injuries as well—and always kept in close touch with the interns working there. He enjoyed teaching them homeopathy by example. When a patient came to the emergency room with the white of his eye punctured by a piece of broken glass, and then after a three-day hospital stay developed an infection in the eye, Copeland prescribed *Rhus tox,* the remedy made from poison ivy leaves. He recorded in his casebook that he had never seen a more "delightful" result. For a woman with high blood pressure as well as bouts of "acute mania," a patient who could never seem to be fitted with the correct type of glasses, he prescribed Sepia, a remedy made from cuttlefish ink. This remedy was used primarily for gynecological complaints, but it helped so much that Copeland began to wonder if it could become an accepted remedy for high blood pressure. For a patient with extensive burns, he prescribed a remedy he had seldom used before: Catharis, a tincture made from the poisonous Spanish fly beetle. (For centuries, the secretions from this insect had been used to remove warts, to lessen rheumatic pain, and, most famously, as an aphrodisiac.)

Copeland, like most doctors at the time, believed that the tonsils "disappear after the age of twenty-five," although he later changed his mind about this. He was in favor of the removal of tonsils if medical treatment didn't help. He often prescribed Belladonna, *Hepar sulf.* (calcium sulfide), or *Merc. So.* (*Mercurius solubilis*), and believed that constipation was a possible cause of tonsillitis, as well as of an infection in one or more teeth. He once said that shingles, the painful rash related to chicken pox, might be caused by diseased tonsils.

His private practice flourished, and because it was at home, it enabled him to see Frances more. But despite "a greater field for work and big fees," New York City and its crowdedness began to bother him. He said he was homesick. He wrote his parents and sister just two years after he took the job that "going there in the first place had been a mistake." He told them that "I confess that I do not grow to love New York as do a good many people. It has its many attractions, but they are the things a tourist sees, and not the every day life of a resident. If we had the theater craze, or the epicurean appetite this would be all right. For people, however, who love a home, a dooryard, real friendship, and some peace of mind, this is not the ideal spot." He said that he found everything too expensive, the competition "tremendously active," "transportation trying," and "the noise and hustle unbearable." In fact, he said "the whole situation was all but impossible." He was even thinking of resigning and returning to Michigan, if they would have him back. He realized now that "the opportunity to do good and to make a living is just as great in Ann Arbor as it is here." New York had taught him "the value of Michigan life." He told his parents that "I believe it is better for all branches of the Copeland family if we return to Ann Arbor." He even missed the local stores. He wrote that "simply because Wanamaker keeps everything from a locomotive to a tooth-pick does not mean that he has any great assortment of each article. You can find more furniture in Martin Heller's in Ann Arbor, more jewelry in Arnold's, and more groceries in Lamb and Spencer."

But homesickness was only part of the problem. Copeland was also upset over the "noise and hustle" of his Board of Trustees. At a specially called meeting to discuss a $40,000 grocery and supply bill, a trustee had shouted at him as if he were a lowly employee, "My goodness! This is terrible! You must find a way to pay this bill!" Copeland stood up in front of all the trustees, men who he thought understood his growing distaste for fund-raising, and said, "If you brought me to New York to raise money to pay bills I wish to resign this month. I came here to spend money, not get it."

In the end, he would not leave because of "circumstances which are now out of my knowledge," he explained. But it was his ambition. The Board of Trustees flattered him and begged him to stay, saying it would be a "calamity" if he went back to Michigan. "It takes a longer time to become known in this great city than in a smaller place," he wrote shortly afterward to a colleague in Ann Arbor; "but, of course, I take it for granted that when success comes, it is of a larger variety than can be attained in a small town."

AFTER THE AMA's relatively secret 1906 inspection of America's medical schools and the criticism that arose because of it, the organization asked the Carnegie Foundation for the Advancement of Teaching to be in charge of an unbiased, independent investigation of all the schools. It was hoped that such a distinguished, fair-minded authority would stop the opposition to inspection. A young educator by the name of Abraham Flexner was put in charge of the project, and he and the secretary of the AMA Council on Medical Education began visiting medical schools in January 1909. (Flexner's pivotal report would be published in 1910.)

Meanwhile, as is often the case when word of an impending investigation is out, some medical schools, especially homeopathic ones, initiated changes. In Minnesota, the Board of Regents abolished the homeopathic school in 1909 and merged it with the standard one. But in Indiana, homeopaths attending an AIH meeting in 1909 were told not to worry about possible allopathic attacks and consolidation, and just to keep adhering to Hahnemannian principles. Homeopaths would confer among themselves whether to go the "Minnesota" way, so to speak, or the "Indiana" way. Debates heated up at most meetings across the country. More often than not, finances were the real concern because so many schools were running out of money and saw consolidation, whether they liked it or not, as the only way to survive. Small homeopathic colleges worried about where they would get the money to keep their physical plants up to date. Tuition could only stretch so far. Some, believing that no one other than the AIH had any authority over them, privately decided to pretend to comply with AMA edicts. They'd just try to fake it.

In the East, "the faithful and efficient" Copeland, as he was now characterized by his Board of Trustees, continued to encourage separate-but-equal medical schools. New York Homeopathic College, like the homeopathic school at the University of Michigan, was respected for its demanding curriculum, and Copeland was determined to make it even better by developing "influence advantageous to the college," even "in circles outside the institution." He was now more than a burgeoning politician, and also one with a growing sense of humor. He wrote a friend in Ann Arbor that "Republicans are so scarce in New York that they are quite a curiosity. Tammany is the boss here."

In early October 1908, shortly after his arrival in New York, Copeland had requested through an intermediary a meeting with Simon Flexner, the older brother of Abraham, who at the time was head of the Rockefeller Institute for Medical Research. Copeland no doubt had in mind influencing not Flexner's younger brother but his boss, John D. Rockefeller, Sr., who was known as a strong defender of homeopathy. Although Rockefeller had given New York Homeopathic College a grant of $26,350 sometime before 1903, he had earlier, in 1901, also given the AMA a large grant of $200,000 for medical research. Copeland's intermediary with Simon Flexner was a doctor by the name of Hamilton Fiske Biggar, who was Rockefeller's personal physician, and a homeopath. Biggar, the acting president of the AIH after Copeland's term ended in 1908, heard back from John D. Rockefeller, Jr. (who unlike his father didn't use a homeopath, but a standard doctor who had been his classmate at Brown) that his father wanted to know "the nature of Doctor Copeland's business with Dr. Flexner," so he "could tell at once whether an introduction would be of value to Dr. Copeland." Biggar, who felt that homeopathy needed what he called "organized evangelization," replied that "Dr. Copeland has no motive besides the pleasure of meeting Dr. Flexner for Dr. Copeland is a gentleman, a profound scholar, and a thorough investigator of anything that pertains to medicine. He is very popular with the medical profession and has held the highest offices that a medical association could bestow." No record exists that a meeting ever took place. Nonetheless, Copeland seemed unaware that the elder Rockefeller had once given money to his school, for in a speech he complained loudly that even though "the richest man in the world" uses homeopathy, "he has never given materially to any homeopathic institution."

Although Copeland persisted with his middle-ground philosophy concerning homeopathic disagreements, he began to use less than middle-ground language. At meetings, he accused some associates of being two-faced and of trying "to carry water on both shoulders" when it came to standard medicine, and said these "supposed adherents" of homeopathy were showing an "aloofness" that could be "evidence of a desire to curry favor with the dominant school." He now called anyone who wanted to join forces with standard medical schools "chicken-hearted," especially in their "silly" efforts to get rid of the word "homeopathic."

Enrollment at New York Homeopathic College (newspaper articles would soon refer to it as "Copeland's school") was not falling as much as it was at other homeopathic schools. Even though in 1909 there were about 60 fewer students than when Copeland began his tenure, out of the total enrollment of 140 future homeopaths, 47 were freshmen. (The Hahnemann College in Philadelphia had only 34 freshmen, and the Boston Homeopathic School had 28. Attendance was also falling at homeopathic schools in Ann Arbor, Chicago, San Francisco, Iowa, and Ohio.) But falling did not mean failing, and a member of the Western New York Auxiliary of New York Homeopathic Medical School said that "the institution will be on solid ground in 2 or 3 years." Yet some doomsday homeopaths felt that, as one wrote in a letter to Copeland, "the recent phenomenal advances in medicine" in chemistry and pathology made it that much harder for the homeopathic schools to scale the high standards. On November 19, 1909, the New York State Board of Charities, which supervised New York Homeopathic College, as well as Flower Hospital Dispensary, issued its annual inspection report, which in many ways helped the institution prepare for the AMA–Carnegie Foundation inspection soon to come. The Board of Charities inspection took place on October 14, 1909. (The AMA–Carnegie inspection would take place two months later, in December.)

A New York State Board of Charities inspection eight months earlier had criticized the gynecological department in the dispensary for having only one table. But the new inspection in October noted that two tables had been added, "and the room curtained off so that three cases may be treated at the same time." The new inspection also praised the cleaning of a yard in back of the college and hospital, as well as the removal of old outhouses. It commended the establishment of a tuberculosis clinic and a social services department, and supplied statistics showing that there had been 4,149 persons treated at the dispensary in August of 1909, and 4,308 in September of 1909. It complimented the arrangement of the dispensary and said the rooms were now well lighted and well ventilated, praise that particularly pleased Copeland, who from almost the day of his arrival had worked hard on improvements. The report also said that treatment was offered in thirteen areas—"general medicine, surgery, orthopedics, lungs, diseases of children, gynecology, eye, skin, genito-urinary, nerves, tuberculosis, nose and throat, ear and physical therapeutic." The inspection placed the facilities in "Class 1," the highest possible category, and noted that the college and hospital "showed practically no defects." Still, Copeland wrote a former associate in Michigan, he had "some serious problems to face, and unless they are solved, the future is not very bright." One major problem was that Flower was run at a loss of $15,000 to $25,000 a year. "We are taking care of a large ambulance district, and are glad to do so, in spite of the fact that this service involves us in a daily expense above any trifling income from this source," Copeland said. The district went from 42nd Street to 69th Street, "river to river," and extended north to 96th Street west of Central Park. Calls were received over a direct police department wire.

"The hospital needs money and can never be any greater until it has increased endowment," he confessed to his parents in a letter. "Indeed it may be necessary to curtail the work to keep within our means. The institution has grown so rapidly that it has outgrown its clothes and we really haven't any money to buy new garments."

SEVEN

"Masters of the Situation"

I N EARLY June of 1910, Abraham Flexner said that poorly trained doctors were menacing America. Copeland clipped the *New York Herald*
article that headlined this shocking judgment, which was based on
Flexner's long-awaited investigation of the 155 medical schools in the
United States. His report, "Medical Education in the United States and
Canada," was contained in a booklet with the unassuming name *Bulletin
Number Four,* published by the Carnegie Foundation for the Advancement of Teaching, but the criticism it contained was harsher than any
criticism that had ever come from the AMA alone.

Flexner found in his travels across the country that some medical
schools had practically no laboratories or lab equipment. He walked into
medical libraries that lacked a single book. He discovered faculty members who claimed they taught at schools but didn't, and instead spent all
their time with private patients. He found schools that were run more as
businesses than as citadels of education, relying on newspaper and magazine advertisements to haul in students. In many schools, nothing was
as it should have been, yet in others, he found nothing but excellence. It
was a rocky road he walked—fairly quickly, it was hinted—over America's training ground for doctors. Far too many medical schools existed in
America, he observed, and certainly too many of them were inferior
ones. "The situation can improve only as the weaker and superfluous
schools are extinguished," he wrote.

His model medical school was at his own undergraduate alma mater,
Johns Hopkins, in Baltimore, Maryland. This was a richly endowed,

innovative institution started in 1893, one that required its students to have college degrees. A high-school diploma and a year of college should no longer be enough to gain entrance to medical schools, Flexner said. (In 1910, nine states still didn't even require a high-school education for acceptance: Arkansas, California, Illinois, Kentucky, Maryland, Missouri, Pennsylvania, Tennessee, and Texas.)

Hopkins boasted a four-year curriculum that combined fundamental sciences, clinical instruction, and, what was relatively new in medical education, research. Flexner, who never attended medical school, wanted all schools to have ample laboratories where experimental research could be conducted. He also cited Harvard, Columbia, the University of Pennsylvania, and the University of Michigan as exemplary. He said that the days of treating medical school like a mere apprenticeship instead of a long and exacting education should end, and he wanted all schools to have a strong teaching connection with a hospital. (Although Johns Hopkins created the term "resident" to describe advanced postgraduate medical training in hospitals, the University of Michigan's standard medical school was the first in the country to build its own hospital.)

Flexner said also that there were too many doctors in the country, and that schools whose standards fell short of his top five should fold. He proposed that the 155 medical schools in existence be reduced to just 31. In other words, he wanted 124 schools to close their doors forever. In time, 61 did; the rest—94 of them—stayed in business. The Homeopathic Medical School of the University of Michigan, with its rigorous curriculum, and New York Homeopathic Medical School, with its equally demanding courses, were among those that kept going. (Other homeopathic colleges that managed to stay open, at least for another decade, included New York Medical College for Women, Hahnemann College of Philadelphia, Hahnemann College of San Francisco, Hahnemann College of Chicago, the College of Homeopathic Medicine in Columbus, Ohio, and those at the State University of Iowa and Boston University.)

Although in its general spirit and in some specific areas, like the need to explore higher standards in medical education, Copeland agreed with Flexner's report (yes, he too believed there *were* too many doctors—but actually, not enough homeopathic ones!), he was opposed to other recommendations, such as making a college degree a requirement for entrance to medical school. He said that Flexner was wrong about this. "Medical institutions are under-graduate institutions," Copeland insisted. The requirements for admission should be no higher than those for admission to a university academic department at Yale, Harvard, Princeton, Columbia, Brown, Michigan, Chicago, Minnesota, Illinois, or Stanford. Medical schools, he stressed, "are training men, not for research work, not for medical writing, not for scientific investigation— they are training men for the cure of the sick, the alleviation of human suffering, and the prevention of concrete, not abstract disease."

Copeland told his Board of Trustees that there were three types of medical schools. Harvard and Johns Hopkins were training "experts working out the causes of disease and preparing graduates who will man the public health laboratories . . . social and preventive medicine is the study of such schools." He said that colleges like Cornell and Yale trained "the rich and learned," and their graduates "are not suited by taste or habits for country life, or the rough and tumble experiences of ordinary household practice. They will seek the centres where great laboratories exist and where culture abounds. Their patients will number university graduates, men of science and letters, art critics, lovers of music." But, he said, New York Homeopathic Medical College was a third type. While it recognized "the place and importance of the other schools," and "respects the erudition of the Cornell graduate" and will "gladly" use the laboratory findings of Johns Hopkins, notwithstanding, he said, "we are training men for the actual practice of routine medicine." He told his trustees that "it is our function to supply the all-around, common, every day, alert, resourceful, general practitioner." That was what the homeo-path had been in the nineteenth century and would continue to be in the twentieth.

Copeland acknowledged that some homeopathic schools "have not been free of shameful standards and unworthy acts." He agreed that Flexner was right to point out "defects in material equipment and record-keeping." He thought that perhaps the medical-school curricu-lum should be increased to five years from the current four, and he went along with the New York State Department of Education (as well as those departments in Michigan and Illinois) in proposing that medical-school applicants must first pass a premedical course and receive a Med-ical Student Certificate before entering medical school. But a college degree should not be a requirement for medical-school admission. Many homeopaths agreed with him, saying that the college-degree path was for the wealthy, and others even suggested that the study of homeopathy should take no more than three years (not four or five).

Copeland favored some form of state supervision, he said, "from the standpoint of the public" for "the protection of the people against charlatans, quacks, and poorly-educated practitioners." (He would later encourage federal control as the "ideal condition" for medical-school supervision.) He reiterated to his trustees that "I recognize the necessity of medical research and the training of abstract scientists." But he also warned not just his board, but the public in speeches, that there had to be "practical" doctors as well, those who "are successful in actual contact with disease." This was important to him, and he reached back to his days in Dexter to explain to an audience of homeopathic educators that he wanted the ideal doctor to be a "pioneer who has learned his woodcraft from actual contact with nature." These pioneers—both the teachers and the student doctors—were "masters of the situation when coping with the novice who acquired his knowledge in the library." And, he said, using the military language he was so fond of, "the doctor from Johns Hopkins is not unlike the artilleryman or engineer, who is not only a trained military man, but one who has had unusual teaching in one of the technical specialties of war science. Likewise, the Cornell graduate may be compared to the cavalry officer. He knows more about military science than his colleagues in the other arms of the service, but he makes a more martial display by reason of his spanking mount." He said that homeopaths "will enter the infantry, less spectacular, but needed in greater numbers and really more important in the long run." This was a telling speech, because Flexner had been extremely critical of homeopathy, saying that dogma didn't belong in the same room as science. Flexner called homeopathy sectarian, and questioned if perhaps in a time of scientific medicine it had any logical defense. (Copeland would later say that scientific medicine had no right to be "contemptuous of homeopathy because it [scientific medicine] was not far enough away from its own dark ages.") Flexner had also been rough on eclectic and osteopathic schools, saying their "so-called" graduates were "half-trained."

During the summer of 1910, an anonymous pamphlet, *What Is Homeopathy?*, made the rounds of standard doctors and schools. (Copeland later said he had been one of its editors.) The pamphlet, which found its way to the offices of the AMA, stated that homeopathy was "entirely based on facts," and "set a true, practical example" as "a branch of positive philosophy," which was a new and novel explanation. The pamphlet said that "all the great operations of nature, those of heat, light, chemical action, etc., and those of the human frame, particularly the wonderful modifications of the nervous fluid, are carried by microscopic, atomic, and infinitesimal movements, almost transcending our imaginations." The homeopaths hoped that standard doctors would read the pamphlet carefully, but few did.

Flexner had stopped short of calling homeopathy (as well as eclecticism and osteopathy) fraudulent; he saved that characterization for chiropractors, calling them "unconscionable quacks." As for homeopaths, he believed that since the number of students at their schools had been on the decline for some time—years before his report—there wasn't much that could be done to improve that situation. He also felt, as the AMA did, that nature would take its course and that these schools would just fade away. He said that basically everything that was of proven value in homeopathy had already been incorporated into "scientific medicine" (by this he meant standard medicine), and belonged "of right" there. He agreed with the AMA that there was no longer any need for separate homeopathic medical schools.

Copeland naturally recognized that Flexner's statements about homeopathy were "of positive damage to the educational institutions and to the practice of homeopathy." The disagreements between standard doctors and homeopaths were now more public than ever before because of the nationwide publicity surrounding the Flexner Report, as it was called in newspapers and magazines. "Flexner has sought to injure us in the eyes of the world by a dogmatic assertion which is unfounded in fact," Copeland fumed. At the same time, he calmed down enough to arrange a brief meeting with Flexner, who told him that "there ought to be but four homeopathic colleges" in America. Copeland needed all his powers of persuasion to protect not only his own college, but also his profession.

He first fired back in speeches around New York State. He decided that "the overshadowing influence of the old school and the daily contact of the student with teachers antagonistic to homeopathy must mould the average mind to a form forever unfitted for the homeopathic system. The way to make shouting Methodists is not to train them from earliest youth in the Catholic Church. Some wise papist prelate said to an antagonist: 'Give me the first ten years of a child's life and you can have the rest.' So it is in medicine," Copeland now preached. "Give a man four years in an old school college and the chances are five hundred to one that he will forever remain an old-school practitioner." He argued forcefully that "the men who control the destinies of medical students determine for all time their attitude toward controversial questions," and told his fellow homeopaths that they would be making "a fatal mistake" if they allowed homeopathic colleges to be "wiped out. The homeopathic fraternity would cease to exist," he said.

At a meeting on October 13, 1910, of the New York chapter of the AIH, he now lashed out that "undue importance and finality" was being attached to Flexner's statements about homeopathy because of "the influence of the powerful corporation employing his services." He followed this attack by explaining that "scientific medicine" could be incorporated into homeopathy because a homeopath was as well trained in science as a standard doctor, but it couldn't be the other way around because a standard doctor dispensing homeopathic remedies was not as well trained as a homeopath. A homeopath needed to learn the kind of exactness that could only be taught in his own school, and Copeland would never, ever, give up the idea of a separate homeopathic medical school. It had been a blow to him that W. A. Dewey, his friend and associate at the University of Michigan Homeopathic College, now believed that the time was right "for one great unified profession of medicine" and that homeopathy should be a compulsory course for all medical students, taught by "masters of the art."

Shortly after making his comments at the AIH meeting, Copeland surprised his audience by accusing a well-known standard doctor who was an authority on botany of plagiarism. He said that Dr. Samuel O. L. Potter had "deliberately and intentionally" stolen material from a homeopathic book and included it in his own medical textbook. He then looked hard at his audience and questioned whether the material that was appropriated from a homeopathic book (without attribution) really "belongs of right to scientific medicine and is at this moment incorporate in it," as Flexner claimed. No. Homeopathy belongs to homeopathy, Copeland said defiantly. He turned to religion for more answers. "Perhaps Flexner uses the word 'incorporate' in a theological sense," he said, "capable of the same doubt as has existed regarding the true nature of the sacrament. Perhaps, from his standpoint, homeopathy is incorporate in scientific medicine immediately its truths are written in the sacred ink of its inspired authors! From my standpoint, however, homeopathy is not incorporate in 'scientific medicine' so called until the authorities in that school and its practitioners actually accept and apply its precepts according to rule. Let us consider, therefore, the records of its scribes and high priests; then, and not till then, can we decide whether or not homeopathy has been absorbed by the older system. . . . I am sure the dream of every homeopathist is that blissful day when scientific medicine shall have accepted 'Similia similibus curentur' as its rule of action and the small dose as the natural corollary. If these are now actually incorporate in the bedside practice of scientific medicine, so far as this speaker is concerned, he is ready to say most joyfully: 'Lord, now lettest thy servant depart in peace.' " But, of course, that was not the case.

At the same time that Copeland was denouncing the standard doctors, he was still in favor of keeping the lines of communication open with the AMA and therefore continued to cultivate the group. On January 10, 1910, he had even invited the secretary of the AMA's Council on Medical Education to lunch. Although a convenient time could not be arranged, the AMA official let Copeland know in a letter that he had "already rated New York Homeopathic College in the council's list of acceptable medical schools." (He did not say exactly which category.) Two years earlier, the editor of the *North American Journal of Homeopathy* had suggested to Copeland (while he was still in Michigan) that they invite the newly elected president of the AMA to speak at the next AIH convention. The editor told Copeland that such an invitation might "improve the relationship between the different wings of the medical profession," something that Copeland was 100 percent in support of, at least privately. The editor hoped that when the "new President of the AMA found himself surrounded by such a band of good fellows as will undoubtedly assemble . . . it might influence him to direct the policies of the AMA upon a little less hardfast lines." He also suggested the board members of the AIH keep him away from "the rabid fellows"—the purists who wanted no compromises and no relationship at all with the AMA. The whole matter of such relations was sticky, requiring the skill of someone like Copeland, who would now say not only that homeopathy was true, but also that "to set aside this conviction would be to surrender a moral principle." He would call upon doctors across the country "to insist that the medical profession ought not be a political machine." As if to prove that he was ready to do this (although he wasn't), he turned to lecturing about the proof of homeopathy.

He said that homeopathy was no longer an experiment, as it was in Hahnemann's time. "Present day methods," he maintained, were proving its validity. He cited an English doctor's recent work with antibodies, the high-molecular proteins that can produce immunity or interfere with it. "Sir A. E. Wright's work is but a confirmation or rediscovery of homeopathy," Copeland insisted. "Working, for instance, with the germs of pus production, he, too, observed the law of similarity. Taking minute quantities of the toxins of the disease producing germs, toxins capable of producing symptoms similar to those caused by the germ, he was able to cure the lesions produced thereby. Not only did Wright rediscover the law of similars, but also, strange as it may seem, he hit upon the century old conclusion as regards the size of the dose." He used $\frac{1}{10,000}$ of a milligram of the toxin. Copeland emphasized science as he almost never had before.

But not everyone was as ecstatic as Copeland seemed to be. One homeopath was miffed that "members of the old school have climbed onto our Band Wagon, and are rapidly learning to drive it." This doctor wanted his fellow homeopaths to "make some concentrated move toward the appropriating and fathering of our own principles." He wanted the old school to stay away.

Copeland, disappointed and angry, had recently heard that there would be no money coming to homeopathic colleges from John D. Rockefeller. The dean repeated words that he said "expressed the thoughts of this affluent patron": that "no homeopathic college has shown executive ability, consistency of therapeutic application, and success by measure of its own ideals and field of operation." Stinging words. He spoke out provocatively, saying that allopathic medicine "deserves no better fate than to pass into innocuous desuetude."

He was fighting as hard as he could, but it didn't seem enough, so once again he explored the possibility of expanding his influence. He was forty-two years old. The Republican bent he had brought to New York was slowly dissipating. Earlier in the year, he had become a member of New York City's Ambulance Board, presided over by the police commissioner. It was a baby step into the city's political world, yet just weeks after his appointment he was already writing a letter to Mayor William J. Gaynor asking that the city's "hospital provisions be overhauled." He suggested the formation of a new department, a Department of Hospitals, and hinted that he could become its head. (Such a department would not come into existence until many years later.) Meanwhile, as was his custom, "the master hinter of his time," as *The New Yorker* magazine would refer to him, took his Ambulance Board responsibilities very seriously, even making time to jot down notes for possible rules to guide medical students on duty: "While serving on ambulance, not to do any talking. Be particularly careful not to tell strangers the diagnosis; make final diagnosis only after patient has been brought to hospital. Not to become involved in disputes with people present at scene of accident, etc."

In the fall of 1910, Frances and Royal Copeland became the parents of a son, Royal, Jr. He looked so much like his Dexter grandmother that Copeland, who now tried his best to spend what Americans were now calling "week-ends" with his family, joked in a letter to his parents and sister that "especially when he laughs, which he does a good deal, we often call him 'grandma.'" He also wrote in detail about his work at Flower:

> This week has been a strenuous one. I was called to the hospital at 9 o'clock Monday morning and found the emergency rooms filled with the victims of the terrible explosion in the Grand Central yards. Twenty of these people were brought to our hospital and most of them had serious cuts about the face and eyes. One poor girl, a teacher of art in one of the high schools of the city had 35 separate and distinct wounds of the face and scalp. I took 75 stitches to restore the tissues and yesterday had to remove one of her eyes. Fortunately, the other is all right and she will have sight. The injury to that one was very trifling. Another sad case was a man who had similar cuts about the face. I removed one eye at once and I do not think there is one chance in fifty that he will have any sight left in the other eye.

After a while, however, he said that he discovered that the man's iris, or curtain of the eye, had been drawn into the wound (received in a previous accident) and had been held there when the wound healed. The eye was thus left without a pupil, or opening. But, Copeland said, he was able to cut through the cornea and remove a cataract that had formed and then draw the iris, the muscle that controls the degree of light that comes into the eye, out through the aperture. A circular opening was made in the iris to provide a new pupil. The iris had, in effect, been reconstituted, and a new pupil had been sculpted. The operation made a headline in the *New York Herald:* EYE BALL SLASHED, HIS SIGHT IS SAVED. Copeland was making news.

That summer, he performed another headline operation: CORNEA GRAFTING FIRST PERFORMED IN HOSPITAL HERE. The *New York Herald* reported on his "daring pioneer work" in which a section of the cornea from a woman with inflammation and failing vision was transplanted to the eye of a blind man. In a preliminary report on the operation, one he had modeled after a similar procedure by a German doctor, Copeland noted that his patient "was a Chinaman, male, aged 26," and went on to explain that "if the surgeon is ever permitted to experiment—and except for experimentation how is the sum total of human knowledge to be increased?—here was a case where one must be fully justified in attempting some new thing." It was the first such operation ever performed in America, and it had been performed by a homeopath, although no explicit mention was made of that fact.

Copeland reported that the corneas in both of the man's eyes had been destroyed, although he said that "strong light focused upon either eye revealed light perception and accurate projection." He said that the woman who contributed her cornea for the transplant had "appeared" at Flower just in time. It was meant to be. Copeland recorded that "the same preparation of each patient as for cataract extraction was made and both were anesthetized at the same time. All was ready then for operating." He used a special surgical knife—"at the top of the shaft is a spring like that of a watch—this is released and the blade rapidly rotates so long as the trigger is kept under pressure." This knife also had a "stop" that prevented it from going too deep into the tissue, although he reported that he "scraped away as much of the uncut deeper tissue as I dared." To retrieve the cornea from the woman, he said that "the blade was sent spinning through the entire thickness of the cornea . . . the disc of clear cornea was tenderly transferred to the first patient and gently stroked into accurate position." Three months after the surgery, which had been witnessed by a large group of surgeons, Copeland said that although there was considerable bleeding and scarring, "the patient readily detects the movements of the hand and has every prospect of form vision." He concluded that corneal transplantation "is an operation which deserves to be taken out of the laboratory into the practice of ophthalmology."

According to Flower's operations book, Copeland also performed appendectomies when no other surgeon was available, as well as adenoidectomies, or removal of the nasal adenoid glands. Once he amputated a patient's left hand, because of an infection, and once performed a "reduction of the wrist bones for a fractured wrist." But the majority of his operations involved the eyes: total removal; dissection of tissue; scraping of tissue; iridectomy, which creates a small hole in the iris; and a fifteen-minute procedure called a "kneedling," which the operations book said was tried four times for "eye cases." (There was no further clarification.)

It was not recorded if any of the patients received homeopathic remedies before, during, or after their surgeries, although for nonsurgical eye problems Copeland often prescribed Calendula, the flowering plant used by all doctors as an antiseptic to aid healing. When a baby with an undisclosed eye ailment was brought to him, he noted that a previous doctor had used bichloride of mercury as antiseptic, and said that it was probable that this treatment was "too strong for the delicate flesh of the baby." He told the mother to moisten a pad with Calendula mixed with four parts of boiled water. Gentle care.

THE FLEXNER REPORT did not mention New York Homeopathic College and Flower Hospital directly, but it did include them in its general criticism of all homeopathic schools. Inadequate record-keeping was charged. Laboratories were found good enough in terms of the equipment they held but faulted for inadequate space—they were overcrowded, sometimes dirty, and often used for multiple functions. Flexner said that both allopathic and homeopathic laboratories in New York City were "clinically unproductive," and needed more "vigorous" teaching-hospital connections. He urged Columbia's College of Physicians and Surgeons, which he approved of, to merge with Roosevelt Hospital. The dean of Columbia said such an idea was "superficial," because "the object of Roosevelt Hospital is to heal the poor and the teaching of medicine is secondary." Flexner singled out Chicago as "a plague spot of the country so far as medical education is concerned."

A later, solely AMA report of an inspection made on an unspecified date in 1911 gives a strong indication of what Flexner discovered at New York Homeopathic Medical College in 1910. The anatomy lab was found unacceptable, with cadavers not only not well embalmed, but with their dissected portions not properly discarded. No room was assigned for animal experimentation. Certain courses, like the study of tissues, were thought to be a waste of time, as the instructor only repeated what the students could read for themselves in a textbook. "The department of physiology is also below the standard of that of the better grade of medical schools," the AMA report complained, and in the same paragraph noted that "there is no evidence of any research work." One of the most damning objections was this: "The department of pharmacology had apparently received very little development and would not compare favorably even with the courses provided in some of the [other] homeopathic colleges." (Still another AMA report of an inspection on November 5, 1914, expressed it even stronger: "There is no modern laboratory course in pharmacology, nor does the school have a well-developed supposedly homeopathic course in drug-proving. In short, conditions in this school seem to have retrograded since the last previous inspection, which was made in 1911.")

Copeland was devastated by the AMA's 1911 report. He had hoped his laboratories could be used "to demonstrate the claims of homeopathy to the world." Even a November 15, 1911, report by the Eastern Inspection District Committee of the New York State Board of Charities indicated that there continued to be physical defects at the college and hospital. Eight specific problems were cited, and within each problem were several additional ones. The first problem was that "the buildings are generally inconvenient in arrangement and lacking in facilities for outdoor treatment and in suitable outdoor recreation space for children and other convalescent patients, except that the roof space is used for children during the summer." Problems two, three, and four mentioned that the bathrooms in the wards were too small, poorly lighted, and poorly ventilated, that the utensil sterilizers in the service room were out of order, and that the laundry facilities were too scattered—in six different rooms. Problems five and six said the exits to the fire escapes were windows instead of doors, as required by the Public Health Law, and that there was no date recorded when the liquid fire extinguishers were recharged. Problem seven cited the generally inadequate plumbing in the entire building and specifically mentioned unsanitary conditions in the porter's toilet. Problem eight read: "The general wards overcrowded."

For a long time, in fact when he first saw what he called "the old plant," Copeland had hoped for better quarters, and after 1911 he began to try in earnest to raise money for a new twelve-story building. The present hospital contained 150 beds and 15 private rooms. Copeland envisioned a hospital with 150 ward beds and 150 private beds, and he was fortunate in receiving a $70,000 gift almost right away, which made him confident that other donations and gifts would arrive in time to make it possible "to erect a building which will cost in the neighborhood of $900,000."

On March 15, 1912, the commissioner of education in New York submitted his report on the curriculum to Copeland. It noted that the total hours of required work "surpass the exactions of the council on Medical Educations of the AMA," which pleased Copeland very much. His students worked hard in sixty-three subjects over four years and did clinical work at hospitals other than just Flower—Metropolitan, Cumberland, and Bellevue among them. The report mentioned that even though the primary purpose of the education is "along homeopathic lines and for the advancement of the homeopathic creed in medicine," instruction is also given "in the theories and practices of other cults in medicine." In fact, out of the sixty-three courses each student took, ranging from anatomy, bacteriology, surgical pathology, and anesthesia to urinary sediments, hygiene, and infant feeding, only eight were specifically about homeopathy. There was also a course in osteopathy. The report recommended that a course in dental therapeutics be added. It cited the lack of "modern volumes" in the library, a complaint that particularly outraged Copeland, who called it "a false statement." He protested that the inspector hadn't looked carefully enough, and "that he began at the top shelf, where the homeopathic publications are filed, and I suppose, because he saw these, he naturally concluded that 'few of our journals could be of particular interest to the student of modern medicine.' Had he gone farther, he would have found that practically every one of the leading journals is found on our shelves." The inspector must have known this, however, because he noted that these "leading" journals "are carefully locked in cases." Copeland conceded this was true, but said that "there is an attendant whose business it is to give prompt attention to any request for access to the case." Still, what was clear was that Dean Copeland left homeopathic periodicals out for the students to browse through freely but put standard journals away in a place slightly harder for them to reach. The Department of Education had a legitimate grievance.

Copeland began having second thoughts about the proposed requirement that students first had to pass a premedical course before being admitted to medical school. In fact, he wrote Dr. Augustus Downing, the assistant commissioner for higher education of the Department of Education, that he was not planning to abide strictly by such a requirement, although he would offer a "pre-medical year to such students as desire special training and to men who expect to practice in states requiring for licensure five years of medical study."

During the fall of 1912, the construction of a new, modified "pavilion"—as it was christened—of one hundred beds began. It was to be a modern, fireproof, six-story building, and besides the interns, it would have one paid resident physician on its staff. The *New York City Globe* would later call it "a private hotel for sick people," because it didn't exactly adhere to Flower's mandate to treat the poor. Still, Copeland was keeping his eye on both his curriculum and his "material equipment." He saw the new pavilion as expanding his hospital's capability to treat all sorts of patients, and, as he wrote in a letter to Dr. Downing, providing an opportunity to add new classroom and library space, including two large laboratories. A second building, for the college only, was scheduled to begin construction in January of 1913. There was also a plan on the table to build a new hospital for charity cases—"and then the plant would be quite complete," Copeland said.

As always, he stayed on amicable terms with those in a position to judge him. He wrote to Dr. Downing that he "owed a debt of gratitude to the authorities in Albany for their aid and support. I wish particularly to mention the brotherly attitude and wise suggestions that you yourself have made from time to time."

The master of the situation was getting better and better at his game.

While he waited for his new buildings and laboratories, Copeland's interest in modern science never faltered. He had smarted when one homeopath told him that there was "too much stress on anatomy in its minutest details, as well as on chemistry, pathology, bacteriology, hygiene, surgery, and diagnosis." Was this homeopath really a doctor of medicine? he asked.

On September 27, 1911, he had clipped an article from the *New York Tribune* about the invention of a new instrument called a calorimeter. He thought that it might have future implications for homeopathy. The machine measured electromagnetic energy—heat—in the calories of a particle. The article said that "the secrets of the human body are being disclosed . . . through instruments which register the energy necessary to breathe, sleep, awaken, eat, walk, think, work, and dream." Copeland said he had been told one of the scientists involved "showed that cheese is much more nutritious and more sustaining to the human body than

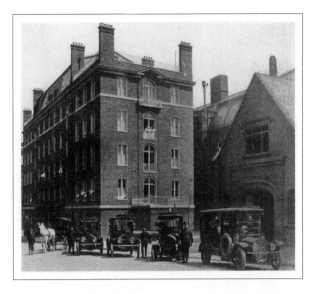

Private "pavilion," ambulances, and garage at Flower Hospital

meat or eggs." He wondered, could an improved version of the calorimeter one day measure energy changes in homeopathic remedies?

IN JUNE 1911, the AMA had announced that "educational propaganda on behalf of the U.S. Pharmacopoeia and National Formulary is in harmony with the work of the AMA." What this language meant was that the AMA was going to stress the U.S. Pharmacopoeia, the official list of recognized drug preparations, as the only legitimate compilation, and was ready to conduct some public relations about it as a means of getting the public to stop using fraudulent nostrums and "irregular" drugs, which also included homeopathic remedies. Once again the homeopathic pharmacopoeia went unnoticed, as it did in an earlier 1895 AMA resolution. In 1911, the AMA also published *Nostrums and Quackery,* the first bound edition of its journal articles on fraudulent products.

The AMA now said that pharmacists, whom they were encouraging to seek "higher education," should not only make an effort to "eliminate sales of nostrums," but should not recommend to the public "medicines for self-medication whether prepared by themselves or not." An article in the standard *Kentucky Medical Journal* called self-medication "an evil practice by a class of people ignorant of the fundamental laws of nature and not capable of comprehending the chemistry of drugs and its relation to the physiological activity of the human body." It included aspirin powder among "the most dangerous drugs," saying that "these tablets are so easy to obtain and so swift in their action that the patient believes he has found a swift and cheap cure." (On January 25, 1911, *JAMA* reiterated that aspirin "should be listed as one of the dangerous drugs.") The *KMJ* article was focused on the fraudulent—e.g., pebbles sold to cure epilepsy or diabetes—but homeopaths and eclectics who read it thought it was also meant as an assault on homeopathic and herbal remedies. The article went on to observe that whatever effects such "time-tried home remedies" had, they were due to "some gratifying psychological effect." This viewpoint signaled a new public approach by the standard doctors in downgrading homeopathy by emphasizing the psychological effect as the cause for its success.

The AMA also recommended in 1911 "the testing, within certain limitations, of therapeutic claims made by manufacturers of alleged new remedies." Homeopathic leaders, including Copeland, were at the time so consumed with raising money and saving their schools that it would be two years before they even noticed and then addressed what they considered the AMA's latest onslaught on their remedies, even though hardly any of them could be considered "new."

That summer of 1911, the AMA had adopted a resolution "that at an early date courses in ophthalmology requiring previous graduation in medicine and one year's work in accredited ophthalmolic hospital and dispensary service shall be established in each medical school possessing the necessary facilities." In other words, the standard medical-school curriculum would now offer advanced ophthalmology courses. (The previous year it had recommended "the formation of a curriculum to better equip medical students and practitioners with a knowledge of infectious diseases of the eye and its refractive defects.") These resolutions were an effort to stem the tide of untrained optometrists and opticians that were flooding American towns and cities. In fact, in 1899 the AMA had passed a resolution saying that opticians not only "were not qualified by their training," but "should not be consultants of regular physicians." Later, in 1911, the AMA, which the year before had discouraged Columbia University from building a school for opticians, "expressed its disapproval of ophthalmologists serving with opticians on boards examining men who have not taken medical courses endorsed by the Association of American

Medical Colleges." It also stated that for an optician to diagnose any condition of the eye was "an infringement on the medical practice laws." In addition, the AMA planned to publish a booklet on "so-called" optometry and its colleges to be sent to all officials of state medical societies in order to "defeat the efforts" of opticians "to enter the medical profession by false pretenses."

Copeland continued to believe that a medical degree was a requirement for any person diagnosing any condition of the eye or any other part of the body. During the fall of 1911, he had given a well-received talk before an educational conference sponsored by the AMA in which he said that he now favored a year of internship in a hospital before a student received his actual medical degree. But, more than ever, he felt the tide turning against his schools.

MAJOR SCIENTIFIC developments continued in the second decade of the twentieth century. In 1910, the first systemic drug, Salvarsan, a synthetic arsenic compound, was developed for the eradication of syphilis and certain other bacterial diseases. (Up to 1910, syphilis had been treated with large doses of mercury, iodine, and arsenic.) The new drug set the stage for the appearance of antibiotics later in the century, as well as for chemotherapy drugs.

Sickle-cell anemia was discovered in 1910. The theory of atomic structure was developed in 1911. Changes in the egg during fertilization were first studied in 1911. The following year, the term "vitamin" was coined by a biochemist who discovered that diseases like rickets or scurvy could be prevented with the addition of "vital amines," or certain organic compounds, to the diet. (The term "biochemist" had been first used in 1903.) Acriflavine, a coal tar derivative, was introduced as an antiseptic for wounds in 1912.

In a speech before homeopaths that year, Copeland was at his most eloquent when he went back to emphasizing the importance of combining the best of homeopathic and allopathic schools. He took a strong stand for vaccinations. Even though he had acknowledged in a letter to his parents in the winter of 1910 that he realized that his sister had "suffered greatly" from "her vaccination experience" (which one is not mentioned), nonetheless, he now believed that "certainly one is much safer to be vaccinated."

He said that "so long as men live they will differ on all questions not actually settled by scientific rule." But, he went on, "we have not agreed as to the importance of the instruction in toxicology and physiological materia medica; indeed, in some circles he is counted almost a heretic who ventures to suggest that the student untaught in these lines has been neglected." He wanted students to learn about all medicinals and herbals, not just homeopathic remedies. He wanted them to know about tannic acid, made from the bark of the winterbloom tree, and witch hazel, from the winterbloom and snapping hazelnut, and tincture of benzoin, a balsamic resin (also used homeopathically as *Benz. ac.,* for gout). He wanted students to understand "historical medicine." He insisted students understand "the thousand and one things that are commonly condemned by our school of practice as unnecessary to apply in the cure of disease." And he wanted students to learn all these things in a way that would make them remain homeopaths, and not become "polypharmacists." He concluded by saying that homeopaths are not "well-grounded unless they are personally familiar with the methods of other systems." He gave his all in this speech, not even caring if to some homeopaths it might seem as if his position was shifting like sand. But in his mind the picture of the practical "cameo-like family doctor" he worshiped included "everything scientific there was to learn about medicine."

Copeland had recently sent his Board of Trustees a confidential memo saying that the college was "trailing behind the procession of medical progress" and that "modern methods filtered in but rarely originated from within." He also said that he had "inside information" that the American College of Surgeons was going "to use its fine-tooth comb" on Flower, along with all American hospitals. They will "rule and demand," Copeland told his trustees. "It is natural to object to new things," he also said, not meaning homeopathy this time, but "modern methods." He told his board that "every innovation is opposed" because people fear inconvenience, and that "modern plumbing is objected to by the rural born."

In 1912, the Federation of State Medical Boards was organized. This national group formally sanctioned the AMA's ratings of medical schools, meaning that homeopathic colleges, at least in terms of licensure, had to accept the AMA's rules no matter what. This presented another crossroads, one they had to tread warily. A few began to think about organizing separate statewide homeopathic medical boards. Copeland was asked to serve on a new AIH committee, "the Joint Conference Committee," which was formed to confer with the AMA on the merits of homeopathic colleges. One dean wrote him, "If all homeopathic colleges would act as a unit, I am sure our efforts might be of some avail and we would certainly win more respect from the AMA." He added that "I have been told . . . to pay no attention to the AMA in any way. I have been told not even to answer their call for various reports, and yet I notice that other deans are anxious to curry favor with the Secretary of the Council of Medical Education and send the called for reports." Copeland was, of course, one of these "other deans." Indeed, he had initiated a "Sub-Freshman" year so his college could meet the AMA's requirements for a Class A school.

There were also murmurs of secession from the AMA's Council on Medical Education. Something had to be done for "self-preservation." (In 1910, the AMA had been in favor of the creation of a cabinet-level Department of Public Health. Opponents argued that "it was being engineered by the allopathic school of medicine to the exclusion of all other schools," and would give allopathy "the power to dictate how all forms of disease should be treated." It would be more than forty years before such a department would come into being.)

Homeopaths now held that impressing the AMA with the merits of their system seemed "useless." A standard doctor who had recently converted to homeopathy called the AMA "gangsters." Some homeopaths thought the AMA would "eventually depose all of our colleges from Class A [acceptable], and as far as possible, to drop them to Class C [unacceptable]." They feared that the end of homeopathic education was getting close. Some A and B (doubtful) colleges discussed merging. One dean even went so far as to say it was hopeless "to resist the onward sweep of the AMA" because homeopathy and allopathy would soon be one "unified profession."

EIGHT

"Losing at the Edges"

O N FEBRUARY 13, 1912, Copeland attended a talk at his state homeo-pathic medical society. He and his colleagues had settled anxiously into their seats but soon found themselves listening intently to their good friend Dr. Horace Porter Gillingham discuss the research being done at the Constantine Hering Laboratory in Philadelphia. This was the sort of lab Copeland had visualized a decade earlier, and it did work that many homeopaths admired, because, as Dr. Gillingham said, it came from "a real workshop, with coordinated departments, including chemical, anatomical, physiological, and pharmaceutical branches, with one or more sub-divisions of each."

Copeland knew that Dr. Gillingham was going to discuss the exciting new work of John G. Wurtz, MD, who had put the remedy Millefolium, made from the yarrow plant—used mainly, Copeland said, "in painless hemorrhages from all mucus surfaces"—through experiments that used "controls" to confirm its effect on the coagulation of human blood and blood pressure. Up to this time, a remedy was accepted as a result of provings by individual homeopaths. Now, for the first time, a "control" was being used; some patients received the remedy and some did not, as a means of showing that the remedy's effects didn't depend on the doc-tor's or the patients' subjective interpretations of the results, no matter how thorough they might be.

Copeland had recently stated publicly that the very nature of homeo-pathic laws might not be explicable. "Life itself is beyond test tube and scalpel," he now said in earnest; "to wander into these fields of thought is simply to lose one's self in an unsolved and unsolvable maze." Still, he was eager to hear Gillingham's reaction to the pioneering work, especially since he had predicted, at the same time he was questioning what might be an "unsolvable maze," that Gillingham's words would probably "fall upon the homeopathic ear with something like the ring of Blessed Hope and Promise of New Life." But they didn't. Copeland and his like-minded colleagues soon grasped that although the speaker was strongly in favor of scientific investigation (that was the "Blessed Hope"), nonetheless, Gillingham had concluded that Dr. Wurtz's findings were worthless (there would be no "Promise of New Life"). The experiments were simply wrong in their premise, Gillingham said, because they involved a complete misunderstanding of the uses of the remedy. He noted that Millefolium's provings "have been relatively few," and that it was well known, as Wurtz had observed in his study, that "the cause of hemorrhages are many and all pathological save menstruation." But Gillingham said that the blood used in the experiments was not the result of a pathological condition and that the patients chosen were "not presenting disease symptoms corresponding to those produced by Millefolium," and therefore "the experiments failed entirely to add to or detract from the reputation of millefolium as a good servant." The experiments did not follow "like cures like." He did admit, though, that its use in the experiment proved that it "will not hasten or retard the coagulation of healthy blood outside the body when drawn from the body artificially," nor will it have "appreciable effect" upon blood pressure. Millefolium did nothing at all for symptoms outside its realm.

Many homeopaths asked if Wurtz's study was the beginning of the end of using laboratory methods to enhance and extend the influence of homeopathy among standard doctors. Not necessarily, these homeopaths said, because Gillingham had said he wanted other laboratories to continue such work, and he wanted such tests "to go slowly." He believed homeopaths had to be even more scientific, and by saying so he meant that they had to apply the methods of classic homeopathic provings. He said that "in the case of Millefolium, for example, to determine its hemostatic value, homeopathically, advantage should be taken of a case of pathological hemorrhage presenting indications calling for Millefolium—the pressure taken before and after the exhibition of the remedy, and the blood to be examined for coagulation time before and after, to be that issuing in the form of a pathological hemorrhage. True," he added, "one might have to wait a long time for the opportunity." But what he was really saying was that there was still no better way than the way of Hahnemann. He believed, as Copeland still did, that "listening to and recording the relief of patients" was often evidence enough of a remedy's legitimacy. Still, Copeland and his colleagues were disappointed that laboratory data had thus far not backed up what they thought to be so certain.

When not anguishing about their remedies or the fate of their schools, and whether or not their graduates would "become contaminated with the free use of hypo medications and all forms of 'shot gun' prescribing," homeopathic leaders tried to get their fold back to business as usual. But another threat was in the air. A "new science," as Copeland called it, had been evolving for a few years, moved along by the AMA. It was called "preventive medicine," and was, Copeland explained, "entirely away from medicine as a system of therapeutics, in favor of the abandonment of drugs." He and other homeopaths saw it not as an application of homeopathic principles involving disease as a whole body dynamic, but as a new attempt to squash their remedies, because the president of the AMA had noted that this "new school" was "one without dogma, gross medications, or absurd attenuations," a direct reference to homeopathic remedies. Copeland said that the AMA was attempting to have everyone live in "a democracy of medicine," something that was worth striving for, but not in the immediate future.

Despite various vaccines, many infectious and contagious diseases were still rampant. Nonetheless, Copeland said that diphtheria was tapering off because of antitoxins, and that consumption was lessening "probably due to sanitary precaution," not because of so-called "preventive medicine." He chose not to acknowledge sanitary precautions as a component of preventive medicine, even though homeopaths were champions of good hygiene, and, in fact, of "preventive medicine." What Copeland preferred to stress now was that the AMA seemed determined to get the public to reject any medications, especially homeopathic remedies, that could possibly cure "that part of what cannot be prevented."

Although Copeland continued to advocate careful use of the vaccines that existed, he, like W. A. Dewey, never lost sight of his faith that certain remedies could be just as helpful. For years, homeopathic remedies had been used as much for protection as for cure. *Cuprum metallicum,* or Cuprum, from copper, was often used to prevent cholera. Chelidonium (New Jersey tea or red root) was used to ward off hepatitis. Pertussin, made of diluted secretions of whooping cough, was used to prevent that disease. Pulsatilla was used for measles prevention in addition to its other applications for eye and digestive problems. Copeland frequently spoke about the recorded provings of Potassium Chloride, or *Kali mur.,* in some cases of diphtheria. *Kali mur.* was a tissue salt often used to treat inflammations of the mucous membranes. He told an audience about one instance: "Fully developed case of diphtheria with the characteristic glandular enlargement, tonsils, uvula, and entire soft palate were covered with a thick, diphtheritic exudation. Deglutition [swallowing] was attended with great pain and accompanied with the utmost effort, and there was exceeding prostration. *Kali mur.* 6X [diluted to the millionth degree] every two hours. The following day, there was marked improvement, and in four days every vestige of the throat trouble had disappeared, and the child recovered rapidly." Still, as if he were not so convinced anymore, he repeated over and over that verification of a single symptom or group of symptoms is one thing, and the ability of homeopathy to cure a given disease is quite another thing. Homeopathy's value "in a given pathological condition" needs to be established by "a cloud of witnesses," he now said.

He began to cite statistics in his speeches, telling one audience that even though such numbers were not always reliable, there seemed to be "no other way of presenting the truthfulness of the superiority of homeopathy." He said that "the cities of Baltimore, Cincinnati, Brooklyn, Detroit, St. Paul, Providence, Denver, Indianapolis, Syracuse, Rochester, Nashville, and Seattle are selected as fairly representing every variety of climate and every phase of therapeutic practice." He said that in 1910 the standard doctors in those cities had "a death rate in measles of 3% and the homeopathic profession lost 0.8%. The mortality rate in scarlet fever was 9.24% for the dominant school and 5.66% for the homeopathic. The typhoid fever mortality was high for both schools," he allowed—22.56% for the standard doctors and 15.15% for the homeopaths. He said that "not only is the death rate very much reduced by homeopathic prescribing, but also the average duration of the disease is shortened." Quoting from an editorial in a homeopathic journal, he said "they who have not tried Homeopathy have not tried to get well." At the same time, the doctor who as a student once observed that homeopathy was "as fixed as the law of gravitation" now confessed, "Personally, I am willing to admit that the theory of similars is not so well founded and certainly is not so demonstrable as is the law of gravitation." And, he added,

"While it may never be beyond the possibility of caviling doubt, yet it offers a reasonable, sensible, convincing, and satisfactory explanation of all therapeutic procedure."

Although his vacillations often confused his fellow homeopaths, as well as his patients, he understood that the times seemed to require clinical experiments, as questionable as they might be. But also he wondered if homeopathic provings could somehow become more up-to-date, something he had thought about since 1901. He had a new idea. He now asked that every member of the AIH "write each month his personal experience with a single remedy in the attempted cure of a patient." He said that "the best we can hope for is the accumulation of enough evidence to convince the individual mind that the proof is sufficient." Short of what he called "unreliable" clinical tests, he reiterated what he had once lectured the class of 1901 at the University of Michigan: "There must be a re-proving of remedies under the direction of expert diagnosticians, expert chemists and expert pathologists." The time was never better for this. The year 1913 saw the development of the Geiger counter, which detected alpha rays, and saw the genesis of the theory of stellar evolution. Coal dust was converted into oil for the first time. The concept of a chemical chain reaction was formulated. Jet propulsion was explained. It was time that the scientific basis of homeopathy was confirmed.

Meanwhile, the AIH now decided the best approach regarding the research question was an aggressive one. This was a surprising tactic for the homeopaths. During the winter of 1913, the AIH directed a request for "a joint investigation of its scientific proposition" to none other than the AMA. The AMA responded positively, and sent this proposal to two laboratories that had been suggested by the AIH: the Rockefeller Institute of New York and the McCormick Institute of Chicago. In June, the AMA reported to its members that "no favorable replies had been received," but it didn't write the AIH about this development until the following year. The AMA then asked the AIH "to suggest other laboratories or some practical plan for investigation." But nothing further was done by either organization at the time. The matter was dropped.

COPELAND now realized that he had better apply his deep faith in education to his own school, and he started to see, as he put it, "the necessity of drilling into the student mind every possible grain of homeopathic materia medica." Even though he would always believe that the best of allopathic medicine assisted homeopathic diagnosis, he wondered if perhaps too much emphasis was being placed on such laboratory advances. Growing evidence in some circles of "hurried prescribing, lax methods, and thoughtlessness" in prescribing protocols had been discussed among leading homeopaths. This "carelessness," Copeland had told his closest associates, was a serious matter for homeopathic educators.

In a typically unconventional speech that he gave before his peers in the fall of 1913, he first announced that his views were "purely personal," and "so far as the New York College is concerned, absolutely unofficial." He said this less because he was afraid to assert his position, and more because he said he didn't want to undermine "the able head of the Materia Medica Department and his associate experts." He then laid out a new curriculum plan that, he said, "appeals to me." It was a four-year plan that highlighted the study of remedies and focused somewhat less on anatomy and pathology.

He said that freshmen should be given "a plain, non-technical explanation of homeopathy" by a teacher with "magnetism" and "enthusiasm." No attempt should be made to use "exhaustive arguments." Afterward, he said, the students' questions should be answered so that "every academic doubt is dispelled." In fact, he added, "as in the German Methodist Camp Meeting system, I would keep at it til the last sinner is converted." But, he said, the freshman should not be overwhelmed, and therefore should study only fifteen remedies the first year.

First on his list was Belladonna, his most frequently prescribed remedy. He also recommended Bromum, made from bromine, a liquid chemical found in sodium, magnesium, potassium, and silver, and which was used for asthma; as well as Cactus, made from the desert plant, used among other things for chest pain; and Cimicifuga, made from the plant of the same name and used to treat headaches or menstrual pain. Copeland also suggested Chamomilla, made from the plant of the same name, used to treat asthma and insomnia; Cuprum, made from copper and used among other things for cramps and breathing problems; Gelsemium, made from jasmine and used to treat headaches, nerves, and fever (he had first learned of this remedy from Dr. Chase); Helleborus, made from a plant also called Bear's Foot, used to treat indigestion and diarrhea; Ignatia, made from the seeds of the ignatia amara tree and used to treat emotional distress; Ipecacuanha, made from the roots of a shrub by that name and used to treat nausea; Lachesis;

Mecurius corrosivus; and his other favorite, Nux Vomica. The final two remedies he proposed were Pulsatilla and *Rhus tox.,* also among his preferred remedies.

Copeland said that he thought students shouldn't attempt their own provings until halfway through the first year. He said, in his distinctive way, that the first year was "too early to give the fruit of the Materia Medica—it is the time to consider the root, merely." During the second year, when thirty more remedies (not named) should be taught, the student would be in a better position "to understand the effects of drugs." He recommended that prescription writing and dosage also be taught at that time, and that the students learn to recognize plants and understand the preparation of homeopathic tinctures. It was critical, he said, that sophomores also learn about "chemical poisons" through experiments on animals performed "in a humane and proper manner." (The following year, the first successful heart surgery would be performed on a dog by a standard doctor from the Rockefeller Institute.)

The new curriculum differed from the usual one in its focus, refinement, and specificity. Copeland had figured out that the cure of disease should not be taught until the junior, or third, year. He felt that the first two years should give the students the fundamentals, and that only after learning these would they be ready for "the turning point": healing disease. He also believed in memorizing, and now wanted all his students to know by heart every aspect of the remedies they studied in their first two years. He said that even if the students never added anything else to the list, he still thought they'd be more successful in their careers "than the most brilliant old school graduate." He said that the senior year must weave together all the elements from the previous three years, and be positive, practical, and useful. If all these guidelines were strictly followed, homeopathic educators would stop weeping "over the degeneracy of the profession." Despite the seriousness of his message, he decided to have a little fun, although some of those listening to him weren't sure at first if he was serious or just "being fanciful," as one doctor asked. What had Copeland said? He made reference to "a 4-hour course on The Psychology of The Soul Of Birds."

DURING the winter of 1913, Copeland was asked by a leading homeopathic medical journal, *Medical Times,* whether or not he was in favor of adding a fifth year to the medical-school program. He answered that he was now in favor of such an extension, provided that it was "devoted to hospital work." Hinsdale, the dean of the Homeopathic Medical School of the University of Michigan had explained in a paper that it was, in fact, a homeopath at Boston University who first advocated this fifth year. Copeland concluded that such a plan would not only benefit students, but improve hospitals as well. In fact, he also favored more hospital inspections, and thought with medical students present such inspections might be even more detailed than they already were, and result in better-equipped hospitals.

But regarding medical-school inspection, the AMA's Council on Medical Education didn't have good news for Copeland's school. Three years after its 1911 inspection, it said that New York Homeopathic was no longer a Class A school. Before its November 5, 1914, inspection even began, the AMA's representative said that a Class B rating was warranted on the grounds that Copeland had told the inspector that courses in physics, chemistry, and biology were not going to be required and that high-school courses in those subjects would be acceptable for admission. Copeland didn't still think that a separate "pre-medical year" should be required, even though he had agreed to go along with it in certain cases. Earlier in 1914, the AMA had ruled that in order for a medical school to have a Class A rating, new students must first have a year of college work. Copeland had always opposed this standard. In any case, the AMA said there were other reasons for the B rating at New York Homeopathic College, and some seemed inexplicable considering Copeland's public stance on them. For instance, the AMA faulted the college for no longer using Flower's outpatient department for the teaching of medical students. (Flower, of course, had been created to complement the college, and students not only used it, but also three other local hospitals. But the AMA believed there was little or no teaching going on.) The AMA also criticized the college for not giving juniors and seniors sufficient clinical training and said they attended too many lectures. Additionally, the AMA didn't approve of the college giving advanced standing to students who had taken courses in osteopathic colleges. (Copeland later said that only one such student existed.) It still faulted the college for not having "a serviceable medical library, not having a modern course in pharmacology, and for not having full-time salaried professors in charge of the laboratories." Things just weren't good enough over at New York Homeopathic, the AMA now said.

Copeland appeared to be all over the map, constantly rearranging his thoughts and, for the first time in his career, somehow floundering. In addition to everything else, he knew that he had to oversee his staff more strictly. He was forty-six years old; his wavy, cinnamon-colored hair was now slightly graying; and he had been the dean at New York Homeopathic for six years. He was not used to so many apparent missteps, although of the nine homeopathic colleges still remaining, his still had the highest enrollment. But, he said, "our college is Class A everywhere except on Dearborn Street, Chicago," the home of the AMA.

ON APRIL 28, 1914, with fighting in Mexico and U.S. troops holding the seaport of Vera Cruz, Copeland wrote his parents, "I do hope the war will terminate speedily. We do not want to fight I am sure." He also wrote them about the state of his health, saying that he had had "an attack of tonsillitis," which he treated with Belladonna, and later with *Hepar sulf.,* made from calcium sulfide. (In the eighteenth century, Samuel Hahnemann had used this remedy to ease the side effects of mercury treatments.)

When World War I erupted in August of that year, 7 million Americans were under the care of homeopathic doctors. There were what Copeland characterized as sixty "strictly-speaking" homeopathic hospitals around the country. Despite the failing health of homeopathic colleges, in all other realms homeopathy was still vigorous; "it is influential and popular," Copeland said.

He pointed out in a speech that "The American College of Surgeons, The American Medical Jurisprudence Society, the law courts, governmental administrative offices, civil service boards, medical commissions everywhere, receive the homeopathic graduates on equal terms with other doctors." He himself had recently been accepted as a Fellow of the American College of Surgeons, which had been founded in 1913 to help keep surgical skills on the highest possible level.

In another speech before his peers, Copeland mentioned what was now a sad fact for him. He wanted, of course, equality, but he didn't want to be absorbed by the old school. Not at any cost. So it was with dismay that he pointed out "there are today more homeopathic graduates in the AMA than in the AIH." He told his audience also that "last month, after full consideration of all it meant, and in spite of every protest, I saw a number of homeopathic graduates move over in a body to the Old School. . . . We have bravely held our own and now are losing at the edges."

The AIH decided it was time to form its own Council on Medical Education, and it would take two years to develop its College Alliance. Homeopaths wanted to take charge of deciding what could or should be the same and what could or should be different in medical education. The AMA had its way of governing, and the AIH would show that it had its way, too. Coincidentally, the College Alliance was launched in Chicago at the exact time that the AMA held its college meetings. Copeland became the alliance's first president, and despite his diplomatic ways, the organization decided to break all relations with the AMA. "The homeopathic college ought to depend upon the homeopathic profession," Copeland now said; "in the last analysis the cause of homeopathy can rise no higher than the loyalty of its practitioners." Privately, he said that he was fed up having "to humiliate his college by crawling on his belly before the AMA." That organization would no longer tell homeopaths what they could or could not do. There would be no more inspections or classifications by the AMA. That era was now over.

In 1914, the AMA, which had 74,235 members out of a total physician population of 143,586 (the AIH had nearly 10,000 members, but by 1917 the number would be down to 3,000), set some guidelines for hospital internship programs. It also established a Propaganda Department, "to gather and disseminate information on frauds in medicine." The AMA continued to vigorously monitor outrageous nostrums, patent medicines, and electrical and other devices. It continued also to watch for false labeling and false statements on both foods and drugs. It encouraged stronger enforcement of the 1906 Federal Pure Food and Drug Act, and hoped that in time a way could be found to stop dishonest manufacturers altogether. "Many people look with suspicion at the motive of the medical profession when they strive to eradicate an evil," a doctor wryly observed in a standard medical journal. The AMA also considered ways to use popular mainstream publications to get out the message about false labeling and false statements. In 1913, it asked *Good Housekeeping* magazine for an exchange agreement—the AMA's journal would encourage doctors to keep *Good Housekeeping* in their waiting rooms, if *Good Housekeeping* would encourage its readers to read the AMA's articles on nostrums and quackery. Since 1912, Dr. Harvey Wiley, the former chief government chemist, had headed the magazine's laboratories, creating

"The Good Housekeeping Seal of Approval." The magazine vetoed an out-and-out "exchange," but did offer a low advertising rate to the AMA, and said that ads in its magazine would encourage readers to buy the AMA's book on nostrums and quackery.

In 1911, the Supreme Court had ruled that the 1906 Food and Drug Act did not prohibit false therapeutic claims, only false and misleading statements about the ingredients in a food or drug. The following year, a congressional amendment to nullify that ruling was enacted, and this outlawed labeling medicines or foods with deceitful therapeutic claims. In June of 1914, when a doctor complained to the AMA that a New York company was claiming that their Mt. Clemens Mineral Water—their "foreign water," he called it in his letter—could dissolve kidney stones, the AMA wrote the doctor that it had never questioned the "value" of the water, only the exploitive features of its advertising. The AMA treaded waters guardedly for the time being; several years later it would not act quite so gingerly.

Meanwhile, Copeland would talk about water and say in speeches that the bottler of waters was "just as important to human comfort and welfare as the food purveyor and the pharmacist." He, too, like the AMA, would also gradually begin to speak out forcefully against quackery, saying it "has thriven in some quarters as never before in the history of medicine." Homeopaths had to join the battle against it, although he didn't think many would want to.

The AMA continued to be concerned about naturopathy. Its Propaganda Department earmarked an October 8, 1914, newspaper story headlined LIKE MIRACLES OF THE BIBLE that said naturopaths had "the surest, quickest, and most reliable means of cure ever offered a long suffering public" and that people on the brink of death were being brought back to life "by modern natural methods of healing." The AMA emphasized that naturopaths were not properly trained and that most schools had "a short school day and an evident carelessness regarding attendance." Their clinics, the AMA said, "are even less adequate than those of the chiropractic schools." Their schools had no labs for physics, physiology, anatomy, bacteriology, or pathology. They had no hospital affiliation. They were simply "fakers," who tried to enter medicine "by the back door." The organization said that one naturopath defended his beliefs by saying, "What we advocate is air, light, sun, water, proper food, and the right mental attitude. That's all anybody needs."

In 1913, another congressional amendment had required that food packages be "plainly and conspicuously marked on the outside of the package in terms of weight, measure, or numerical count." In 1914, the Supreme Court issued its first ruling on food additives. It was very tame because products with certain additives such as nitrate were still allowed on the market, but the government was now obliged to show the harm done by them. That year, the Harrison Narcotic Act required that drugs containing narcotics must be prescribed by a doctor. Slowly but decidedly, bad foods and bad medicines were getting the boot. The AIH still didn't heed Copeland's call to get involved in combating quackery, and the following year, once again, homeopathy became a target of the AMA.

During the winter of 1915—the year that Einstein's general theory of relativity was announced, the first transcontinental phone call between Alexander Graham Bell and Thomas Watson was made, the bacteria causing dysentery was isolated, and aspirin was put on the market in easy-to-take tablet form—George Starr White, a California homeopath who was a member of both the AIH and the AMA, read a paper called "Magnetic Meridian in Diagnosis and Therapeutics" before his local homeopathic medical society. The paper, which he told Copeland in a letter was "the culmination of a life's work," described a new way of diagnosing and treating illness using special magnets and colors, plus oxygen and sometimes water. A process called "air-column percussion," which used a vibrating column of air "to outline and locate any organ of the body," was also part of White's method. He told Copeland that in the past year alone he had "diagnosed over a thousand cases and not one diagnosis has been found wrong when checked up by every known laboratory method." He went on to report that by his method he can "diagnose tuberculosis as early as its very inception, and the patient can be treated by the indicated color and oxygen vapor inhalations, along with magnetic meridian adjuncts." He also said that he could "detect gonorrhea in a patient even if they contracted the disease fifty years ago . . . the same is true of syphilis, cancer and other diseases." (Hahnemann wrote about the use of mineral magnets in the sixth edition of his *Organon of the Medical Art*, published in 1842, saying that they can "act as powerfully and as homeopathically on our life principle as actual so-called medicines." Nonetheless, Hahnemann remained apprehensive about using anything other than "the positive actions" of the north and south poles of magnets, and said their electrical energy was "little proven.")

During a clinical demonstration he was giving in Chicago, Dr. White was arrested by the State Board of Health of Illinois for practicing medicine without a license. The AMA, which had known about White's work and considered it unscientific and of no clinical value, praised the arrest, which was based on a technicality, because White was actually only demonstrating his technique and not "practicing" it, as the authorities charged. White was fined, forced to cut short his nationwide speaking engagements and return to California. The following year, the Los Angeles County branch of the AMA charged him with teaching and practicing sectarian medicine. He was also charged with being unethical for publicly disclosing his membership in the AMA, i.e., causing embarrassment to the AMA. The organization was concerned about other so-called diagnostic devices, like an "electro-cranial" machine and a metal cylinder that was plunged into water at the same moment electrodes were connected to the body.

White began a letter-writing campaign to enlist the support of leading homeopaths to prove that his teachings, as well as those of eclectics, were not sectarian, but rather "a specialty in drug therapy." He disclosed also that the AMA had told him it would "allow" him to remain a member if he resigned from the AIH. But, he told Copeland and others, "I would never give up an old friend for a new one, and neither would I resign from any association of good standing to meet the whims of another association." As for that other association—by which he meant the AMA (which had recently denounced aspirin again, saying now that it "produces a mental condition similar to that found in the morphine habit")—White said that "I am not the first nor the last one whom they will attack . . . [and] try to muzzle and impede honest, independent medical progress."

In 1915, the AMA's Propaganda Department fought hard against what it considered the cruelest, most heartless form of medical fraud: cancer cures. It said that ordinary olive oil was most often the "cure" offered by quacks, and wrote that "it seems to be a recognized rule of quacks and nostrum manufacturers that the more hopeless the disease the more worthless and the more expensive should be the treatment." A patent medicine called "Enzymol, made from 'animal gastric juices,'" was promoted as a cure, as was a medicine later shown to contain only what the AMA called "bowel washings."

The AMA was particularly incensed by one doctor it had been following since 1909, who was "still loose," it said, and "depraved and dirty" for exploiting cancer victims. He claimed to have a remedy that he advertised as "a most wonderful, strange, but fortunate combination of several medicines, easily obtained at any large drug store." Many times over the years, this doctor had been indicted for fraud, and federal authorities had stopped his mailings, but after being fined, he would resume his business under another name. He was always able to avoid prison. The doctor in question, S. R. Chamley, of Los Angeles, was a homeopath, which further infuriated the AMA.

Hahnemann believed that cancer was caused by the psora (part of the hidden miasm) and was an itch that was the consequence of a negative spirit. Most homeopaths believed that finding the right remedy to restore the body's balance in a disease such as cancer was very difficult but not impossible. Although Copeland, who maintained "the deadly cancer 'germ' can not enter healthy tissue," didn't know of a true homeopathic cure for cancer, he had often lectured that one was possible. He talked about certain cancers disappearing "after a single dose of Phytolacca in an appropriate dilution." *Phytolacca decandra,* or pokeweed, is an herb that had been used for centuries for glandular problems, and its root was often used as a stimulant for the heart as well as to treat breast tumors. In 1911, a doctor at the Rockefeller Institute in New York, a graduate of Johns Hopkins, had circulated a controversial report saying that certain cancers were caused by a virus. Both allopaths and homeopaths were dubious, but also intrigued, as they also were the following year when a French doctor said he had been able to grow a microbe of cancer—a discovery, he said, that could eventually lead to a vaccine for the disease.

The naturopaths believed that cancer could be cured "by natural processes without medicine or surgery." An associate of Copeland's once asked him to save and send to him all the soiled bandages used on cancer patients at Flower, because he wanted to prove that cancer was caused by an excess of certain minerals in the body—phosphorus, chlorine, and nitrogen. Later, Copeland began to think that "long continued irritations," like corns and calluses, "may be a factor in the development of cancer."

ON FEBRUARY 12, 1915, the United States Public Health Service distributed a booklet entitled *The Limitations to Self-Medication: Uses and Abuses of Proprietary Preparations and Household Remedies.* Although it was basically meant to deter the use of unscrupulous patent products, its definition of a "remedy" included homeopathic ones, which the U.S. government was now for the first time acknowledging as fraudulent. The booklet was widely circulated by both the Public Health Service and the AMA. Standard doctors (especially those who were still angry that homeopathic remedies were getting such a big share of the market) hoped that by closing ranks with a government agency they were closer than ever to what could be homeopathy's last gasp.

In 1914, members of the Homeopathic Medical Society of New York had heard a talk by Dr. Charles Duncan on a form of self-medication that made the AMA breathe fire. This was called "autotherapy," and it was being used, Duncan said, "by many physicians of high standing all over the country, some holding distinguished positions in colleges and hospitals." It was a treatment that used the body's own fluids to deal with obstinate problems not helped by established homeopathic remedies. A properly diluted specimen of the patient's urine was said to initiate a correction of the body's chemical balance, as was a drop of diluted blood, pus, spit, tears, or ear discharge. Autotherapy was thought to aid the body's immune system, and even to be a way to eventually eradicate cancer.

The New York homeopaths said it posed no more danger to people than vaccines, and recommended its use in general practice, even though it could—and would—be misunderstood by some people. After all, Duncan said, "many of our best therapeutic measures were at first misunderstood, denounced, and won recognition slowly." Autotherapy's basic principle, the minute dose, "is the beacon-light today of experimental and preventive medicine," he lectured. Patients were reported to have recovered from acute appendicitis, bronchitis, and even compound fractures. In one autotherapy case, a patient had been cured "of a persistently recurring ivy poisoning by drinking the milk of a cow that had been fed poison ivy." There was evidence also of autotherapy's positive effects in veterinary medicine, curing infections in horses and dogs.

Copeland's attitude toward this treatment was not wildly enthusiastic. He remarked simply that "theoretically, the principle is sound and the evidence presented shows that, in many cases, the practice is successful." In a report to his state society, he and some other leaders commented that the treatment needs "further elaboration and precision in the size of the dose and the interval between doses," and noted that it was good that it seemed "free from the taint of quackery and charlatanism." This was not exactly a red-letter endorsement. Indeed, a year later when Copeland received a letter from Duncan asking for a letter on his behalf for a Nobel Prize, Copeland wrote a colleague that "Duncan's effort to obtain this distinction seems to me to be absurd; at the same time, of course, I would gladly assist any homeopathic brother in any of his laudable undertakings."

But he did not write a letter.

In 1916, with war still raging in Europe, Americans tried to console themselves—work themselves up, really—with the jazz that was sweeping the nation. The 101,208,315 citizens in the country needed to brace themselves for more than world war: On January 24, the Supreme Court had ruled the income tax constitutional. People would have to pay up.

During the summer months of 1916, a polio epidemic had torn through New York City, as well as many other large cities, although New York was hit the hardest, with over 8,900 cases and 2,400 deaths. Polio affected primarily children. The viral disease had no cure, and no one could figure out how it was transmitted. (The virus itself had been identified eight years earlier, in 1908.) Lack of sanitation was blamed, rats and other rodents were blamed, stray cats and dogs were blamed, milk was blamed, sugar was blamed, water was blamed, and new immigrants were blamed. Copeland said polio was "a low power" infection, adding that "how it travels is uncertain," although he was sure it was "not from personal contact." New York hospitals were overwhelmed with sick, paralyzed, and dying patients. Flower opened a small polio ward and admitted and treated 40 cases, later reporting that it had seen 24 complete recoveries, 10 partial recoveries, and only 6 deaths. (The following year, an inspection found the polio ward "in no fit condition to receive any patients.")

The epidemic, which lasted for six months, was partially controlled through isolation and quarantine. Some vaccines were tried, but all failed. One homeopathic remedy was widely used, *Lathyrus sativus,* an herb also known by the names chickpea and grass pea. The usual dose was 30C. Many immigrants also wore camphor (used homeopathically in cholera) around their necks as a preventive and a cure.

The stress of dealing with the epidemic, in addition to his own recent poor health, and that of his wife, who had been sickly since the stillborn death of a daughter, Alice, led Copeland to resign once more as dean of the college. He was especially peeved at the controversy that had erupted after he had tried to find a university affiliation for the college. He believed now that such a partnership could help the school get a Class A rating. But foes of such a plan accused Copeland of "underground diplomacy" and trying to be "the one-man power," and an affiliation never happened. He no longer felt that he could lead both the school and the hospital. He wrote an associate that "Mrs. Copeland is quite ill, but is getting along as well as we could expect. Personally, I have had an acute empyema of the antrum [probably an ulcer] and have had an uncomfortable time."

As unwell as he was (he mentioned to a friend that he also had what he called "an infected face," most likely impetigo or eczema), it didn't stop him from writing an angry letter to the Postal-Cable Telegraph Company for failing to send the full text of the message he had sent his parents in Dexter about the baby's death. "I consider this a heartbreaking and outrageous violation of taste, good ethics, and good business," Copeland lashed out.

In time, as the couple's health improved, and Copeland simmered down, the trustees of Flower convinced him, as they had done earlier, that they needed him to do both jobs and that he could do both jobs. He rescinded his resignation.

He was also yearning secretly not for a respite from the challenges he was facing, but rather for a new adventure. Solace through work always helped him. His father-in-law had once told him that "a change of work is rest."

NINE

"But One of Many Methods
of Treating Sickness"

Shortly after America entered World War I in April 1917, Copeland found something more he could do; he decided to try to create an army base hospital and serve in Europe. At first, the director general of military relief was reluctant to give Flower Hospital permission even to draft a hospital unit because of misgivings about homeopathy, but finally he was persuaded by a group of AIH officials, and as Copeland later elaborated, "homeopathy had its chance and rose nobly to its privileges and opportunity." Hospital Unit "N" was born. It later became United States General Hospital No. 5 at Fort Ontario, New York.

The faculty of New York Homeopathic College decided it couldn't part with Copeland as its dean, especially so soon after getting him to stay, and voted to ask another doctor to head the unit. Copeland accepted his fate with great disappointment, although Frances of course was glad to have him stay on the home front. In the end, more than 1,900 homeopathic doctors were commissioned in the army and navy during the war.

Although he was upset not to lead the first homeopathic medical unit given all it represented to him, and others, as confirmation of the value of homeopathy from at least one arm of the government, he carried on with his practice, his school—"the sanctuary of his faith"—and his hospital. He helped console himself by renewing his commitment to his responsibilities, even introducing the idea to his colleagues that all

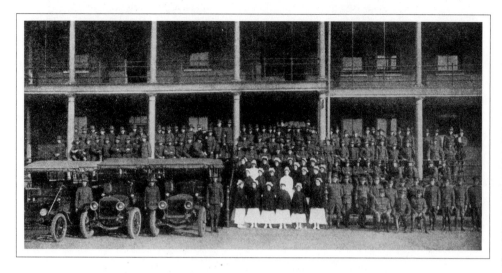

Hospital Unit "N," October 1917

homeopathic colleges have "a Rally Day, or Pentecost, or Hahnemann Day"—he didn't care what it was named—to celebrate their "mines of riches" and "the advanced work of their laboratories."

At the same time, he decided to explore another medical path, one he had never actually taken but which had interested him ever since it came on the scene in 1896: naturopathy. He was particularly interested in the achievements of his fellow Michiganites, the Kellogg brothers of Battle Creek. For over a decade, according to a brochure he kept in his college office, their "sanitarium system," which had "more than one hundred offshoots . . . in different parts of the world," treated "chronic invalids" with special diets, disciplined hygiene, and exercise. John Harvey Kellogg, MD, one of three brothers, was the staff physician. As Copeland himself explained in a speech he gave in 1910, "Kellogg considers disease only in relation to metabolism, and, standing in the high place of liberal medicine, broad and unsectarian, proclaims to all the world that the vegetable diet is the one and only cure for suffering humanity!" Americans had heard of the benefits of specials foods since the 1830s, when Sylvester Graham (he originated the cracker named after him, as well as granola and cold breakfast cereal) lectured about eating too many spicy foods and drinking too much whiskey and coffee. Like Kellogg, Graham advocated a vegetarian diet. He believed that the only worthwhile drink was cold water.

Kellogg also used hydropathy (water treatments), electropathy, radium (radioactive cures), and mechanotherapy, which involved the use of a vibrating chair. He was obsessed with the bowels, and maintained that 90 percent of disease started in the stomach and/or the bowels. His patients often used his special bowel machine, which could pump as much as 15 gallons of water through their systems. One of the uses of the intensely vibrating chair was to activate the bowels, but it was also meant to cure headaches—when it was not bringing them on with its painful agitation.

Copeland, who said that "physicians are all agreed that constipation and fermentation in the colon and lower bowel are largely responsible for loss of efficiency, for discomfort and lowered vitality," wrote to Kellogg that he and his wife were interested in visiting his sanitarium overnight when he was in Chicago on business, even though Battle Creek was a 167-mile train ride from Chicago. As Copeland told Kellogg, a number of his New York patients had stayed at Battle Creek and were "enthusiastic." Dr. and Mrs. Copeland wanted to see things for themselves. Copeland said that he was told that every patient admitted to the Battle Creek Sanitarium—"The San," it was called—"has a most careful examination, blood count, chemical analyses of the excretions and secretions." Like homeopathy, naturopathy was not loath to benefit occasionally from scientific advances, an aspect that appealed to him, and unlike most naturopaths, Kellogg had a medical degree.

As well as wanting to observe the health program, Copeland was intrigued with the entrepreneurial aspect of Kellogg's venture. Alongside the doctor, surgeon, dean, lecturer, and politician was a businessman longing to try his wings.

The AMA had been concerned about Dr. J. H. Kellogg's brash salesman brother, Frank J., ever since 1909, fifteen years after another brother, William Keith, or Will, had created corn flakes. The AMA was troubled by Frank's products—Kellogg's Safe Fat Reducer; Sanitone Wafers, "The Greatest Nerve Vitalizer Known"; Kellogg's Brown Tablets, for bladder weakness; and Kelloids—and said they were fakes. The AMA reported that "advertisements in newspapers and magazines bring to Kellogg the necessary mailing list; follow-up letter and advertising circulars do the rest," adding that " 'Kellogg's Safe Fat Reducer' used to be known as 'Kellogg's Obesity Food.' It is not a food and never was, hence when the Food and Drug Act went into effect and falsifying became illegal as well as immoral, the name was changed." The AMA disclosed that a government laboratory showed that the preparation contained toasted bread, poke root, and thyroid gland. Poke root was a laxative. The AMA concluded: "that the prolonged administration of thyroid gland will sometimes bring about a marked reduction in weight is true but its use even under skilled medical supervision is fraught with danger. It is little less than criminal that ignorant quacks of Kellogg's type should be permitted to distribute indiscriminately drugs that have the potency for harm that is possessed by the thyroid preparations." In fact, overdosing on thyroid could induce a heart attack or stroke. The AMA also criticized C. W. Post, one of Kellogg's former patients, when he invented his own versions of some of Kellogg's foods. Post concocted Postum as a cure for coffee neuralgia, and Grape-Nuts as a corrective for appendicitis, malaria, and tuberculosis.

Copeland learned a great deal from his visit to the Kellogg sanitarium, although the powerful bowel machine didn't appeal to him. But he soon began talking about another procedure he had read about called an "internal bath," in which "water passed through a short tube, just long enough to reach the free space of the rectum, will find its way by its natural flow into every part and crevice of the bowel." This procedure, Copeland believed, "avoids the bearing-down sensation which follows rapid injection," adding that "modern life and eating tend to intestinal stasis. This is a misfortune and every effort should be made to correct, as far as possible, by example and education, every evil effect of civilization. . . . The evil effects coming from the absorption of the poisons developed by intestinal putrefaction are not limited to physical symptoms. There may be the most profound effects upon the nervous system and even upon the brain." Indeed, he mentioned that some doctors in Trenton, New Jersey, had found "the absorption from an infected colon is the chief cause for functional insanity." Copeland stressed that "had the colon been kept clean, there could never have arisen a pathological condition sufficient to undermine the mind itself."

The AMA kept up its watch on naturopathy in general, saying the practice, "in common with all the cults, consists in treating all its victims by the same method, without bothering to diagnosticate the cases." It continued, "The 'naturopath,' like others of similar ilk, realizes the value of the psychic element and will administer treatment in the shape of unusual diets or unaccustomed exposures, such as cold enema or dips, or the application of heat, or some other so-called natural method of treatment. If the victim happens to improve, either because of, or in spite of, the treatment, he (the victim) tells everyone about the marvelous treatment and the wonderful results. If, on the other hand, the victim is either not benefited or made worse, he tells no one about his foolishness in having trusted a charlatan."

The AMA's Council on Medical Education had nothing but contempt for what it referred to as the "imposters" who ran schools for naturopaths, even some "nondescript Doctors of Medicine" who said they had attended reputable colleges. The AMA found that naturopathic schools had "a fly-by-night character," with vague entrance requirements that allowed almost anyone to enroll. Most students were told that when they finished their course work they would "get a beautiful diploma but not a degree." The schools were faulted for not having a single "scientific apparatus for the clinical diagnosis of a variety of common illnesses." Licenses were practically nonexistent, except for a very few naturopaths who had graduated from medical schools and held MDs. The AMA reported that many naturopaths bought bogus diplomas and licenses, and were told in a brochure that "there are many ways in which you can practice drugless methods without a license. One of them is to work under the supervision or direction of a medical physician. Or you can work in a sanitarium or institution." They were encouraged to call themselves "health builders," or "health specialists," because there was no law preventing such titles.

THERE WERE only six homeopathic colleges remaining in 1918. New York Homeopathic was one of them, thanks to Copeland's continued leadership. Across the country, there were a mere 580 homeopathic students in schools in New York, Philadelphia, Boston, Chicago, Columbus, and Ann Arbor. (There were 12,925 standard medical students in the United States.) Most new students decided to follow the John Hopkins model, and if they decided to use homeopathy at all, to learn about it later. And most also later joined the AMA, not the AIH. The AMA's Council on Medical Education now required two years of college prior to entrance, a guideline that only a few homeopathic schools followed.

The AIH's own Council on Medical Education inspected the six homeopathic schools and gave certain distinctions to several: Philadelphia and Boston had the best-equipped hospital facilities; Philadelphia's Hahnemann excelled in "the character of the curriculum," as well as in its outpatient department, library, and "all around equipment." Columbus, Ohio, had the best pharmacology and homeopathic work. Michigan's lab received high praise. New York Homeopathic was not cited for any special recognition, although it was noted that it charged the highest tuition for four years' training—$955.00. (The other schools ranged from $438 for resident students at the University of Michigan to $812 for students at Hahnemann in Philadelphia.)

The small number of students enrolled in the homeopathic colleges, where medical education was still basically the same as it was in standard schools (except for admission requirements), generally didn't even call themselves homeopaths after graduation. The AMA considered this circumstance as nature taking its course, the phasing out of homeopathy so there could be that "one science of medicine" it had wanted for years. (By 1919, most states had only one medical board, with only six states continuing to have separate homeopathic ones.)

Yet homeopathy was still popular in the nation. The health departments of many corporations were entirely homeopathic: the General Motors Company, Montgomery Ward (which sold patent medicines, much to the AMA's dismay), the General Electric Company, the National Cash Register Company. Copeland, highly visible around New York City and much in demand as a speaker, remarked to one audience that he had "no desire to be bitter or unkind," but he simply did not believe that "the diverse practices of the dominant school show a remarkable degree of scientific exactness." Only homeopathy did. "For a given set of symptoms, no matter where the homeopathic physician was educated, or where he may practice, be it in Maine or California, the Dominion of Canada or the British Isles, 'from Greenland's icy mountains, from India's Coral strand,' the remedy selected will be the same," he said.

But Copeland was getting fidgety again. He would soon celebrate his fiftieth birthday. "It isn't so bad to be fifty," he wrote in his Bible. "One no longer worries over many things—things by the way, that rarely happen. We are here to do the best we can and what matter whether one is thirty, or forty, or fifty! There is always strength for the task and for new tasks, too. To serve and for the privilege of serving—these are rewards for passing years. 'The Lord is the strength of my Life: of whom shall I be afraid?' "

Seven months before the formal end of the World War on November 11, 1918, a new task came to the dean (some colleagues whispered that he had petitioned for it). On April 29, 1918, he was appointed health com-

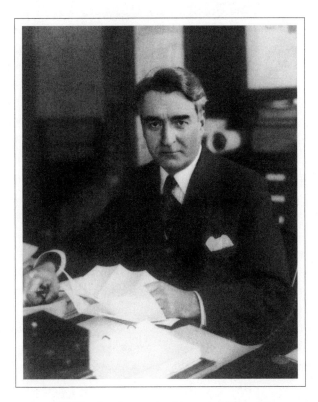

Copeland as the new health commissioner of
New York City, 1918

missioner of New York City, a job, he said, that had "almost unlimited power" and a budget of $7 million a year. Copeland immediately became a good Tammany Democrat as well. He later told a reporter of a chance meeting at dusk in New York City Hall Park with the current mayor, James J. "Jimmy" Hylan. The reporter wrote that "the Mayor shook his fist under the nose of the astonished physician, when Dr. Copeland had at first attempted to decline the mayor's request that he become health commissioner of the greatest city in the world. 'As Mayor of New York, I believe that I have the right to draft any man for any big service this city needs in wartime. You serve!' His Honor insisted—and Dr. Copeland did serve." Copeland, however he got his job and wherever the offer was made, had a new challenge that combined his love of medicine and his love of politics and history.

New York Homeopathic Medical College would finally have to do without him. He would seem to many people to be leaving homeopathy behind him, but he wasn't. Even though he would soon hardly ever say that he was a homeopath, he continued to keep Hahnemann close to his heart. But usually he now said, with the majority of homeopaths, that he was simply a physician. He was a doctor. He would still lecture to homeopathic groups, and would apply homeopathic principles in every area under his control, observing Hahnemann's dictate that some kinds of ill health are brought on by "prolonged deprivation of things that are necessary for life." Hahnemann also wrote in his *Organon* that certain diseases are caused by people who "suffer lack of exercise or open air," and "live in unhealthy places, especially marsh areas, reside only in cellars, damp workplaces or other confined quarters." Copeland followed these ideas as he took public charge of the health of New York City residents. He said that "a health commissioner who disregarded pest-infested and disease-breeding basements would not be worthy of the name."

At fifty, Copeland was, in many ways, exactly the homeopath he always wanted to be. He began to act as if medicine were a "unified profession." More and more he avowed that homeopathy was, as he wrote in *A Reference Handbook of the Medical Sciences,* "but one of many methods of treating sickness." It had its limitations. Copeland finally crystalized his belief—the belief of most moderates—that homeopathy was a specialty of medicine, just one method (a word he had used from the beginning of his career) of getting people well. This was his core belief when he stripped away the religious and historical rhetoric, when he pruned the flowery imagery, and stood alone before a mirror and saw a country doctor who believed in science and scholarship, with some political power thrown in.

Still, he never stopped believing that "the duration of diseases concerning which we have pretty accurate knowledge of their natural history, can be materially shortened and the suffering of the patient alleviated" by the use of homeopathic remedies. "Hahnemann," Commissioner Copeland wrote in an article, "placed homeopathy squarely on two facts or two classes of facts; on one side the facts of disease, the subjective and objective symptoms of the naturally diseased patient; on the other side, the facts of the remedy." He concluded, "These two classes of facts he made to serve for the premises of a scientific therapeutic application." Facts.

He started writing his farewell speech to his coworkers and students at New York Homeopathic on the back of an envelope while he was in transit from one place to another in his new job. Jotting ideas on scraps of paper while he was in cars, trolleys, and trains became a necessity. He also sent the same letter to different relatives, friends, and associates: "I have been so overwhelmed, first by the sudden call to assume this office, and then by the many burdens of its administration. . . . In the spirit of service and with the help of my friends, I will 'carry on,' 'doing my bit,' by trying to keep the city free from contagious, infectious and pestilential diseases."

And right at the beginning, he had to face a crisis: an outbreak of influenza. Little did he know at the time how momentous it would be. When the flu first began to appear in July, Copeland told New Yorkers and his staff of 4,000 employees that there was no real danger of an epidemic. He kept up his reassuring talk until the autumn, when it became clear that a disaster was most likely at hand, a disaster that would be worldwide. "Every great war has been followed by a marked increase in epidemic disease," he would later point out.

An attempt at making a vaccine faltered; it contained, according to Copeland, "the germs of the various types of pneumonia and the several forms of streptococci, as well as the influenza bacillus itself." He warned that "it must be frankly admitted that its use is largely experimental," and, in fact, when it was tested, it didn't seem to work at all.

He hired emergency workers to deal with the sick. He created a "Sanitary Squad," made up of sixty policemen, who, he said, "used the highest degree of detective knowledge" to protect New Yorkers. He put the buses and subways on a special schedule to reduce crowding, and thus contagion, and he also saw that the cars had proper ventilation. He knew that sick people traveled the subways but, he said, "you might as well try to cut off the main artery of the body as to close the subway." He forbade spitting on the floor, platforms, or sidewalks, and put up signs everywhere. He asked mothers to avoid getting chilled, and to stop wearing thin satin slippers outdoors. He recommended that they wear woolen understockings and said the practice would also help prevent arthritis. He said parents should avoid kissing their children. He advised isolating the sick person in a separate room, if possible. He urged restaurants to use paper cups instead of glasses.

He was pressured to close schools and theaters, but wouldn't. He thought children could be better monitored by teachers and nurses in the confines of schools, and said the schools were often less crowded than the tenements—and warmer. He also believed that biting winds contributed to the formation of deformed ankles. In 1916, a "set-back" law had been put into effect, making it a requirement that buildings be a certain height and include commensurate setbacks for light and air to get through. But quarters were still constricted because of multiple people—four, five, or even six—living in a single room. Copeland said that "any physician will tell you that the greatest disinfectant in the world is sunlight. . . . Our grandmothers knew the story when they used to put the bedding out on the line to sun."

Most people who didn't die from the flu waited out its symptoms with bed rest, sometimes sugar and turpentine, burned brown sugar, brandy or whiskey, quinine, digitalis, and aspirin—all prescribed by standard doctors. Copeland did not recommend whiskey in the prevention or treatment of the flu, although after the National Prohibition Act—the Volstead Act—was passed in 1920, he diplomatically "urged stores to keep whiskey in stock, exactly as they keep other drugs in stock," and asked the prohibition commissioner "to cut red tape, as far as may be possible, and to facilitate the efforts of such physicians as are in the habit of depending upon whiskey in the treatment of pneumonia." But during 1918 and 1919, at the height of the pandemic, as it became, he recommended that patients take castor oil as a laxative; take magnesium citrate to promote healthy bones, muscles, and nerves; soak their feet in hot mustard water; and drink hot lemonade. It was most important, he said, that patients "avoid patent medicines."

Many homeopaths used Gelsemium, Eupator (agueweed), and Bryonia to treat flu symptoms. In large doses, Gelsemium, the poisonous climbing plant, can cause paralysis, but used in minute doses it can help breathing and fever. Eupator was used by American Indians for malaria, and centuries before that for ulcers, dysentery, liver disease, and chronic fevers. Bryonia had remained one of Copeland's longtime favorite remedies for coughs and inflammation. New York Homeopathic Medical College issued a detailed four-page "Influenza Bulletin" that recommended more than forty other remedies, depending on the symptoms. On its list were such things as Aconite, the poisonous plant used for infections; Allium (red onion), used for discharges from the nose and eyes; Antimony Potassium Tartrate (*Antim. tart.*), to loosen phlegm; and Spongia, made from the sea sponge, for coughs, laryngitis, and heart disease.

Copeland himself, it was said, contracted the flu, and worked straight through it. Like many doctors, he didn't heed his own advice to rest. "I sat in my office for six weeks," he later told an audience; "I had only one meal in my house during that time. I watched the death rate go up and

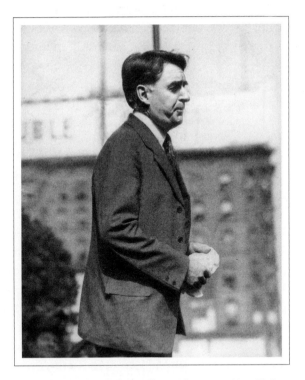

Standing in front of the Liberty Theater in New York
City. Handwritten on the back: "Notice handkerchief.
He is suffering from the Epidemic he is trying to
stamp out."

up. I went to Calvary Cemetery and saw a new grave in every lot and 400
dead bodies in a building at the rear of the cemetery waiting to be
buried. I went out and got a steam shovel and men off the street. We dug
trenches to bury the dead."

He told the *New York Times,* "We did a number of unconventional
things, and we did not do several conventional things that were done
elsewhere," like closing schools and all places of public assemblage,
including some stores. Without any fanfare, Copeland did close certain
small "hole-in-the-wall" theaters, which, he said "were breeding grounds
for the disease." But he said that in general his goal was "to keep this city
from going mad on the subject of influenza. My aim was to prevent
panic, hysteria, mental disturbance, and thus to protect the public from
the condition of mind that in itself predisposes to physical ills." (Hahnemann wrote about such conditions of the mind.) Copeland told an

interviewer, "I found that movies kept the minds of the people off the subjects of the flu and death. To combat sickness successfully, a doctor has to be something of a psychologist. He must keep his patients cheerful and optimistic."

In every way, 1918 marked the beginning of Copeland's intensely unconventional—indeed, unique—service to homeopathy in America. He followed its principles but did not shout that he was doing so. Yet most things he did as health commissioner were in the name of homeopathy, even if they were not disclosed as such, or remarked upon by his colleagues and contemporaries. And everything he did for homeopathy promoted the bold and confident politician he was becoming. Newspapers were already hailing him as the next governor of New York.

Copeland boasted that the city's death rate was lower than that of other big cities; for instance, at the end of the first month of the epidemic, mortality rates were higher in Boston, Philadelphia, and Baltimore. "We fared better than did the rest of the world," he said. A public health report said that over 48,000 people (out of 6 million) succumbed to the disease in New York City between the fall of 1918 and the summer of 1919. (In a later speech, Copeland said that 2 million had the disease and 35,000 died. He would eventually be heavily criticized for deflating the mortality rate, although it remained true that in terms of percentage of total population, New York did come out better than any other city in the nation. Many years later, he said that he had "learned that in the great East Side, New York, where there is the greatest crowding, the death rate among babies is the lower than it is among the homes of the wealthy of this great city. This is because the Jewish mother is the best mother in the world.")

In testimony he gave in Ann Arbor on behalf of his alma mater to stop the consolidation of the two medical schools, he commented that after the flu crisis he "immediately put forward a private inquiry to see how the homeopaths got along." Copeland, who kept a small apartment in Ann Arbor while he was the New York City health commissioner, told his former colleagues that "the contrast between the two schools was startling. There can be no doubt that the superiority of homeopathy in a purely medical condition is just as great as it was fifty years ago," he said. He didn't provide any statistics, just saying that the difference was like "night and day," although Dean Hinsdale reported that "one instance will be illustrative of the many experiences of homeopathic physicians throughout the country," that of the families of the 8,000 employees of

Montgomery Ward & Company. Hinsdale said that only homeopathic remedies were used there during the pandemic (he did not say which ones) and that one lone death occurred. He also reported that the July 1919 issue of the *Journal of the American Institute of Homeopathy* had disclosed that of 88 homeopathic doctors treating a total of 26,795 cases of "epidemic influenza," there were only 273 deaths.

W. A. Dewey, Copeland's friend at the University of Michigan, believed that many of the deaths from influenza were the result of overdoses of aspirin, which, he said, causes "violent palpitation of the heart, deficient respiration, and weakness approaching unconsciousness," as well as "eruption" on the head, face, mouth, and throat, and "disturbances in the sensory centers, vision and hearing"—in fact, "sensitive nerve tissue is paralyzed." Dewey firmly believed it was a drug that should be classified with opium, heroin, and cocaine, and that when it was combined with quinine, as it sometimes was, it became "distinctly poisonous." He, Copeland, and the AMA were in agreement about its dangers. Many people bought aspirin tablets, he said, in packages of 100 or 500, and took them by the dozen. (There were many reports of counterfeit aspirin, contaminated with talcum powder, being sold.) Dewey quoted a doctor in Kansas City, Missouri, who observed that aspirin tablets "were swallowed by tons last winter by hysterical people who went beyond all advice in self-medication. . . . Many persons were in bed from the prostration of the drugs taken instead of from the 'flu.' " Dewey also criticized the overuse of Digitalis during the flu pandemic, saying it "poisons the heart and the circulation," causing "the heart to drive more blood into the lungs already overcrowded." This "routine treatment has undoubtedly been responsible for a considerable part of the excessive mortality" during the flu pandemic, he concluded.

In time, Copeland would become convinced that most deaths "were really due to the secondary pneumonia, to the complication, rather than the influenza itself." He said that "studying the problem it struck me that the cold rooms of late October, rooms in which the weak convalescents lived after leaving their beds, were responsible for the complicating pneumonia. Next came the question of how to remedy the evil of cold houses." He decided to prepare an amendment to the Sanitary Code, requiring that all landlords furnish heat of a certain temperature, even though his attorney told him such a ruling would never stick. But the commissioner of health insisted on going through with the measure, and he got it. Sixty-eight degrees was the minimum. The

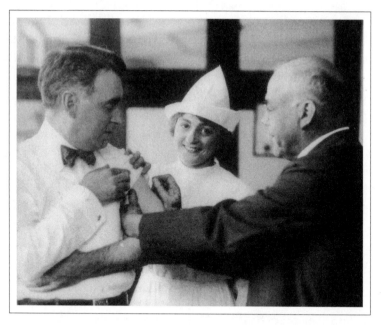

Copeland receiving his smallpox vaccination, July 28, 1920

amendment was practically unenforceable, but it was on the books, in plain sight.

Copeland confronted many other diseases during his tenure. Typhoid was a continuing problem, and he quarantined all immigrants suspected of having the disease. It was not unusual for him to quarantine a shipload of 1,700 passengers for as long as twelve days. All incoming vessels and the clothing of the crew and passengers were routinely disinfected. Barbershops were inspected for lice. An infestation of fleas in Greenwich Village confronted him. To ward off bubonic plague, or "the black death," his Sanitary Squad made sure all ships had rat guards, and the Health Department laboratories made regular examinations of waterfront rats. Copeland was worried about smallpox, too (New York had about twenty cases a year), and he urged people to get vaccinated, and then revaccinated after "six or seven years." He said that vaccination was "the only preventive remedy against smallpox"—calling a vaccine a "preventive remedy," was a new term he began using in his public addresses.

In speeches around the city, he now spoke of a plan he preferred above all others: inspecting all immigrants not at Ellis Island but "on the other side," before they left for America. "There should be a mental, a physical, and a moral examination," he said, "so only those really fit should be allowed to start for this country." He also had a theory about the work of immigrants. "There should also be an industrial examination," he said, "that those fitted, for instance, to be farmers, should be sent where they would be contiguous to the soil, and not allowed to become peddlers and button-hole makers in the city." These plans were never implemented.

In 1919, he became concerned about contaminated milk, particularly after a strike by the Dairymen's League that year. Copeland was appointed by the governor to be chairman of a milk commission to study the issues. In fact, after this appointment he announced he was leaving his job as health commissioner (it was even reported in the newspapers) but once again, as was almost a ritual by now, he was persuaded—this time by the mayor—to stay on the job. He became a champion of babies and children as a result of his work on the milk commission. He urged parents to be sure their children had regular meals and adequate sleep. He thought children should not become overexcited—especially by watching too many movies. He became an advocate for safe foods and made sure the inspectors of his Food and Drug Bureau performed meticulous investigations at factories and the New York ports. Thousands of prosecutions were launched. His inspectors found dozens of harmful products—glue in ice cream, rotten fruit in a jam factory, worms in chocolate candy, cockroaches in mince. Copeland became determined to safeguard New Yorkers. Health Is a Purchasable Commodity was a slogan of his department. "We can purchase health by buying pure food," he said.

He was also alarmed about drug addiction and worried that the prohibition law would cause people to turn to opiates if they were deprived of alcohol. In fact, he predicted that cocaine would become the drug of choice for millions of people unless something was done about conditions. He set up a clearinghouse and a clinic for addicts and blamed standard doctors (although he didn't identify any by name) for prescribing so many habit-forming drugs. He noted that in one six-month period three standard doctors had prescribed over a million and a half opiates. Such numbers did not startle homeopaths, who knew that even twenty years into the twentieth century, allopathic doctors still gave out far too much medicine, medicine meant only to suppress symptoms and not get to the source of the real trouble. By stressing the harm done by opiates, Copeland hoped, he might encourage people to begin to think twice about using them. "From 25,000 to 100,000 addicts are in our city now," he told the Grand Jurors Association. "And there is not one serious crime committed but is done under the influence of a drug. I know of a corner in this city where I can go and sneeze and where a package of morphine will be brought to me for sale."

On January 9, 1919, the acting commissioner of health of the City of Cleveland, Ohio, complained in a letter to the AMA that Copeland's "propaganda" about keeping theaters open during the flu pandemic was being used in a publicity campaign by the National Association of the Motion Picture Industry.

Copeland was now officially in the files of the AMA's five-year-old Propaganda Department.

The Cleveland official wrote that "crowds of any kind are to be discouraged," and the AMA replied that it wished its journal could do something about the matter, commenting that "what else could be expected of such a Commissioner?" Sarcasm, which the AMA generally used only in private letters, in-house memos, and occasional jottings on the margins of articles it collected for its files, would become in the 1920s and onward the AMA's final weapon against homeopaths. It did little else because it felt that homeopathy was either out, on its way out, or tolerably incorporated into standard medicine. The AMA would stay interested in Copeland throughout his career, and because he was the only leading homeopath to have a propaganda file of his own, the AMA began to judge homeopathy by his conduct.

Unlike many homeopaths, Copeland didn't become a member of the AMA, although he tried to remain on cordial terms with the group. It is not known if he was aware that the AMA was leery of him. One AMA letter to a correspondent asking about his credentials answered with one terse line: "Dr. Royal Samuel Copeland is *not* a member of the AMA, and, as far as we know, has never claimed to be." The organization tried its best to restrain its hostility, and when asked in another letter to describe the American Institute of Homeopathy, it said that the group "corresponds in the homeopathic field to the AMA—in other words, it represents the membership of the best men in homeopathy." High praise.

Soon after starting Copeland's propaganda file, the AMA marked a page from the *Bulletin of Pharmacy* that contained an announcement of "a metallic health phone cap" that "intended to embody a highly effective germicidal protection against stray germs and infections and to prevent the accumulation of dust and dirt in telephone mouthpieces, which physicians now agree were a dangerous but heretofore unsuspected source of spreading infection during the recent influenza outbreaks." What prompted the AMA's interest was a photograph of Copeland that accompanied the announcement. It showed him using a telephone with the phone cap. Standard doctors were unconditionally opposed to doctors appearing in any advertisements and considered it unethical behavior displayed only by quacks. The AMA report on Copeland mentioned that not only were all the phones in his New York department equipped with the devices, but that the commissioner had "started a nation-wide educational campaign" saying the phone caps might prevent a recurrence of the flu. Although he had helped form the Ann Arbor Brick Company in 1903, and didn't actually enter the phone cap business, the "educational campaign" is the first instance of his budding health-related entrepreneurism, a way of life that had fascinated him ever since he had observed the Kellogg brothers in action. Such undertakings as theirs would come a little later, but meanwhile Copeland enjoyed and valued the attention advertising and publicity brought him.

Many citizens wrote letters to Copeland asking health questions. They wanted to know whether a chiropractor could clear the face of pimples. No, he answered. "Is a red nose indication of intestinal trouble?" one woman asked. Copeland replied that indigestion was probably the cause of the red nose. When someone asked about ulcers, Copeland said the condition required "careful dieting, but an operation is often indicated." A man asked about the cause of shingles, and Copeland said they were caused by abscessed teeth or gums, diseased tonsils, and "female" disease. Someone asked about ways to gain weight. Copeland's main interest in weight was getting women (more than men) to lose it, and, in fact, he had conducted an experiment on fifty women who collectively "rid themselves of seven feet of waistline and half a ton of weight" at the end of their "training period." When a man asked for a remedy for hard calluses on the soles of his feet, Copeland first told him to soak his feet in warm water every night and then crossed out that answer at the bottom of the letter and wrote a new reply telling him to go to a school of podiatry. Up until 1911, podiatrists, then called chiropodists, learned their craft by apprenticing with an experienced podiatrist. In 1911, the first school for podiatrists was started in New York City—at first only one year of high school was required for entrance to the eight-month course; then gradually, over many years, it became a four-year course requiring a college degree, an entrance exam, and a residency program after graduation.

Copeland answered many of his correspondents with a form letter that contained no specific advice, just an acknowledgment that the letter had been received. This was generally used to answer the many sex-related questions he was asked, especially those about "that dreaded disease called Spermentoria, a nervous disorder," that one seventeen-year-old boy said caused him and others "a wasting of seminal fluid by nocturnal emission." But Copeland relished personally answering most of the letters he received. Years earlier, when he was still living in Michigan, he had spoken to a group of recent medical-school graduates and told them that "much may be accomplished for homeopathy, it seems to me, by an occasional press or magazine notice." And so, in 1920, after he had gained prominence as health commissioner, he jumped at the opportunity when he was asked to write a nationally syndicated column for the Newspaper Feature Service, which later merged with the Hearst King Features Service. "It's time to do away with the mystery of medicine," he told an audience in Jackson, Michigan; "the people should be informed. The newspapers now gladly publish articles upon diseases . . . and I have the privilege of speaking every day through the columns of the news."

The column, "Your Health," was an immediate success. He never once mentioned the word "homeopathy." He met and became a friend of William Randolph Hearst, often called the "Barnum of Journalism." "Your Health" quickly caught the eye of the AMA, which, according to Copeland's son, denounced him for "encouraging self-dosage" and for "degrading the medical profession." (In the letters to doctors and patients that the AMA collected in Copeland's propaganda file, the stock response was a careful "Dr. Copeland's syndicated health articles are, in our opinion, nearly always scientifically sound.")

Some of the columnist's "self-dosage" advice involved using lemon juice to soften the skin of the hands, face, neck, and arms; for nail care; as an "effective" shampoo and a tonic for the scalp; as a "harmless" brightener of blond hair; and as an aid in brushing the teeth. Copeland also recommended using lemons for the treatment of scurvy (caused by a lack of vitamin C) and for beriberi (lack of vitamin B1), bedsores and other wounds, and rheumaticism. He wrote that "lemon baths, such as Queen Wilhelmina of Holland has adopted as a daily procedure, are recommended as a means of preventing rheumatism by keeping the skin clean and healthy." Other "self-dosages" included "one of the purest foods than can be eaten"—an orange. They not only "regulate natural functions," he wrote, but "smooth the road to recovery."

He had less and less time for his private medical practice, yet he found the time to write a movie script on health subjects, which he hoped would become part of a series. The project never worked out. By 1921, his was a household name. He was enjoying his success as a public official and writer in a large city. His health column had over 11 million readers, and his office received nearly 10,000 letters a week. His requests became more brazen, too, as when he wrote a general he knew in Washington that "I observe by the press that the President will be in New York in the middle of April. You will find on inquiry that it is not an uncommon thing for the President or the secret-service people to communicate with the Police Department, asking that in the assignment of men, certain ones be called upon to guard the President while in the city of New York. Our mutual friend, my Body Guard, Denis J. Mahoney, Shield No. 102, will be broken hearted if he is not delegated to guard the well-being of the President of The United States."

On November 21, 1921, Copeland's mother wrote him from Dexter that it had been announced in the *Detroit Free Press* that the two schools of medicine at the university had finally merged. "This means no more teaching of homeopathy," she wrote, adding that the school of homeopathy "has lived now longer than you thought it would when you decided to go to New York." This revealed that he knew all along that consolidation couldn't be avoided in his home state. His older sister, Nellie, who was an English teacher at Central High School in Ann Arbor, where she now lived, remained the adoring sibling when she wrote her brother, "but I am so glad you are not there [in Ann Arbor], though, doubtless your splendid powers could revive its life." Her last phrase would resonate for Copeland, especially in the early 1920s, when scientific developments included new techniques in brain surgery; discoveries about the blood, nerve impulses, the functions of the kidneys, heredity, the stratosphere, magnetic fields, X-rays, and isotopes; and the first use of insulin for the treatment of diabetes. He would need the "splendid" powers his sister attributed to him to keep alive the public's interest in and need for homeopathy.

Despite letters and pleadings from the friends of homeopathy (including a threat that legally and morally the Ann Arbor property was meant to be used only for homeopathic purposes), the homeopathic medical school was "wiped out," as Copeland wrote in an angry letter for the record to the president of the university. He said that "the Regents have made a grievous mistake. They have taken a detour which will give the university a rough and disastrous ride. . . . It was an untimely and unfortunate added burden to homeopathy." Hinsdale, too, wrote that "to defend the right of oneself to future existence is not always easy or pleasant, but, to defend a principle in which one has faith is a task to inspire. Today homeopathy is as true and unerring in its foundations and end results as it was in the beginning." And yet by the mid-twenties, the only homeopathic medical schools left intact were Hahnemann in Philadelphia, Hahnemann at the University of California, and New York Homeopathic Medical School.

Moderate homeopaths like Copeland (considered an invisible homeopath by his colleagues, especially since he never wrote about it in his columns) all still agreed that their way of medicine had been advanced by chemistry and physics, and that homeopathy had had "a tremendous influence upon medical thought . . . and that medicine today is upon a far saner basis than ever" because of this influence. They also understood that most standard doctors used at least some homeo-pathic remedies, that many leaders in standard medicine "recognized the pertinence of homeopathy," and that standard medical-school texts con-tained many pages of homeopathic therapeutics. Pharmacies were reporting the sale of increasingly large quantities of homeopathic drugs to nonhomeopathic practitioners. Homeopathy was on the brink of joining the mainstream.

But most homeopathic educators, instead of helping to ensure that professors of homeopathy became a permanent fixture in all medical schools across the country or helping to provide graduate education for students, moped in their cities and towns, and mourned the decline of their separate schools.

TEN

"Hitch Your Cart to a Star"

COPELAND kept a newspaper article his mother had sent him close by on his uncluttered desk at the 150-year-old white clapboard house that he had recently bought in the Ramapo Mountains, near Suffern, New York. The three-story house on Haverstraw Road overlooked a man-made pond, formed, Copeland said, "by throwing a dam across a tiny mountain brook." The landscape around the house was radiant with flowers, bushes, and trees. A small white gazebo had been built close to the pond, which was often used for ice skating during the bleak, Michigan-like winter months.

"Life consists of a series of contradictions," the article started out. "When one is young—opportunity, success, wealth and glory lie away off somewhere. The urge is to leave home." He had done that, and he had achieved a great deal in his fifty-four years. "You may leave Dexter, but Dexter will never leave you. . . . Dexter is you, and you are Dexter," it went on. Copeland, who had named his country house Dexter Manor, wholeheartedly agreed with this sentiment. Despite his success, he still considered himself the boy from Dexter who had some good luck, and his hometown was "always in his heart and near the surface of his mind."

The Dexter of 1922 looked very similar to the Dexter of his youth, with cows and pigs still roaming freely. "You had to keep your premise well-fenced to keep the cows out of your yard," Copeland's father, Roscoe, had told him in a reminiscing letter. "Some of us on the council thought it was about time to quit making our village a cow pasture," he wrote. Eventually, a herder was hired.

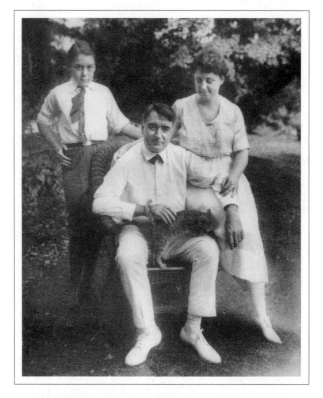

Royal, Frances, Royal Jr., and pet cat at Dexter Manor,
circa 1922. During the flu pandemic, Copeland wrote
that the "fondling of pets is not a good practice."

There were more stores and new churches in the downtown area—the Pentecostal Church, St. Andrew's Lutheran Church, a spacious pharmacy with a soda fountain, a men's-only clothing store, a millinery store, a dime store called the Racket Store, the New Dexter Ice Cream Parlor, which advertised "vanilla and chocolate ice cream 50 cents a quart delivered free anywhere in the village," and the Dexter Service Garage. Ford Model T's, Dodge roadsters, and Hudsons were spotted along Main Street, which was newly planted with shade trees. There were still canoe races on the Huron, grand parades during holidays, community picnics, watermelon-eating contests, and beard pageants, which crowned a "king of the brush." The old bandstand in the park had been torn down because its structure was no longer considered safe. Bus service between Dexter and Ann Arbor had begun in 1921. A windmill, built to pump water from the millpond to surrounding lots, had been replaced with an electric pump. Roscoe Copeland, who didn't drink, had been convinced to join the "red ribbon movement," which, he said, "did not believe in prohibition, they were trying to dry up the saloon by moral persuasion." The movement "did a lot of good in its day and it had its day," he wrote, adding that "there's a red ribbon pledge hanging up in the school house that your mother helped make." (In 1928, Royal Copeland would restore Dexter's original post office—"a priceless relic"—and name it after his grandmother, and his stillborn daughter, Alice. "The only condition I attach to this proposal is that I may be permitted the personal use of the building when I am in Dexter," he requested, adding that he loved the town "as I never have any other place.")

Copeland's childhood homeopath, Dr. Edgar Chase, had remained in Dexter until 1905, when he moved to Ann Arbor, where he continued practicing medicine until 1926. By 1922, Dexter had several doctors (it is not known if they were homeopaths) and dentists serving the area.

Copeland's life was increasingly a series of contradictions. He could be a romantic; he could be a realist. He could be scientific; he could be mystical. He could be natural—"a regular guy," he liked to say; he could be calculating. He could be secretive; he could be public. He could be Dry—for prohibition; he could be Wet—against prohibition. Sometimes he could be a Democrat and sometimes a Republican. He could give a speech representing one position, and end the same speech completely reversing his position. He could announce that he respected Christian Science, as he once did, and then tell the AMA, "Personally I am terribly opposed to the medical pretensions of Christian Science, yet I must admit that many apparently sane people piously accept what to me is the height of absurdity." He could even appear to be in favor of homeopathy on the one hand and opposed to it on the other. Some doctors had no idea whatsoever where he stood. Was he a moderate? A purist? A "mongrel," as James Tyler Kent might have called him? An *allopathic, regular, standard* physician?

He would try to illuminate part of his nature in a speech: "The true physician is not only the moral and spiritual guide of the patients who place their mental and physical welfare in his hands, but in similar things he should be the guide of the community or Nation as a whole." He believed he was a true physician, and thus shouldn't confine his energy and intelligence just to his individual patients, but should try to reach the masses. He should be a lawmaker, in fact. He would soon get another opportunity.

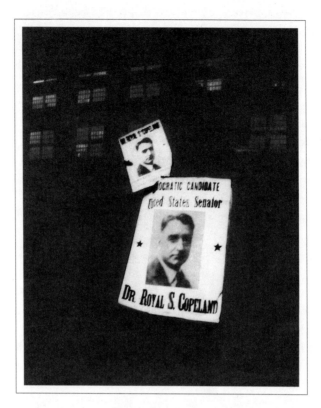

Doctor Senator, 1922

"The American people are peculiar," he told a reporter. "A man no sooner makes good on one job than they try to advance him to another." He said that "he was drafted, with but an hour's notice, to run for the Senate of the United States." It almost happened that way.

In 1922, his new publisher friend, William Randolph Hearst, was feuding with the current governor of New York, Alfred E. Smith, over Hearst's plan to run for the Senate. Smith point-blank refused to have Hearst on the ticket. The Democratic boss, Charles F. Murphy of Tammany Hall, wanted to remain on congenial terms with both men, so he suggested that perhaps Hearst's pal Royal Copeland could run instead, even though many people believed that he was still a Republican. Copeland on the ballot was meant as a mollifying gesture, one that was unthreatening to Hearst and acceptable to Smith. Hearst went along with the plan, since there was no way he was going to be able to run for the office. Copeland's honorary campaign manager was Franklin D.

Roosevelt, who was between jobs, having served as assistant secretary of the navy from 1913 until 1920, when he ran unsuccessfully as the Democratic candidate for vice president.

No one expected Copeland to win the senatorial election. But he did, with a 281,000-vote majority. His fame as health commissioner, his health talks in lecture halls and often on the radio, his weekly health columns, plus his continued work with the Methodist Church around the state, had made him a highly regarded man. The "true physician" could now help guide his nation and, in his words, "fight for the plain men and women of these United States," in what was called the most exclusive club in America—the United States Senate.

HE FELT right at home in Washington in terms of his natural surroundings, for just as scenic Dexter had been designed so all the houses received sunlight, Washington, D.C., dominated by the Potomac River that runs through West Virginia, Virginia, and Maryland, had been designed to be a pleasing city, with wide streets and abundant trees.

Copeland decided he would keep writing his health column, legislator or not. (Many of his campaign posters had shown "Dr." in front of his name.) He wrote to all the newspapers that carried his column, "I do not consider this a 'job' in the ordinary sense. This is the pleasure I get out of life. To stop it would be to deprive me of the sweetest things in my life. I am glad that my new undertaking will not interrupt the writing of my articles and answering the letters of those who write me about health matters."

He came to be relied on for any work he was called upon to do as the junior senator from New York State. His "new undertaking," as he called it, would take him many places, and in his first year in office he was on the Immigration, Naval Affairs, Education and Labor, and District of Columbia committees (he was called the unofficial mayor of Washington). Right away, he saw the chance to continue advocating on a higher level the need for better public health standards. When he was given the chance to speak on the Senate floor, he had no compunction telling his new colleagues that the air in their chamber was vile, and, in fact, that the chamber was "the vilest ventilated room in the world." He said "the only sunshine comes through the heavy ornamental glass-paneled roof." Three months after taking office, he told an interviewer that being in the Senate was "like having malaria." He once described the Washington he had wit-

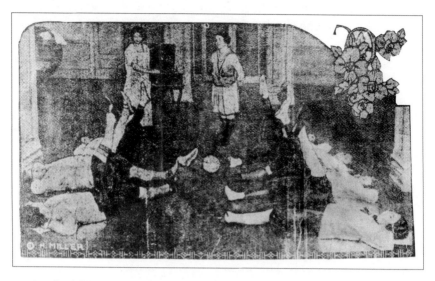

Copeland felt that women should exercise together. One of the prostrate women (not specified) is his wife.

nessed on a visit in 1898, and how it contributed to his desire "to rid the city of its horrible breeding places of dirt, disease, crime." Ignoring the spaciousness of the avenues and the leafy foliage along them, he said that "the streets were ugly—old and unsightly buildings on each side of Pennsylvania Avenue. Sixteenth Street was a road of horrors, a stately mansion, and right alongside, a tumble-down shack unfit for human habitation."

Over time, he criticized his colleagues' lack of exercise, and their poor eating habits: "Fat has replaced muscles, including the heart muscle." (Copeland, himself, remained slender and sleek.) Some members eventually stopped listening to him, a predicament he had never experienced before, and over time he became known as "the great anesthetist of the Senate." The pages began to call him "General Exodus," because his colleagues made a beeline for the cloakroom when he got up to talk. But this didn't stop Copeland from talking about the things he cared about. During the summer of 1922, he became the very visible chairman of the AIH's Bureau of Sanitary Science and Public Health.

Yet even if he bored his Senate brethren, they all liked him. "There's nothing up-stage about him. He can always be reached and he is ready with any assistance he can offer," a reporter said of him, adding, "they call him 'Doc.' When any of them are taken sick, he is often called in consultation." And he was extremely well liked by the senators' wives, who read

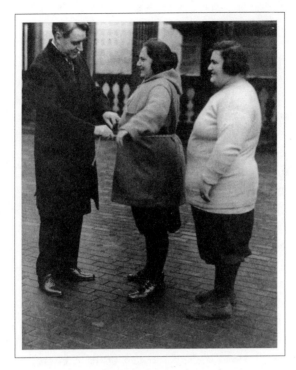

Senator Copeland believed that most women were
overweight and needed more exercise and
discipline in their lives.

his health columns avidly and were familiar with his recently published
book, *Over Weight? Guard Your Health,* which was directed at a female
audience. In the year before his election, Copeland had written that he
was in favor of short skirts for women because they were "more hygienic"
than long skirts that picked up filth from the streets. Short skirts also gave
women freedom, as did low heels. He approved of thin silk stockings and
low-necked gowns as well. He was in favor of bobbed hair—it was "more
sanitary . . . and better for the scalp." The women of Washington—
indeed, the whole country—approved of Doc Copeland's modern views,
especially after having won the right to vote in 1920. Copeland believed
that most men overdressed, what with their wool socks and high collars.
He also believed that mothers overdressed their babies.

Mrs. Copeland made friends easily. She said that "President Harding's life came to a close just as we were elected to office. The first official
duty of The Doctor was to go to Mr. Harding's funeral. Then came the

Coolidge administration . . . Mrs. Coolidge added much to my own happiness in Washington." The Copeland home was always filled with Washington luminaries.

The new junior senator refused to dress the part. He didn't wear the usual black fedora his fellow senators did, or the double-breasted frock coat, or the black or white string tie. Instead, he wore dark suits or a cutaway and striped trousers. Still, with his silver-rimmed spectacles and temples of now-white hair, he looked like the distinguished elected official he was.

He opened shop across the street from the Capitol in the Senate Office Building and began "to do something for the public good," as a profile of him entitled "Copeland Has the Floor" plainly put it. He and Mrs. Copeland rented an apartment at the new and fashionable Shoreham Hotel, which overlooked the nearly 3,000-acre Rock Creek Park, a preserve full of vines, mosses, hills, rapids, wildflowers, and forest timber. The Shoreham's Renaissance-style lobby and interiors full of cherry wood furniture were grand and casual at the same time. "We decided that the hotel, with every comfort, would lessen our worries," Mrs. Copeland said. She liked also that the hotel could arrange her frequent parties, sometimes held on the roof terrace, where "Rock Creek Park sent up a perfume with the night breeze," she wrote in a letter to her mother-in-law.

With his surefire intelligence and curiosity, Copeland quickly learned the ropes. He saw early on how the Senate was run and how to get things done in the committees, even as a freshman. (Over time, he would be on the Appropriations, Commerce, and Rules Committees. He would help pass a federal probation bill, ask for an amendment to the income tax laws, request improved immigration laws, oppose the St. Lawrence seaway, and even get into a fistfight with another senator over a proposed army bill.)

He said that his "training of a physician fits him in many ways for the activities of political life." As senator-elect, he said in a speech that "the concerted movement to stamp out cancer should have the support of our national legislature at every point." (He was hoping for the discovery of a vaccine.) At the same time he promised to involve the government in getting rid of every infectious and contagious disease known to man, and to talk about the hygiene of sex. He wasn't going to be prudish about the topic.

In the months before his election, he had carried on with his attraction to advertising, ignoring the fact that the majority of doctors con-

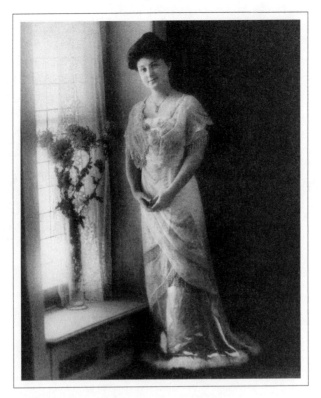

Mrs. Royal S. Copeland

demned such practices. An article in the Minnesota State Medical Association's journal spelled it out—"the quacks all depend on it." But Copeland was fascinated more than ever by the publicity and excitement an advertisement could evoke. It was bread he was endorsing right before the election, not any patent medicine or hygienic gadget. It was Bond Bread. His picture was next to an advertisement in the *New York Tribune*, and the text announced, "Pure Food means health. The Bond behind Bond Bread is an epoch-making guarantee of purity. It offers a plan which should be adopted by every food manufacturer!"

The AMA considered advertisements by medical men and women unethical under any circumstances whatsoever. But Copeland didn't. A few years later, in a speech before the annual convention of the American Bakers Association, he glowed as he told his audience that "in the country, the Sunday night meal and many other body building meals consist of nothing but bread and milk. In every crockery store, they used to sell

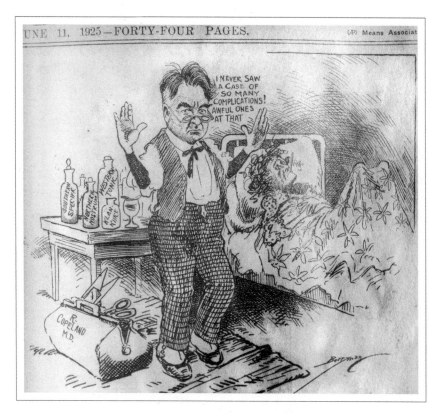

Dr. Copeland treated the world as his patient.

'bread and milk sets'—a plate, a bowl and pitcher. I wonder how many city folks ever heard of such an idea. Truly, bread is the staff of life." And he meant it—the attitude was part of why he spoke out for bread. He claimed that "the famous brands on the market now" were actually better made than the homemade kind because "the flour is made by standard methods of properly blended wheat," and the "temperature and humidity is better controlled." It is not known whether he was paid by Bond Bread to speak in its favor. In any case, he didn't feel it was wrong to be a spokesman for a product he considered so exemplary, and he saw no resemblance between his ads and the ones considered misleading under the Pure Food and Drug Act of 1906. The maverick was on the rise.

During the winter of 1923, Copeland, as a member of the Committee on Education and Labor, investigated medical "diploma mills." The committee was determined to rid the country of phony medical degrees and diplomas that could be bought for a price, especially by naturopaths.

The only way to be a doctor in the United States was through attendance at an accredited medical school that issued a legitimate diploma upon completion of all requirements. Copeland had never been a nonconformist when it came to medical regulations. He also believed, as he told the graduating class of the North Carolina State College of Agriculture and Engineering in the spring of 1923, that "next to doctors, farmers are the poorest business men in the world." He now wanted that to change.

His emerging progressive political leanings had begun to soften his feelings about standard medicine's use of the term "preventive medicine," and he no longer saw the concept as necessarily hostile to homeopathy. He told the North Carolina students that "the doctor of the future will prevent disease. His every energy will be devoted to heading off disease. Preventive Medicine will be his chief concern." And, he underscored, "without health there can be no wealth. Health is fundamental to commerce, to culture, and to national prosperity." But, the grandson of a farmer cautioned them, "let us hope no graduate of today will devote his life to money grubbing and to selfish acquisition." The country was still in the throes of the Teapot Dome scandal, in which the secretary of the interior had profited from illegal oil leases. Still, Copeland told the graduates, "Hitch your cart to a star." Just as he had done with homeopathy, though some people believed his was hitched to power.

The senator continued to assist his father, who had complained bitterly about the noisy whistle-blowing at the train crossings in Dexter. Copeland immediately wrote the president of the New York Central Railroad about the problem and was assured it would be "corrected." He also found the time to advise his mother about the building of a garage and to assuage her concern that it might "overshadow the house." "I suppose it is natural to worry about such things," the senator wrote in a letter. "I believe, however, if windows were put in front, in the second story, it would take away the bleak look the garage will give." He loved immersing himself in such details.

"I am going to breathe in the pure air of New York State," he lectured his associates on the eve of a congressional vacation. "I am going to do horseback riding. . . . I am going to walk through the fields and woods. As my muscles grow hard, I am going to climb mountains. . . . I am going to read some good books and go to the movies. . . . I am going to drink creamy milk and lots of pure water."

· · ·

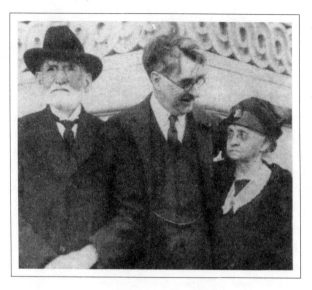

The new junior senator from New York State particularly
enjoyed showing his parents around Washington, D.C.

THE AMA had had water on its mind for many years, as did a large
number of Americans. But now the AMA began to question seriously
the content of mineral water, which had been used around the world for
centuries to fight infection and promote healing. (In 1890, a homeopathic remedy called Sanicula had been proved. It was made from the
salt in a spring located in a town in Illinois.)

"The exploitation of some mineral waters is almost as fraudulent as
that of the exploitation of 'patent medicines,' " the AMA's Bureau of
Investigation said. Its attention had been drawn to a mineral water called
Chuck-Muck-La that claimed to have broad healing powers. The distributors alleged that its secret formula went back to a primitive Indian tribe,
even though it was not used by physicians until 1827, when a spring was
found near Pensacola, Florida. The water was advertised with the slogan
"Tastes Good—Does Good," and was said to cure indigestion; ulcers;
diabetes; bowel, kidney, liver, and bladder troubles; gallstones; kidney
stones; open and running sores; all skin diseases; blood troubles; and
rheumatism. Hundreds of testimonials came from around the country.
In 1910, a man wrote that the water permanently cured his varicose veins.
In 1913, another man wrote that after ten days of drinking the water, his
severe bowel problems vanished. In 1916, a woman wrote that 5 gallons of
the water had cured her skin rash. In 1922, another woman wrote that

she and her brother were cured of headaches and that "while I was at the springs a lady was there who was cured of a facial cancer in six weeks." The testimonials went on and on, and the AMA's reaction was that if the water could do all it was said to have done, then "it would have received considerable scientific recognition," which it hadn't. It said it was quackery, and its claims "preposterous," adding, "That many people are greatly benefited by drinking high-priced mineral waters in place of ordinary city tap-water is due to the fact that they drink more water. There may also, of course, be a psychic element."

In 1907, a cure-all product called Bioplasm had particularly irked the AMA; it was made from the "digestive and ductless glandular organs of calves," with milk sugar added. The AMA sometimes found it hard to see any difference between this nonhomeopathic substance that contained milk sugar and "real" remedies that contained milk sugar. The majority of homeopaths still refused to address the question directly because they were sure their patients would understand what was what.

In 1910, another deceptive water had been brought to the AMA's attention. This one, "pushed in New York especially," was called Radam's Microbe Killer, and was found to contain "ordinary hydrant water," ash, sulfuric acid, or oil of vitriol, a corrosive used at that time in tiny doses as an astringent. In 1919, a water called Barium Rock Spring Water, which was said to cure diabetes, was found to contain not a single grain of the element barium, a toxic earth metal. (At the same time, a drink called Fruitola, which was advertised as a cure for gallstones, was found by the AMA to contain only olive oil and anise flavoring.)

The AMA went after waters containing lithium, a metallic element that was said to remove kidney stones and aid in the treatment of rheumatism, gout, nervous disorders, menstrual problems, and malarial fevers. These waters had proliferated in the country since the late 1800s, and were touted as "the new elixir of life." The AMA had received hundreds of complaints and had applied pressure to have any reference to lithium removed from the labels. In 1910, the Department of Agriculture had sued the Buffalo Lithia Water Company for misbranding, saying, among other things, that the "water contained only one grain of lithium in 10,000 gallons." The department condemned what it referred to as the uric acid fallacy, that the water had distinctive elimination features, and was particularly outraged that the label read "Guaranteed under the Food and Drug Act, June 20, 1906." On February 21, 1914, Buffalo Lithia Water was forced to change its name to Buffalo Lithia Springs

Water, the name now representing its origin (Buffalo Mineral Springs, Virginia) and not its content.

In the late fall of 1921, the again-renamed Buffalo Mineral Water asked the AMA to run an advertisement in its journal, but the AMA refused, telling the advertising agency that the water had been "criticized rather unfavorably" in its pages. The agency pleaded with the AMA to change its mind, saying that *Harper's Magazine, Literary Digest,* and the *Chicago Tribune* had accepted ads. In a postscript, the agency noted that "this advertising has also been accepted by the *Journal of the American Institute of Homeopathy* and the *Journal of Osteopathy,*" not realizing that mentioning this was the kiss of death.

During the winter of 1924, the AMA learned that Copeland had appeared as an expert witness for Buffalo Mineral Water and was in favor of keeping "lithia" in its name. The AMA wrote in a letter that Copeland, "who represents scientific medicine (heaven save the mark!) in that most August body, the United States Senate," said that without lithium, the lime content of water produces, among other things, cataracts. The AMA said that with a senator mouthing such thoughts, was it any wonder the public also "fell for such things as . . . chiropractic?" (Copeland believed that "without silica and lithium, potash, and a dozen other chemicals, the daily needs of the human system are not provided for as they should be.") But the AMA was reluctant to criticize a U.S. senator directly in the pages of its journal, so Dr. Arthur J. Cramp, head of the Propaganda Department (to be called the following year the Bureau of Investigation), asked a friend at the Indiana State Medical Association to publish the criticism in its journal instead. "You are running a journal that does not have to keep silent for reasons of state," Cramp said. The editor wrote Dr. Cramp that he "would take great pride in publishing an exposé of the foolishness of Dr. Copeland . . . who certainly makes some bad breaks as a doctor . . . in his hectic career." But he suggested that Cramp write the exposé himself and publish it anonymously in the Indiana journal. Cramp agreed. It is not known exactly what he wrote, but he characterized his submission in a letter as "snappy enough to have some interest, but not vicious enough to cause Copeland to hunt you with a shotgun." Aside from not wanting to get into a war of words with a senator, *JAMA* was also reluctant to denounce Copeland because among the testimonials for the old Buffalo Lithia Water was one from a "Professor of Clinical Surgery, University College of Medicine, Richmond, Virginia, and ex-President of the American Medical Association."

. . .

IN 1924, twelve people, some of them doctors, formed a new group called the American Foundation for Homeopathy. Its objective was to offer postgraduate courses in homeopathy to doctors, as well as to continue to familiarize the public with the benefits of using its remedies. The foundation wouldn't try to establish schools, but rather would offer expert lectures, create and establish a library, raise funds, and encourage research.

The organization first began in California, a year earlier, in 1923, when two doctors used a $10,000 gift "from a grateful patient whose life had been saved through homeopathic remedies" to try "to preserve homeopathy for other generations." The doctors believed they needed to exert some paternalism over the present situation. That same year, the American Association of Homeopathic Pharmacists was also founded, to offer research support and to help promote excellence. Neither group addressed the questions of patent medicine, fraudulent foodstuffs, or water.

Science was continuing to advance. Specifics about the application of radio waves were discovered in 1924, as were details about the luminosity of stars. Insecticides were now available in the nation. The following year, in 1925, the formation of oxygen was understood, discoveries about the nature of anemia were made, the role of the spleen was explicated, and, most important, quantum mechanics, the definitive mathematical formulation of the theory for atoms, was developed. Doctors and scientists everywhere marveled at the progress. Homeopaths, especially the purists, continued to brood. Where did they fit into this world?

"Because the old school has opposed our teaching in the past, would any one dare now to withhold it arbitrarily from being reincorporated in their curriculum of extended education?" the California branch of the American Foundation for Homeopathy asked. This was an important question, because embedded in it was a strong wish to be part of "the mechanism of modern medical education" without giving up the homeopathic ideal. Still, the foundation said, "The only thing that does not change is change." Yet it was not talking about scientific change as much as economic change, and primarily blaming the loss of their colleges on lack of sufficient funding.

The foundation wanted to offer independent course work but not within the framework of any standard medical school. It said that even though "the old school has repeatedly acclaimed Hahnemann's genius as reflected in the discoveries of the twentieth century," maintaining a separate existence was necessary because "homeopathy deserves the best setting that a generous world will allow." There was little talk anymore about how to bring homeopathy into the twentieth century, and the AIH had not revisited plans to present the scientific evidence of homeopathy.

Still, some homeopaths put their faith in the work of a German nurse, Lilly Kolisko, who, in the early twenties, began researching the effects of homeopathic dilutions of metallic salts (sulfate of iron, nitrate of silver, nitrate of lead) on the development of plants. Her observations over a period of many years were connected to the cosmic force theories of a philosopher-educator, Rudolf Steiner, who created a movement called anthroposophy, which was viewed by its followers as a science of the spirit. Kolisko's experiments involved astronomy, light, the moon, space, and a spiritual vision. There was not a "standard" bone in her body.

But most homeopaths were busy with their own practices, and were content to let things be. They were used to being in the minority, and some even believed it was better that way. The moderates were literally indistinguishable from standard doctors.

In 1923, the AMA had started *Hygeia,* a magazine for the general public. Now everyone, not only doctors, could read articles on "irregular" medical treatments, aids, and products. The following year, the AMA began a regular series of radio programs for the general public in the hope of further educating them about detecting medical fraud. Two years earlier, in 1922, it had formed a "committee to study the entire question of sects in medicine." It was fed up with homeopathy, osteopathy, and every other kind of "pathy" it regarded as a cult "with an exclusive dogma or sectarian system." It decided, once again, that there had to be just "one standard of educational qualification," but that now, "if necessary, each case should be carried through to the United States Supreme Court where the merits of the situation will be cleared up." Homeopaths were still welcome as members, of course, as long as they didn't preach what they practiced or belong to the AIH.

The AMA resumed its attacks on other sects as well. In 1923, it said that members should not associate with osteopaths, that it was unethical to do so, although if a member did come into contact with one in a clinical setting, the member couldn't be disbarred from membership in the AMA "in the absence of action by their component society." (The onus

to disbar was put on the regional medical society.) In two other complicated decisions, the association ruled that "a registered physician who
graduated from an osteopathic school" and who met all the requirements
of the law in receiving a license couldn't be expelled from a county
medical society without cause. In other words, a standard doctor who
decided to try osteopathy and went to school to learn about it was probably going to remain a member of his regular society, but maybe not.
About allowing osteopaths and chiropractors to work in "regular" hospitals, the AMA said that hospitals have "the legal right for reasons sufficient to the board" to refuse privileges of the hospital at any time to any
practitioner regardless of his so-called school of practice." Hospitals
could reject osteopaths and chiropractors. The AMA said also the hospital had the "moral right" to refuse to accept "objectionable people"—i.e.,
osteopaths and chiropractors.

The AMA's Propaganda Department received a letter asking about a
magazine called the *Hygienist,* and Dr. Cramp explained in his reply that
its editor was an osteopath who was against proper medical legislation
and therefore the magazine was "simply the mouthpiece of his anti-
medical views." Cramp was also very critical of Copeland for writing an
introduction to a book, *Right Food: The Right Remedy,* published in 1923,
because its author was a chiropractor.

By 1926, the AMA increased its pressure on sects by announcing that
"the approval of certain chiropractic schools by the U.S. Department of
Labor . . . is to be condemned as encouraging quackery." It also
announced that hospitals allowing any "drugless" practitioners on their
staffs were no longer on the approved list of the AMA. The AMA also
decided that for the protection of the public the term "doctor" should be
restricted only to doctors of medicine and doctors of dental surgery. No
one else had the right to use that designation.

In 1924, the AMA issued a new definition of a sectarian, saying that as
applied to medicine, it was someone "who in his practice follows or
claims to follow a dogma, tenet or principle based on the authority of its
promulgator to the exclusion of demonstration and experience." Up to
that point, the AMA had continued practicing benign neglect on homeopaths, allowing them to be members, but now its attitude changed.
There had to be "demonstration and experience"; there had to be science.
In fact, the AMA said also that "under no circumstances should a regular
physician engage in consultation with a cultist of any description."

The AIH, the IHA, and the American Foundation for Homeopathy stayed silent. They didn't try to defend themselves in any way, mostly because they didn't consider themselves cultists. They had their own organizations and their own way of doing things now, even if most of their schools had closed. Their beliefs were active and alive. They didn't really need the AMA, though those homeopaths who belonged to it didn't agree.

Copeland began leaving "homeopathic" out of his Senate biography. He had graduated from "The University of Michigan Medical School." He had been president of "his national medical association." He had been the dean of "New York Medical College." His colleagues in the AIH were mystified.

During the winter of 1924, Copeland cosponsored a bill that would prevent the public from being victimized by manufacturers of fake vaccines and serums "for which impossible curative claims are made." The *Chicago Herald and Examiner* reported that the bill was introduced as a result of "startling revelations" in *Hearst's International* magazine. (It was not written by Copeland, but by one Norman Hapgood.) Sponsorship of the bill, which was in the form of an amendment to the Biologics Control Act of 1902, was Copeland's first foray into the national arena of safe foods and drugs. Three years earlier, in 1921, the AMA, which had once recommended that pharmacists needed to be well educated, had gotten serious about helping to develop pharmacy as a respected and licensed profession. (It had allowed reputable pharmacists to be "pharmaceutic members" in 1903.)

On May 17, 1924, *JAMA* ran a brief item that mentioned Copeland's introduction of a bill for the establishment of a bureau of medical research within the Department of the Interior. This bureau "would investigate the chemical and biologic processes that underlie the functioning of the organs of the human body." In addition, the bureau "would be required to 'devise means of controlling the bodily processes, to determine the physical properties of materials where a knowledge of these materials may be of advantage to medical science.'" This basically meant that the government could get into the business of managing bodies, as well as of testing "materials" such as homeopathic remedies. Copeland also tacked onto his bill "an elaborate program for the purchase of a 100-acre tract of land in the vicinity of Washington, D.C., on which buildings shall be erected at a cost of not more than $1,000,000." Presumably, these would be laboratories. The Senate was not impressed, and the bill was dropped.

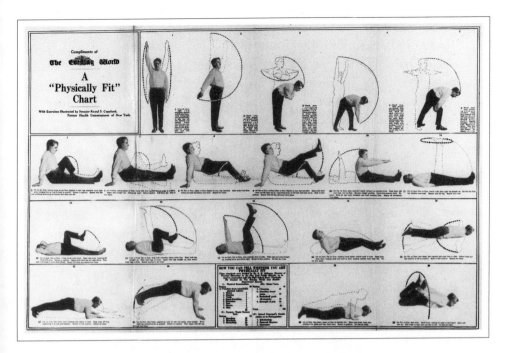

Copeland performed what he preached.

Nonetheless, in his usual, almost nonchalant way, Copeland also let it be known that there was already talk of his being a candidate for president of the United States at the 1924 convention. At first, it was said half-jokingly. The senator was firmly behind Alfred E. Smith, governor of New York. But his candidacy did find some support, including that of his friend and boss, William Randolph Hearst. Yet in the end, a conservative lawyer from the state of Virginia, John W. Davis, was chosen on the 103rd ballot as the nominee to oppose President Calvin Coolidge.

In 1924, Copeland once again became a published author with the appearance of *The Health Book.* It was an outgrowth of his health columns, and it even included exercises for fitness, demonstrated by the senator himself in a series of dramatic photographs: The senator, dressed in dark pants, an open-collared long-sleeved white shirt, and shiny black shoes, on his stomach, head up, palms resting on the floor, then reaching back to grab his ankles with his hands. The senator sitting up, then lying back and arching his back while at the same time raising one leg at a time. The senator, flat on his back, hands at his sides, doing knee bends.

He worked long hours, often staying at the huge mahogany desk in his Senate office until 2 A.M. To amuse himself, he once wrote a song describing his stamina: "It's always getting-up time with me. It's always getting-up time with me. No matter how lazy other people may be, it's always getting-up time with me." Copeland was so busy with such a variety of projects that he became one of the few officials who posted office hours on the door of his suite.

SOMETIME in 1924, Copeland met Bernarr Macfadden, a well-known naturopath. They met when Macfadden was a house guest of Copeland's colleague and mentor, Minnesota Senator Magnus Johnson, who had been an early booster of the short-lived Copeland-for-President drive. Macfadden had first gained fame in 1898, when he began publishing a five-cent magazine called *Physical Culture,* which brought together his interests in bodybuilding, a vegetarian diet, and the natural treatment of illness. He particularly believed in fasting as a cure for all diseases.

Eventually, he launched other publications (*True Story, Movie Weekly, Muscle Builder,* and *Dream World* among them), until Macfadden Publications, with its own six-story building on Broadway in New York City, included not only dozens of magazines, but books, encyclopedias, and even a daily newspaper, the *Evening Graphic,* which some people dubbed "the Evening Pornographic" because of its explicit photos (many faked) and overall sensationalism. Over time, Macfadden would write 150 books, develop many businesses—including Physical Culture City, a health spa—and establish the Bernarr Macfadden Institute for Training. Along the way, he would be nicknamed "Body Love," by *Time* magazine, found a religion he called Cosmotarianism, marry three women, mistreat his children emotionally and physically, get arrested several times for obscenity, and be acknowledged as the Prince of Quacks by the AMA.

On April 1, 1924, the AMA replied to a letter from a doctor at the Mayo Clinic in Rochester, Minnesota, saying that "Macfadden is one of the largest advertisers among that group which comprises the self-styled drugless healers." It concluded, "Macfadden, apparently, rejects even the most axiomatic facts of medical science, and persistently blackguards the medical profession." The AMA received many complaints about him: "The Macfadden stuff is pouring in by every mail," it told one correspondent. Macfadden is "dangerously ignorant," the AMA said. "If there is a better ballyhoo artist in the United States than Macfadden, I don't know of him," Dr. Cramp wrote. The AMA was concerned about every-thing Mcfadden did, and didn't do: He told the parents of a child suffer-ing from diphtheria to ignore advice about the disease affecting the heart and to encourage the child to run around. He was opposed to all vacci-nations, with one result being that there was an outbreak of smallpox at one of his "healthatoriums" in Chicago. He manufactured his own min-eral water, which he said brought about "wonders." He worked with a questionable eye doctor named W. H. Bates, and together they encour-aged "a new course of eye training" to cure people of errors of refraction without using glasses; the training involved exercises as well as exposing the eyes to intense light. Macfadden and Bates considered glasses "eye crutches."

During the early winter of 1925, another eye doctor suggested to Mac-fadden Publications that it market phonograph records made from his successful body exercises. This eye doctor was now a United States sena-tor. Mcfadden Publications, however, turned down the chance to "take over the records," because, as it explained to Copeland, "we would imme-diately antagonize several concerns who are now advertising their records in our magazines and who have spent many thousands of dollars with us." Mcfadden suggested that the senator "interest some mail-order firm in the proposition . . . perhaps an arrangement could be made where you could be paid a royalty on each set of records sold." This is precisely what followed. Copeland made a deal with the Advertising Record Corpora-tion in Cliffside, New Jersey, to manufacture 3,000 sets of phonographs of the Copeland health exercises, which would be advertised for sale in all the newspapers that carried his health column. The company, which wrote the senator in New York and addressed him as Dr. Copeland, not Senator Copeland, also suggested that "the proposition should be sold to the business managers of the newspapers by means of a good strong initial letter accompanying the consignment of records . . . and the newspapers should also be supplied regularly with a series of news stories featuring the records in a great variety of interesting ways and dealing with the prob-lems of the fat woman, the scrawny woman, the child, and all the other angles that would readily suggest themselves." It was balm to the budding entrepreneur in the senator.

Earlier, during the fall of 1925, Copeland, whose beloved mother had died that summer, helped a Dexter cousin who was marketing a product called the Malar Pile Remedy. Copeland wrote the solicitor general of the Post Office Department on his behalf to make sure, as he worded it, that its "attitude" toward the remedy would be a positive one—i.e., that it could go through the mails legally without a fraud problem. The solicitor general, however, told Copeland that he couldn't get involved in the matter. Another friend later told him, though, that there probably wouldn't be a problem if the ads for the product told the "exact truth" and weren't misleading. The cousin, who asked Copeland to invest in his product, said that it would be "foolish" for his publicity campaign not to say that the remedy had "miracle powers," so he would limit his publicity to just three states (Ohio, Indiana, and Michigan) and keep it out of any high-priced publications. He said his ads would run only in certain small rural and/or foreign-language newspapers, and he maintained that despite such methods, honesty was his highest priority. Copeland did not invest.

But he did look around and make some other investments that year: a controlling interest in the *Nyack Daily News* (his country house was located nearby); a business to be called Camp Land, Inc., to operate the Royal S. Copeland Camp for Boys, "a high-class camp for general health improvement"; Royal S. Copeland Restaurants, Inc., which was going "to teach people how and what to eat"; and property in Key West, Florida, of which he said, "Key West is bound to become the most popular winter resort of America." Later, he would buy a Spanish-style beach house in Venice, Florida, and a dark wood and stone three-story house in Mahwah, New Jersey. Also he became the president of the Fordham National Bank in the Bronx. His longtime secretary explained to a constituent that "the Senator's venture in banking will not curtail his political activities."

The junior senator from New York seemed to be on a roll. A member of the Sullivan County Democratic Committee told him, "I believe there is more real money in the camp business than any other line of endeavor that I know of." Copeland agreed, but also felt that a close second was the restaurant business. As he wrote potential shareholders, "When I was Health Commissioner of New York every restaurant in the City came under my jurisdiction. I was struck by one outstanding fact. I believe it will be equally obvious to you. It was this. The most important business centers of the City lacked sufficient good restaurants to feed even the men and women there every day." Copeland wanted the patrons of his restaurants—and he envisioned a chain of them—to be served wholesome food. "The better the food the longer they will live." Then he added, "The longer they live the longer they will patronize us!"

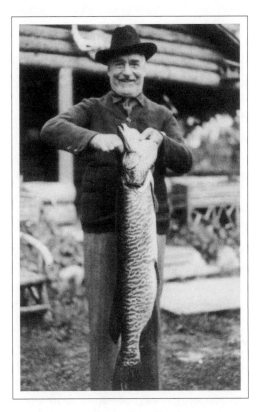

Copeland and big catch in Florida, circa 1930

He got involved in every detail concerning his camp and his restaurants. The camp was to be built on a farm not far from Dexter Manor. Copeland created a long list of necessary additions and improvements to the property, from dormitories, barns, and a garden to roads, an electrical system, and a stone crusher. However, midway through the financing of the restaurant business, with many fine points already worked out, he withdrew his name "because of complications," he said. (He had received criticism for using Senate stationery for his negotiations.) By November 25, 1925, his secretary in New York was telling potential vendors and applicants for employment that "nothing active is being done in the restaurant work." By December 11, the restaurant was turned over to its general manager, although 4,000 shares were given to Royal Copeland "in appreciation of the Senator's services in helping to get the plan underway." At Copeland's request, his name was removed from all corporate papers. Shortly afterward, he said in a speech that "before a great many years roll by, the restaurant will have almost entirely taken the place of the home kitchen in Metropolitan life."

In 1925, the senator also started the Copeland Service, Inc., which offered "a complete analytical laboratory service for foods, drugs, pharmaceuticals, cosmetics, and health products," including advice on labels so that they would conform to state and federal regulations. The manager was to be Ole Salthe, the director of the Bureau of Food and Drugs when the senator was health commissioner in New York. The nature of the business made Copeland a little jittery because of possible conflict-of-interest issues, but nonetheless, like all his other businesses, it followed the letter of the law. Still, he was prudent in going through the marketing material and made certain changes to avoid putting himself in a compromising position. For instance, on the cover of one brochure, he removed his full name, so the words would read only "Copeland Laboratories Founded in 1925," and in the text he again removed his name, plus any reference to "drugs," so that it read that his laboratories were "a consultant service for food products," rather than food and drug products. (This was probably as much a concession to homeopathy as it was to his public role in the fake vaccine and serum congressional bill.) But the brochure still "advertised" the full Royal Copeland name because the senator's son, Royal Jr., was listed as a chemist, "formerly with Food and Drug Administration," on the advisory staff. At the time he was fifteen years old, and in high school.

Copeland continued endorsing products. The New York *Daily News* of May 4, 1926, carried an advertisement (and picture of the doctor) captioned "Dr. Copeland's Advice Always Helpful." The advice was for "frail, thin men and women who yearn for strength, vigor, and vitality," to take McCoy's Cod Liver Oil Compound Tablets, which were sugar-coated. (In a letter to one of his cousins around the same time, he recommended Walpole's Cod Liver Oil as the "best brand.") He allowed his name to be used in a newspaper advertisement for a food store in Pittsburgh. No explanation exists as to why he chose this particular store, but he said, "Donahoe's Fifth Avenue Store is my idea of what the ideal food store should be."

He seemed far away from medical practice and homeopathy with these current pursuits, and his hunger for publicity seemed to be getting stronger. Yet he remained an effective lawmaker in many areas—immigration, farming, the income tax, probation laws, and court reforms. He went out and about frequently, in and away from Washing-

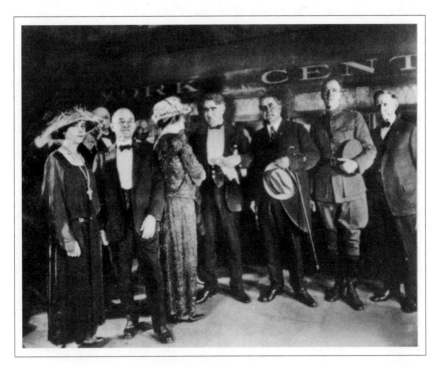

Time for dinner on a train

ton—dinners for the New York Letter Carriers Association, the Butchers and Packers Supply Association, the Italian Pharmaceutical Association, the Mexican ambassador; a speech before a podiatry group; a minstrel show in Suffern. His appointment book was always filled to brimming. He even found time to entertain the senior class from Dexter High School, and to dress up as Santa for a children's party. Although he no longer saw patients in an office, he continued to speak before homeopathic gatherings. In fact, at the Southern Homeopathic Convention, delegates wore COPELAND FOR PRESIDENT ribbons on their lapels.

By 1926, the year he proposed that the Library of Congress appoint a scientist (it didn't happen), as well as the year there were further developments in quantum theory and macromolecular chemistry (areas that would have implications for homeopathic principles), he knew exactly what he wanted to do when he grew up in the United State Senate. He wanted to concentrate on strengthening the 1906 Food and Drug law. In doing it, he'd hitch his cart to his first and only true star (besides himself)—Samuel Hahnemann.

ELEVEN

"As the Wing of a Bird Fits the Air"

In May 1927, the AMA further consolidated its efforts to outlaw sects by deciding that every state medical society now had to cooperate in keeping "irregular practitioners" from receiving any official recognition whatsoever. More than eighty years had passed since the term "irregular" came to mean anything other than standard medicine, the only "regular" medicine.

The AMA's Bureau of Investigation continued to follow Copeland, by clipping articles by and about him. (In 1926, Copeland began his own file on fraudulent medications and other quackeries. He also introduced a bill to authorize a psychologist to measure the brains of members of Congress, in what he called "anthropological psycho-physical and statistical examinations." No measurements were ever taken.)

On December 16, 1926, the AMA reported that Copeland had praised a patent medicine called Magic Materia Medica, and had been quoted in an advertisement as saying that the product "has wonderful healing powers." It was claimed that the medicine was made from an unidentified rock that contained radium and was said to cure cataracts, hay fever, rheumatism, diphtheria, stomach and kidney troubles, boils, pimples, cuts, bruises, and "old sores," and was also "an excellent eye wash, stopped bleeding immediately, strengthened the eyes, and removed corns and blisters." (The AMA's lab found that it contained three substances: dried lime nitrate, which was used to make gunpowder; dried chloride of lime, used as a disinfectant or a bleach; and "a small amount of sodium iodide," or plain salt.)

Copeland announced that the ad was unauthorized and that he had never praised the product. Eager to maintain good relations with the AMA, he wrote the association that "the statement is so ridiculous" that the organization "must have known that it was in no sense a quotation from him." But the AMA knew no such thing. In fact, Dr. Cramp wrote the editor of *JAMA* that "from other material in our files, we have no reason for such an assumption." Included was this example:

> In Dr. Copeland's own daily health column, over his own name, we find such statements as these:
> > Miss V.C.—question: Will olive oil grow hair if used on the face?
> > Dr. Copeland's answer: It might possibly.
> And this:
> > G.W.M.—question: What effect had grapefruit on the system?
> > Dr. Copeland's answer: It produces acid in the system.

The AMA also seemed to know in advance about Copeland's plans for a radio program. Dr. Cramp wrote, "We also have in our files the evidence that the National Broadcasting Company, which owns the Red Network System, is going to put on, if it has not already put on, a 'Dr. Royal S. Copeland Hour,' and that Copeland is to broadcast a series of lectures on pure foods." The "evidence" was a letter dated October 6, 1927, from the network to a food manufacturer soliciting its business as a sponsor of the broadcasts. The network told the company that Copeland's lectures on the nutritive value of foods would be given every day from 10 to 11 A.M. and that the senator would answer some questions on the air and answer all others by mail. In addition, the network said that these letters "will not only bear the name 'Dr. Royal S. Copeland Hour' but also the names of the sponsors." The AMA was particularly irked by this latter "inducement," as it called it, that the sponsors would have their names on what could amount to thousands of letters a month. Free advertisements.

Two of Copeland's sponsors, when the radio program officially started in 1928, were Fleischmann's Yeast and a laxative called Nujol. Listeners heard what they often referred to as soothing "old style country doctor" wisdom mixed in with a healthy dose of plugs for the products. Such blatant promoting (he even recommended the use of a certain type of mattress) brought Copeland flak from more than just the AMA. He was censured by some colleagues in the Senate, and by some newspapers. However, it didn't interfere—none of his advertising or business deals did—with his being reelected for a second term in 1928, when Franklin Delano Roosevelt was elected governor of New York and the Republican Herbert Hoover was elected president. (Copeland had worked hard on former New York governor Al Smith's behalf for the office.)

Copeland had plenty of advice for presidents, ex-presidents, and would-be presidents. He believed that all ex-presidents should automatically enter the Senate so the country could still benefit from their experience and training. He said in a speech that President Wilson's death in 1921 "must be regarded as much a casualty of the World War as that of any veteran who died from wounds or exposure." He went so far as to say that "temperament shows and controls, whether the man lives in the White House on Pennsylvania Avenue, or in a story and a half house on Huron Street in Dexter." Even though he said that former president Calvin Coolidge "wanders like a lost soul," Copeland praised him for taking a nap every afternoon and the new president, Hoover, for "getting up early, taking himself seriously, and plodding through his work." "It all depends on temperament," he repeated. "Life is what we make it and we make it what we are willing to have it."

On February 9, 1927, Copeland had given a speech before Congress about farm relief. "Mr. President," he began, "happiness is the most elusive thing in the world, but I doubt if there can be happiness in any home where there is economic distress." He went on to say that "the farmer is the victim of economic unsoundness," and by that he meant that because of the Tariff Act of 1922 the farmer was forced to pay a tax on materials essential to his job—"products which he must buy in order to operate his farm." Copeland said it was "unfair and unsound" that "there is a tax on all kitchen knives, butcher knives, and carving knives," and that the farmer even pays a tax "on pliers, pincers, nippers, files, and rasps of all sorts." He circled around the many issues, attacking and condemning his colleagues, saying finally, "I want to ask this question of any fair-minded man living in a great city: are we not willing to assist the farmer?" In his long speech the resounding answer was yes, yet in the end he announced he was in favor of the tariff so the farmers could be given an "equal chance" in the economic world, and because "it is necessary to protect American labor against cheap labor abroad." So the actual answer was no. "It all depends on temperament," and his was one that played both sides and could be one thing at the beginning and the complete opposite at the end. He "played" homeopathy the same way.

During the summer of 1927, with farming still on his mind, Copeland decided to go into the poultry business. He asked his former health department colleague Ole Salthe, now the manager of Copeland Services Inc., to run it for him and named the business the Dexter Poultry Company. Salthe had been head of the New York Live Poultry Commission Merchants' Association after leaving the Health Department, and had helped control an epidemic affecting poultry across the country. He knew poultry and knew how to handle and feed it, and Dexter Poultry advertised that it would sell freshly killed poultry "of the highest grade . . . free from contamination." A leaflet for potential investors and customers said that one of the biggest problems Salthe and Copeland had to deal with in New York's Health Department "was the correction of the evils in the live poultry industry." Now the two men had found a way to both correct the evil and make a profit. By the fall there was a subsidiary, Ole Salthe's, Inc., for kosher and retail operations, with six stores already up and running. "We can give you poultry as fresh as you could have if you lived in a sunny farm house," the company advertised in flyers. Copeland monitored its operations from Washington, letting Salthe run the day-to-day affairs in New York. However, Copeland was not against exerting his influence when it was needed, as he did when he wrote the current New York City commissioner of health a letter asking for a temporary permit "for the finest poultry-slaughtering establishment I have ever seen, and I suppose as a matter of fact, it is the finest in the world."

For a long while, Copeland had also been concerned with the hazardous substances used in cosmetics and hair dyes, ingredients such as benzol, wood alcohol, lead, mercury, and arsenic. And so, in the fall of 1927, he proposed a National Cosmetic bill to outlaw the use of such substances. (That year Congress passed the Caustic Poison Act, which provided warning labels on corrosive substances, such as lye, packaged for household use.)

Copeland read passages to his Senate colleagues from a best-selling book, *Your Money's Worth,* which urged better controls on cosmetic products. Poisonous lipsticks and face powders containing carbolic acid were a lurking danger. In seventy-four reported cases, permanent disfigurement to the mouth and face resulted, and in some cases, death.

His cosmetic bill was strongly opposed (as similar proposals had been), and opponents cited figures, based on an article in *JAMA,* that estimated there was only one unfavorable reaction in every 150,000 hair-dye treatments (which, opponents argued, was comparable to reactions people sometimes got from shellfish or strawberries). The bill lingered in committee, awaiting another that a beauty journal characterized as "sponsored by the AMA." In fact, the AMA would be 100 percent behind the concepts and intentions of all drafts of a cosmetics bill, as well as bills on food, drugs, and therapeutic devices. The organization would object only to the inclusion of dentists, pharmacists, midwives, chiropodists, osteopaths, chiropractors, naturopaths, "and other similar practitioners of the healing art" in the definition of "medical profession." Homeopaths were not named directly.

A durable bill was years away from passage, but Copeland persisted in his efforts and at the same time continued to indulge his craving for publicity. He allowed his name and picture to be used in the advertising of a mineral water called Pluto Concentrated Spring Water, which focused its many promises for cures on one main symptom: constipation. But what the AMA didn't seem to realize or notice was that Pluto water contained five homeopathic remedies. Copeland didn't mention this, but it is surely one of the fundamental reasons he endorsed the water. Pluto contained small amounts of Sodium Sulfate (*Nat. sulf.*), a Schussler tissue salt used to control water in the body; Magnesium Sulfate (*Mag. sulf.*), another salt remedy used for muscle and nerve improvement; Calcium Sulfate (*Calc. sulf.*), a Schussler tissue salt used for blood cells; Sodium Chloride (*Nat. mur.*), a Schussler tissue salt for emotional problems and colds; and Magnesium Carbonate (*Mag. carb.*), a mineral first proved by Hahnemann for the treatment of constipation. In its criticism of Pluto, the AMA said that the concentrated form of the water purported to be ten times as strong as regular water. It was condemning, without saying so directly, and probably without realizing it, homeopathic dilutions. The AMA said that there was "positive fraudulency" involved, and that testimonials for the water's medicinal properties came only from "bucolic statesmen and romantic old ladies." One "bucolic" statesman was, of

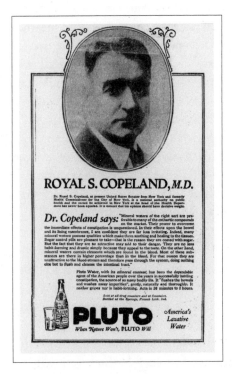

Few people knew what Copeland knew, that
some water he peddled was more than H$_2$O.

course, the homespun but debonair senator from New York, who had
once estimated that he had worn more than 10,500 carnations in his lapel
since 1908, when his "romantic old" wife first pinned one on his coat.

DURING THE summer of 1929, the AMA noted that the fourth graduating class of the American School of Naturopathy held its commencement exercises in Los Angeles on July 17. Twenty-three students had
completed their studies in three months. According to the dean of the
school, as quoted in the AMA's report, the students "managed to get
some ideas" of the following subjects: anatomy, physiology, histology,
bacteriology, pathology, diagnosis, chemistry, toxicology, hygiene, sanitation, chiropractic analysis, and technique. In addition, he said that the
students had "listened fairly attentively to the many stories" that the
dean had told them about his "practical" experiences. It was no wonder
the AMA was unnerved. This wasn't medical school. This was, as the

AMA wrote, "a recurring problem," despite the fact that many of these schools were in the process of dying "a natural death." Two years earlier, in 1927, the AMA had reported that there were five schools of naturopathy, and "all of them teach chiropractic" as well. (Another report said that there were twelve naturopathic schools; the exact number was difficult to obtain, the AMA explained.) It was common knowledge that many of the fifty chiropractic schools in existence taught naturopathy, too. The AMA reported that "the chiropractor may easily become a naturopath by taking a 3-month 'postgraduate' course in one of the naturopathic schools." The AMA said that the faculties of the schools were rarely—and barely—trained: an insurance clerk was a professor of pathology at a naturopathy school in Connecticut; a pants-maker started his own school of naturopathy in an unnamed state.

The AMA also reported that some chiropractors began to manipulate their patients' eyes (and skulls), believing such techniques could improve vision. The idea for this probably evolved from a procedure that had gone out of favor at the turn of the century, that of placing tiny stones under the eyelids.

The AMA was also bent on condemning something called "Iridiagnosis," also known as "Iridology," which was a theory that all diseases could be diagnosed by looking at the eyes, a concept that went back to the first millennium before the birth of Christ. Most iridologists believed that a patient's entire medical history could be detected by reading signals in the eye. In 1927, the AMA had written that such beliefs were "preposterous" (now its favorite pejorative) and had "no scientific basis." It had been troubled about this since 1911, when it reported that a bogus professor from Kansas said he could treat heart trouble, eczema, tuberculosis, ovarian tumors, and numerous other diseases "through the eyes." His specialty was "hard cases" that, he said, "regular doctors" could not handle, and his remedy was a secret eye water that the AMA said contained sodium chloride, a trace of sulfate, and sugar. Minus the sulfate, this was actually *Natrum muriaticum,* or *Nat. mur.,* the homeopathic remedy used for anxiety, depression, and colds. It was not supposed to be used as an eyewash.

Americans were still longing for medicines that could help them recover from their illnesses faster. Many, in desperation, still tried the hundreds of crude, deceptive patent medicines the AMA and others (like Copeland) were desperate to get off the market. Concoctions with odd names such as Agmed contained unnamed ingredients said to cure diabetes and urinary problems. DDD was supposed to cure everything from gangrene to diabetes. Zendajas claimed to cure arthritis and other ills. And there were Von's Pink Pills, for ulcers, and Dr. Town's Epilepsy Treatment. All with unknown ingredients. All worthless.

Most people tended to cling to the homeopathic remedies they had used for decades and had been obtaining for a long while now from both standard and homeopathic doctors. In a speech before the Missouri Institute of Homeopathy in 1931, Copeland emerged, calling Hahnemann "the greatest savior of physical ills."

Yet nothing about homeopathy was changing, and everything about "physical ills" was changing. In 1928, Alexander Fleming, a Scottish biologist, had discovered that a mold called *Penicillium notatum* was an effective treatment against bacterial infections (although it would not be for thirteen more years that this first antibiotic, named penicillin, was proved safe in humans). The structure of the cholesterol molecule was first understood in 1928. In 1929, brain waves were tracked and the sex hormone estrone was found in urine.

Medicine was living in a new world. So was American society, after the Stock Market Crash in October 1929. "Distress is everywhere," Copeland said in his speeches. His own assets were not in jeopardy, except for a $4,000 banknote he had demanded two months earlier, in August. He had resigned from the Fordham Bank in December.

He spoke often about the Depression, remaining an optimist, arguing that even though millions of citizens were partially or totally unemployed, "this is a time when clear thinking is needed. To fall into a panic of fear may bring disaster to a sick nation, to a sick world." Like many others, he said "it was not the gold standard that did it, it was the breaking faith with the gold standard." He fought with his colleagues for the "stabilization of business and relief of unemployment." He shared the view that to believe American credit was "inexhaustible" was "a delusion."

THE AMA monitored *The Royal S. Copeland Hour*, mostly through correspondents who wrote in about statements he made during the show. When the AMA heard that Copeland was making diagnoses and prescribing over the airwaves, it decided that since he appeared not to be practicing medicine anymore (it wasn't quite sure about this), "any advice that he may give to individuals over the radio, or elsewhere, presumably is without financial gain on his part and does not give him an unfair advantage over the practicing physician." It was the "unfair advantage" phrase that was the most telling because, aside from everything else, it revealed the AMA's rivalry with and resentment of any nonstandard medical activities. To the AMA, Copeland was always a senator and a homeopath. Later, the AMA answered a correspondent inquiring about Copeland by saying that "every physician is, of course, supposed to be bound by the ethics of his profession, but some disregard these in seeking personal publicity for some of their individual theories or in lending their names to the exploitation of 'patent medicines.' " The statement echoed the more direct one the organization once made that "Royal never overlooks a good thing." From 1933 to 1935 the AMA issued stronger condemnations of radio advertising related to medical preparations, now calling such broadcasting "evil."

In July 1929 the AMA criticized the American Red Cross (which had been founded in 1881) for permitting its nurses to take care of patients under the care of osteopaths and chiropractors, and a few years later would lament that a more durable way to bring "cult practitioners under rational supervision and control" had to be found. (In 1936, it singled out osteopaths, and said there had to be a more aggressive approach toward them "lest the standards of medical practice be lowered." It also began to include optometrists "among irregular practitioners.") It again condemned the use of the word "doctor" "for commercial purposes," and recommended that "correction of the evil be left to action before the Federal Trade Commission." (The foundation for the FTC was begun in 1887 with the creation of the Interstate Commerce Act, which was designed "to apply technical expertise and a semi-judicial and less partisan approach to the regulation of complex affairs." In 1914, the FTC was created "to prevent unlawful suppression of competition.")

In a speech before Congress, Copeland spoke passionately about not giving the Federal Trade Commission such powers as the AMA wished it to have, and said that the FTC "was created to assume the role of commercial umpire rather than guardian of consumer welfare." He said that he was willing to compromise, "by leaving the Federal Trade Commission control of false advertising that was purely economic in its aspects." But he wanted a stronger Food and Drug Act, and he didn't want the FTC involved "in the purity and wholesomeness of our food and drug supplies." He said that "the Food and Drug Administration has built up a competent scientific staff. No such staff exists in the Federal Trade

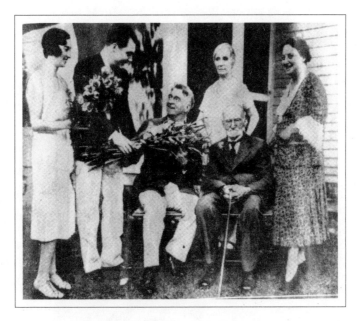

Copeland family reunion, 1932

Commission." He didn't want the FTC to have any authority over health matters. (The Food, Drug, Insecticide Administration had been formed in 1927, becoming the Food and Drug Administration in 1930.)

The truth was that Copeland didn't like many government agencies, although he did agree there should be a National Institute of Health and was pleased with its establishment in 1930. After Roosevelt was elected president in 1932, Copeland performed his usual flip-flop—first he seemed to be a New Dealer, then he didn't, and in the end he voted with the Republicans against most of Roosevelt's objectives, including devaluation of the dollar and the expansion of the Supreme Court. But as much as he was opposed to the New Deal, he never hesitated to join its efforts if it could help him reach his own goals.

ON FRIDAY, April 29, 1932, Copeland stood up in the Senate and gave a speech on water—radioactive water. He began by saying, "Mr. President, this week marks the one hundredth anniversary of the acquisition by the United States of the Hot Springs Reservation," which was in Arkansas. At first, he seemed to want to talk less about the curative powers of the springs (both as a drink and something to dunk oneself in) and more

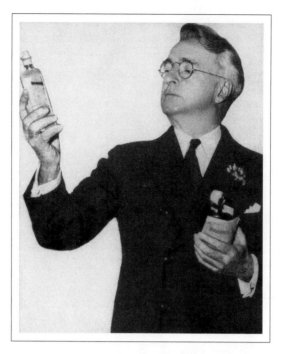

The senator holding unidentified bottles of medicine

about a bill he wanted to introduce, a bill to protect the public against fraudulent waters. But once having mentioned such a bill at the beginning of his speech, he never brought it up again. Instead, he concentrated on the effect of radioactive water, which he thought of as a medicine. (Twenty-three years earlier, in 1909, radium combined with a "gelatine" solution had been used successfully to treat a malignant tumor.)

Copeland said that he wanted to help end the confusion that existed over the ingredients in the water. Some radioactive waters contained radioactivity from radon, the gas created by the decay of earth and rocks (which was okay and not considered dangerous at the time), and some from radium salts, the metallic element derived from uranium (which was not okay, and said to cause cell damage). Most important, Copeland said he wanted to find out if the waters were harmful in any way— especially after the headlined death of a man who drank some water containing radium salts. Copeland said that he had a strong intuition that radioactive springs were not going to turn out to be dangerous in any way because people in Europe had been "taking the cure" for decades, and besides, such springs had been in existence since the time of the Romans. He also quoted an unnamed American doctor who said that any benefits from the springs were both psychic and "due to hygiene," a theory he didn't agree with. He told the Senate, "I hold in my hands" a copy of a scientific report on radon and its use in chronic rheumatism, written by a professor of "experimental medicine" at the Paris municipal hospital. Copeland said that some very famous French doctors agreed that "radioactive waters are considered as giving decided therapeutic results, and that it is impossible for radium deposits in the body to result from regularly drinking such waters . . . [and] like any medicament, such waters should be used in certain doses, and not indiscriminately." He added that it went without saying that the waters should be used under the direction of a physician, and then he spoke as a homeopath: "Practically every drug used by the medical profession is a poison if used in large doses." He also spoke as a homeopath when he called for the health commissioner of New York to duplicate the work of the Parisian doctor, because "nothing short of convincing clinical data, collected under the direction of our own institutions, is likely to remove completely the loss of confidence in all radioactive waters," and he wanted confidence restored. "It is a terrible thing to have the morale of the Nation broken down," the senator said. (There is no record of any follow-up tests performed in New York or anywhere else.)

Copeland found his chance to begin to boost the country's morale when, on June 12, 1933, as chairman of the Senate Commerce Subcommittee, he introduced the Tugwell Food, Drug, Therapeutic Device, and Cosmetic bill before Congress. Copeland's cart was now hitched to a bill named after Rexford Guy Tugwell, a member of Roosevelt's "brain trust" and the assistant secretary of agriculture, soon to be undersecretary. Tugwell believed that the time was now right to strengthen the existing Pure Food and Drug Law because of technological changes in marketing and production that made the old bill outmoded. There was better and faster train service, a growing air transport industry, improved canning and packaging procedures, the advent of home gas and electric refrigerators, and the beginnings of frozen foods. Tugwell was the man to promote an improved bill, and he had the president's ear. Copeland knew a good opportunity when he saw one, and he was in the right place at the right time.

Despite its pedigrees, there was enormous opposition to the bill, even more than was anticipated, and after two revisions it got left in commit-tee. The problem was not only extensive pressure from manufacturers, trade associations, and advertising companies, but also Copeland him-self. He was a problem.

Not only had he opposed certain provisions of the bill (he felt it gave the Federal Trade Commission, as well as the secretary of agriculture, confusing and inefficient powers to control certain products and/or false advertising and labeling), but he was also a cause of other people's oppo-sition. Some members of Congress, as well as leaders in the nonlegisla-tive community, including John Dewey of Columbia University, Rabbi Stephen S. Wise, and Freda Kirchwey of *The Nation* magazine, asked a question of Copeland: "How can the American consumer be assured of fair dealing when the chairman of this committee, we are informed, is receiving pay in behalf of a nationally advertised product, the claims for which would be adversely affected by the terms of this bill?" They said Copeland ("who is and has been employed by manufacturers of dubious drug products") was peddling Fleischmann's Yeast, a sponsor of his radio show. The product, America's first commercially produced yeast, was used to make bread, of course, but it also had medicinal uses—for ane-mia, constipation, and ulcerations.

Copeland's critics said that his compensation for backing yeast ("a high fee") was a violation of the criminal code if it involved intent to affect the pending legislation, adding that "while intent cannot in this case be proved, there is clearly a violation of the spirit of the law." As they wrote in a public statement, they were particularly offended that "at the end of the first day's session, Copeland went from the hearings to a broad-casting studio to speak on behalf of Fleischman's Yeast." They all agreed, too, that "Dr. Copeland has taken excellent advantage of the opportunity thus afforded him to emasculate the original bill." What they meant was that there didn't seem to be enough protection for the consumer in terms of all foods and drugs, and Copeland seemed to prefer it that way.

Copeland defended himself by saying that his intentions were being distorted. He went on the offensive, declaring that "the consumers of this country are being raped. The housewives of America will be the vic-tims of evils that will be felt by every home in our country." When a movement arose to oust him from chairmanship of his subcommittee, he explained that "there were subtleties to be understood."

One of the multitude of phrases Copeland (who didn't lose his position) wanted eliminated from the Tugwell bill was one calling for "general agreement of medical opinion." He said that "in the first place there is no such thing as 'general agreement of medical opinion.' " He continued, "In the second place, 'general agreement of medical opinion' is simply a rewording of the phrase 'consensus of medical opinion' which was concocted by the Food and Drug Administration with the aid and assistance of the American Medical Association in order to avoid the necessity of proof in litigated cases of actual therapeutic value, or lack of value of any drug in question." (Homeopathy would lose out here, since there was no "general agreement" as to its benefits.) Copeland went on to say that "there is no recorded case in legal history where there has ever been established a 'consensus' or 'general agreement of medical opinion' on any subject." This particular objection was Copeland's first tentative step toward his as yet undisclosed goal of protecting homeopathy; by deleting that phrase, he was paving the way for homeopaths not to be dismissed automatically by standard doctors, but to have the chance to prove in a court of law that what they did had "actual therapeutic value."

On the Tugwell bill, Copeland would not be a rubber stamp. He would risk being misunderstood. He would go where he needed to go, even if it took him several more years to get there.

BY THE mid-1930s, medicine had seen more wonders. In 1932, a year after new findings allowed geologists to gauge the age of the earth at roughly 2 billion years, a German physician, Gerhard Domagk, discovered that sulfa, a synthetic chemical, could cure streptococcal infections in mice. He eventually used it on his daughter, who was deathly ill with such an infection, and it cured her. "Chemotherapy" treatment had been launched.

It took time for the drug, called Prontosil, to catch on because there were continuing fears about its safety and effects; but once it did, sulfa, or sulfanilamide, revolutionized medical care, especially after President Roosevelt's son, Franklin Delano Roosevelt, Jr., was prescribed it and its use was said to have saved his life. The acceptance of sulfa as a treatment for bacterial infections brought about a decline in the use of mineral waters, both as a drink and a cleanser. It also brought about a decrease in the use of homeopathic remedies.

The early thirties saw the development of an elementary electron microscope that could magnify cells four hundred times. Things not seen before were now visible. A vaccine was developed for yellow fever. The neutron particle was discovered, as was a rare particle called a muon, which was a subatomic relative of the electron.

In 1933, the AMA wrote a Mexican doctor that "the true simon-pure homeopathy in the United States is as dead as a last year's bird nest." The following year, it told another correspondent that "homeopathy is rapidly dying out." In 1935, the AMA's Council on Medical Education and Hospitals announced that "sectarian" institutions were no longer on their approved list. And that was that, as far as the AMA was concerned. Homeopathy was over. There was only one science of medicine. A "unified profession." Homeopathy and the other "sects" were shut out. Sulfa drugs and the future they represented were in, although toward the end of the decade the AMA would begin to worry about what it called the drugs' "indiscriminate sale over the counter" and to condemn their use unless prescribed by a doctor.

In 1932, Morris Fishbein, the editor of the AMA journal, had included a chapter on homeopathy ("an unprovable theory") in his book *Fads and Fallacies in Healing: An Analysis of the Foibles of the Healing Cults, with Essays on Various Other Peculiar Notions in the Health Field.* His views now represented the views of most standard doctors.

He began by debunking Hahnemann's proving on cinchona bark, or quinine, by saying that it was worthless, since we now know "that malaria is caused by a plasmodium which gets into the blood through the agency of the mosquito." He criticized provings in general, too, singling out how inconceivable it was that "one decillionth of a grain of table salt was found by an imaginative prover to produce on himself 1,349 symptoms." He wrote that "like cures like" wasn't even that original, and that the idea of disease having anything to do with the spirit was "preposterous." In a section titled "The Death of Homeopathy," he began by arguing that "publicity is a powerful tool." He continued, "Students who observed the gradual decline of homeopathy began to seek regular schools; in fact, many a young man who had been doctored in his early youth by a homeopathic physician was advised by that very physician not to enter a homeopathic college. The fact is, indeed, that homeopathy died from within."

Copeland, when he was dean of New York Homeopathic College, agreed not that homeopathy was dying, or was dead, but that there was trouble "from within" its ranks. He had tried to address this aspect early on, but it seemed that he could never get the attention of his fellow homeopaths. Fishbein turned the AIH's definition of a homeopathic doctor on its head and argued that by saying that "all that pertains to the great field of medical learning is his, by tradition, by inheritance, by right" (in addition to having a special knowledge of homeopathic therapeutics and observing the law of similars), the group was offering homeopaths an excuse "to prescribe 'old school' drugs in old school dose" and that this was a concession of inadequacy and failure. He faulted homeopathy as a whole for standing still in the face of all that science had discovered, although he acknowledged that some individual homeopaths were using the new breakthroughs in their practice of medicine. He concluded by addressing a concept that was new in 1932—"the placebo," a substance having no pharmacological effect, but given to pacify the patient. (The word actually goes back to the sixteenth century and derives from the Latin for "I shall please.") Fishbein wrote of the homeopaths using "regular" medicines, vaccines, surgery, and advanced testing, asserting that "it came down to this: that a homeopath was just like any other physician" (with which Copeland wholeheartedly agreed) "except that he gave what were essentially nothing but placebos in minor conditions" (with which Copeland wholeheartedly disagreed). Copeland never stopped believing that the remedies worked because the selection process was so exacting, and that when selected properly, "the remedy fits the disease as the wing of a bird fits the air."

Fishbein conceded, but very indirectly, that homeopathy taught scientific medicine the value of milder medicine, just as he also conceded that "perhaps osteopathy has taught us something by its stress on massage," or just as Christian Science "has made itself valuable by showing the value of suggestion in conditions affecting the mind." But, he concluded, "others such as chiropractic . . . teach only the ease with which delusions may be foisted on the public. The history of homeopathy is distinct and peculiar. It records the propounding and acceptance of a theory which, in itself wrong, nevertheless influenced the steps of a beginning science into paths that were right."

ON MAY II, 1935, six months after Copeland had been elected to his third term as senator, the AMA ran the following gibe at his expense in its journal:

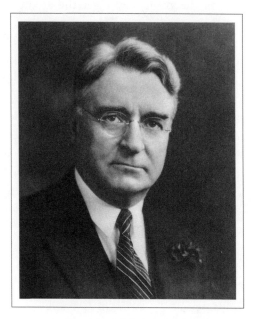

An official Senate portrait, circa 1935

BLINDNESS, CHRISTIAN SCIENCE AND
SENATOR COPELAND

"The Senate proceeded to consider the bill (S2153) to provide for the prevention of blindness in infants born in the District of Columbia. . . .

"*Mr. Copeland.* Mr. President, there is an amendment on the desk of the clerk which I desire to suggest to the bill.

"*The President pro tempore.* The clerk will state the amendment.

"*The Chief clerk.* On page 3, line 15, after the word 'physician' and the period it is proposed to insert the following:

'*The provisions of this act shall not be construed to apply to persons treating human Ailments by prayer or spiritual means as an exercise or enjoyment of religious Freedom.*' "

"*The President pro tempore.* The question is on agreeing to the amendment.

"The amendment was agreed to.

"The bill was ordered to be engrossed for a third reading,

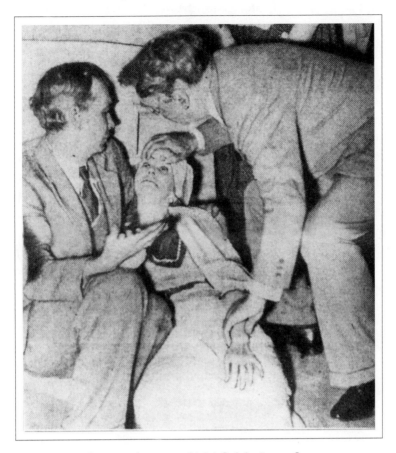

This time, the senator (right) fled the Senate floor,
to help an ailing woman in the gallery.

read the third time, and passed." *Congressional Record, April
15, 1935, pp. 5860–5861.*

"And so the Senate of the United States, on the motion of
the Senator from New York, Royal S. Copeland, a doctor of
medicine and at one time commissioner of health of the city
of New York, recognized 'prayer or spiritual means' as legally
sufficient protection against ophthalmia and blindness in
newborn babies."

Copeland was immune to being poked fun at, although he was in a
more somber mood since the death of his father the previous year, at

ninety-six, an extremely old age for the time. His father, as much as his mother, had always been right at the front cheering him on through the years. Roscoe Copeland called his son "a man of destiny."

Copeland's mind was still focused on trying to find a reliable food, drug, therapeutic device, and cosmetic bill to get behind. In fact, he was already working on a new version. The man of destiny didn't have to wait too long. With enormous and intricate politicking, a version he approved of was passed by the Senate on May 25, 1935. It was an extraordinary victory. The bill was sent to the House of Representatives but was delayed in the House Committee on Interstate and Foreign Commerce for more than a year. Yet, as Copeland explained, "Government is a complicated thing. I don't care whether you are in the legislature or on the Board of Aldermen. The real work is done in the committees."

One of his Senate biographies noted that "Dr. Copeland is a typical representative of what industry, perseverance, and the ability to acquire friends can accomplish."

TWELVE

"A Very Great Advance"

T HE AMA had plenty to say about the stalled "Copeland bill." An editorial in its December 31, 1935, *JAMA* said that the bill had too many "loopholes and evidences of weakness in its administrative provisions, particularly with reference to drugs, including 'patent' " ones, and urged the house subcommittee to "develop a bill free from such defects." The AMA reported that "for drugs, three private organizations are to have similar authority; namely the United States Pharmacopeia Convention, Inc., the American Institute of Homeopathy, and the American Pharmaceutical Association." The American Institute of Homeopathy? *What?*

Copeland had sneaked in his dream, his beliefs, and Hahnemann's vision. To do so had been one of his objectives all along. *The Homeopathic Pharmacopeia* could become part of the new law. Homeopathy could become "legal."

For thirty years, it had been in the back of his mind to attempt to do this, and it was one of the reasons he acted the part of an invisible (or hidden) homeopath. He had managed to slide his pharmacopoeia into the bill quietly and seamlessly, and even as the AMA criticized its inclusion, it at first did so with abstruse language about how drugs and devices (read homeopathic remedies and drugless healing) will have no "standards of soundness and potency." Later, in its twenty-four-page analysis of the bill, the AMA was not so abstruse: "So far as is known, the fact that the Pure Food and Drug Act of 1906, for the past thirty years, has not officially recognized *The Homeopathic Pharmacopeia* has caused no trouble. No edition of that pharmacopeia has been published since 1914.

What motivates the proposed recognition now of such an archaic volume it is impossible to understand. The situation is not improved by the provision that an agency not named in the bill, but easily identified as the American Institute of Homeopathy, is to be authorized to publish from time to time 'supplements' to this pharmacopeia."

The AMA concluded that Copeland's bill would "tend to facilitate the fraudulent practice of drugless healing, favoring particularly chiropractic," and that "osteopaths, naturopaths, optometrists, chiropodists, and midwives" would be allowed to assert their "medical opinion." The AMA strenuously objected that drugs or devices "not supported by demonstrable scientific facts" would be accepted in the bill as true. In other words, homeopathic remedies would be acceptable and "true" under the law if the Copeland bill passed the House in its present form. Homeopathic remedies would receive legal status as legitimate drugs. (In fact, both homeopathic and standard drugs would benefit from the bill, even though there were no requirements that the drugs be effective.)

The burden of proof for the safety of products now lay on the manufacturer, a critical change. The remedies, as listed in *The Homeopathic Pharmacopeia,* wouldn't need to undergo testing for safety and performance, because if they were listed they were considered safe. All the manufacturer had to prove was that the drug was listed in either pharmacopeia and formulated according to its standards. New drugs were required to have "adequate testing" before going on the market, a directive that didn't affect homeopathy, since most of the remedies were not new and had been in use for years. It seemed as if Copeland had succeeded in doing, as a fellow homeopath once said he would, "something militant, and at the same time, diplomatic" for his cause, a cause most other homeopaths believed he had abandoned long ago.

The AMA struck in every direction it could, especially at an amendment concerning misbranding that Copeland had added (and obtained unanimous consent of the Senate for), which was basically a further safeguard for homeopathic remedies. The amendment stated, "Much criticism has been launched at this provision on the ground that it applied to innocuous drugs for which extravagant therapeutic claims are made and which thus indirectly impair the patient's chance of recovery through his postponement of proper methods of treatment. The language does not relate to such products"—outright fraudulent products, that is. The amendment went on, "It applies only to potent drugs which are per se harmful unless properly administered" (i.e., specific standard medications and homeopathic remedies). The AMA argued that "a drug not in itself inherently dangerous, may, under the provisions of this bill as construed by the Senate committee, be lawfully labeled and advertised for the scattering of 'lumps in the breast,' although by its use diagnosis and rational treatment are delayed and the patient dies of cancer when an early operation would have saved her life."

Despite the AMA's qualms, homeopathy had found a savior in Royal Copeland. Meanwhile, in the May 30, 1936, issue of *JAMA,* the director of the AMA's Bureau of Legal Medicine and Legislation had even more to say. Dr. William Woodward urged his readers to write and telegraph their senators and representative not to pass the bill in its present form. (President Roosevelt had said somewhat cryptically that the bill "produces, I fear, a contrary result.") Woodward called the bill "unsound and deceptive," and reiterated that "midwives, osteopaths, chiropodists, chiropractors, pharmacists, nurses, optometrists and others of similar types are not members of the medical profession" and thus do not constitute the "medical opinion" necessary to assume responsibility for the purity and integrity of drugs.

While the bill remained in committee, the Bureau of Legal Medicine asked the American Naturopathic Association (ANA) to help in a survey it was conducting in 1937 on the qualifications of naturopathic schools. (The following year, the National Association of Naturopathic Herbalists of America was organized, giving the AMA even more to worry about.) Although the AMA said the ANA offered very little assistance, the AMA managed to find out on its own that "there was no school in the United States that confined its teachings to naturopathy, but that naturopathy was just something extra thrown in with a chiropractic course or with a general course in drugless healing." The AMA decided that "the designation 'naturopathic' seems to be another meaningless name or tag under which a lot of self-styled drugless physicians with very little knowledge of the care and cure of human ills get before the public as being qualified to practice some recognized branch of the healing arts."

The year before, the Medical Society of New York published a booklet on the attitude of standard doctors to chiropractic theory. A professor of anatomy at the University of Michigan said the doctrines made no sense and that surgery was the only means of treatment for the conditions that chiropractors said they could heal. Dr. Harvey Cushing of Yale said, "There is no pathological basis for the theory of chiropractic, and it is silly to allude to it as a science." Doctors at Columbia University, the

Mayo Clinic, and the University of Pennsylvania used words like "nebulous," "vague," "charlatanism," and "a real danger." The AMA would determine that, "without exception, all the chiropractic schools are business institutions run for the profit of their owners. Most of them fairly reek of commercialism."

The AMA later acknowledged that the "one or two homeopathic schools that are still in existence"—Hahnemann in Philadelphia and New York Homeopathic—"teach modern medicine rather than homeopathy." "Modern" meant teaching all the up-to-date scientific facts. This had always been true in those two schools, of course, as it had been with many of the other homeopathic colleges. But Hahnemann and New York Homeopathic were now almost completely indistinguishable from a standard medical school, a circumstance that gratified Royal Copeland, his public stance on separate but equal homeopathic colleges notwithstanding.

AMERICANS CONTINUED to ask for nonstandard means of healing. In the mid-thirties an English homeopath, Edward Bach, MD, devised what he called "the first precise system of soul healing based on medicines extracted from the flowering parts of plants." A bacteriologist, Bach used "mother tinctures" to create thirty-eight remedies meant to affect emotions. They included crab apple, for shame; holly, for jealousy; honeysuckle, for homesickness; pine, for guilt; wild oat, for uncertainty; impatiens, for impatience.

Many people started using the word "aromatherapy" after it was first adopted in 1937, even though the healing properties of plant and flower oils and vapors had been known for centuries, and aromatherapy was an ancient technique. Eclectic teas made of seeds and herbs continued to be popular in the country, especially after the introduction of tea bags in 1904. In 1936, the AMA was queried by a high-school teacher about a tea called Lion Cross Herb Tea. The teacher was told that the tea contained the following ingredients: anise, coriander, caraway, fennel seeds, peppermint, senna, ash, *Rhus rad.* leaves, licorice, altnea root, saffron, Arnica, Calendula, lavender flowers, peach, sassafras bark, couch grass, and juniper berries. "Such a mixture as this is usually called a 'shot-gun' mixture," the AMA reported, "which is about what the name implies, hoping that one of the ingredients will bring about a desired or anticipated result. Undoubtedly, the chief effect of this stuff will be that of a laxative and a diuretic, the senna furnishing the former and the couch grass and juniper berries the latter." The AMA said that "there are many people, especially among the ignorant, who are strong for herb teas; if they can make a brew that will move their bowels and stimulate their kidneys, they think the product must be good." (Herbal medicine, which used full-strength herbs as therapy, was still prevalent, although not as favored as the teas.)

Other less benign teas also concerned the AMA, and anyone else interested in curbing unquestionably fraudulent products. "Photo-Synthetic Tea" and "Flowering Herb Tea" were made up entirely of ground-up weeds. Many more teas contained alcohol (not mentioned on the label) or iodine, petroleum, and chalk, also not noted on the labels. (In 1897, the Tea Importation Act had been established to monitor the quality—not the safety—of imported teas.)

Copeland used what spare time he had, "those few odd moments," doing what he loved to do when he wasn't talking or politicking— namely, write. In 1935, he had published *Doctor Copeland's Home Medical Book,* advertised as "a new kind of health book." It revealed his controversial and contradictory nature as no other publication by him had before. He didn't say he was a homeopath (just as his newspaper columns didn't), although in a few cases he recommended certain widely used homeopathic remedies—for example, suggesting Belladonna be given for hives and other skin troubles, or Aconite for earaches. He also suggested that "vapor of chloroform relieves some ear aches as if by magic." He was combining what he considered the best of both schools of medicine. Most of his medical suggestions involved common (and mellow) standard remedies, including many herbals. For asthma, he recommended a hot footbath, drinking strong hot coffee, or the inhalation of "fumes from burning blotting paper which has been dipped in a solution of saltpeter" (potassium nitrate). For chills and cold, he suggested drinking hot unsweetened lemonade. For cramps, he advised tincture of ginger and/or essence of peppermint ("well-diluted"), or sometimes a soapy enema. For toothaches, "oil of clove." For cuts, mercurochrome or iodine. As always, he recommended avoiding aspirin, saying its constant use was "dangerous." He was opposed to cathartics, as well, saying they were too "violent." He prescribed as a doctor, not necessarily a homeopath. Above all other advice, he insisted that the reader should "consult a doctor who will prescribe in proper dosage." The latter was an important consideration because Copeland didn't believe in—and never had believed in—prescribing homeopathic remedies without first seeing if they "fit" the symptoms of the patient. He had always followed this rule as much as "like cures like." He advised that "regarding your health train yourself to accept as gospel what your doctors tell you." In other words, let the doctor see your symptoms and prescribe, preferably homeopathic remedies.

Home remedies, he wrote, can often "do more harm than good." "Early attention" from a doctor "may save serious trouble." A cold, he wrote, "should be recognized as a warning. It is one of Nature's danger signals." And, he also counseled, "do not neglect an ear ache. Consult a doctor as soon as possible." As for pain, especially nerve pain, he wrote, "keep in mind that the seat of trouble could be somewhere else than in the spot where it seems to be located. For example, there may be a pain in the sole of the foot when its exciting cause is in the middle of the body."

He stressed that infections were the result of germs and often advised readers to see their family doctors about vaccines. He said that "although we have made great advances in our knowledge of antiseptics and modern surgery, in certain places there is amazing ignorance of their importance. There are persons who place spider webs, cuds of tobacco, or soot on fresh cuts. I have heard of some who still employ raw oysters, salt pork, or boiled onions as a means of 'removing the poison' from an infected wound." He was in favor of looking into "the recent use of vitamins" in certain infections, and was in favor, especially during the winter months, of taking haliver oil and/or cod-liver oil for vitamin A. He believed that "the circulation of the brain is influenced by toxins or poisons," and, he wrote, "fever is regarded nowadays as the body's natural way of ridding itself of infection." He now hypothesized that the tonsils might be what he termed the "gateway of admission for germs of disease" and, like many doctors, often recommended the surgical removal of the tonsils. Still, he said that "although no one can escape contact with germs, the body is armed with powers of resistance to disease." And, he concluded, "while we do not know all about these powers, if they are intact and kept so by right living, right eating, and observance of proper rules of hygiene, the body can fight off all the germs it is likely to meet." He said the strength and forms of germs depend a lot "upon the degree of weakness of the human tissue." He spoke "homeopathically," without using any of the classic terms. He didn't need to. For him, homeopathy was firmly embedded in American medicine, and had become part of the mainstream.

In general, the *Home Medical Book* was more a description of various illnesses than anything else, and, more often than not, if Copeland wasn't telling the reader to seek out a physician, he was recommending naturopathic remedies—rest, cleanliness, cold or hot compresses, fresh air, sunshine, and "plenty of water."

The few remaining homeopaths, most of whom were purists who followed strictly the treatment of each symptom separately, as well as the use of extreme dilutions and shakings, didn't understand Copeland's point of view, and they were particularly offended by his saying in the introduction that the purpose of the book was "to tell in simple language how to relieve pain and what to do to prevent or to cure some of the many ailments which are likely to invade every home . . . advice, which if followed, may add years to your life." How could the word "homeopathy" not be uttered in this instance, they wondered? But Copeland was not going to single out *any* specialty of medicine. As he said, he was writing for "this age of scientific understanding." He also rankled homeopaths in his concluding section, called "Right Living," when he said that "there are cults and schools of thought teaching that everything depends on the mind and its operation. There is much that verifies this belief. Of course, I cannot go as far as many of my friends." Yet he did attribute illness to the miasm (once again without saying so directly) when he wrote that Christian Scientists "talk much about 'error.' While I may not use the word in quite the sense they do, yet I believe it to be true that most of our illnesses come from wrong habits or wrong acts of some sort. In short, they have their origin in error."

What Copeland had accomplished was to bring homeopathy into twentieth-century science.

AFTER THE publication of his health book, and in the midst of his most important crusade—the still-unsettled drug bill—Copeland decided to write a book about education and character-building. (He would also soon be appointed chairman of the Senate's Committee on Crime. One of his ideas was to assemble the American equivalent of Scotland Yard—local police forces with intricate command structures similar to those of the FBI.)

Copeland had always managed to spend time at his Suffern house, where, in the summer, he now generally dressed all in white, a fad among fashionable men, and he always took Senate and other work with him, when he wasn't reading, fishing, horseback-riding, and occasionally mending fences, the real fences that bordered Dexter Manor.

Education had always been a preoccupation. He enlisted the help of a junior-high-school principal in Washington, and after they had finished a first draft together (she did most of the work and considered it her book), Copeland approached the John C. Winston Company, the publisher of his *Home Medical Book.* The publisher sent the book to some experts for evaluation. The news was not good. "The first part of the manuscript by Copeland is an amateurish approach to the problem conceived in the old-fashioned rubric of doing good," one report said, adding that "the author advertises his approach in terms of his background, especially in medicine and through his radio advertising in other ways. He apparently is in bad taste in introducing this personal note. The very first paragraph of his first chapter begins by personal advertising, and the same element is introduced from time to time." The manuscript was also criticized for lacking "specific facts," for being "unrealistic," for being based on "wishful thinking," and for taking "too negative" an approach. Another report praised Copeland's ideas (he believed that America's greatest social problem was juvenile delinquency) but said the writing itself was "sadly bungled" and that it was "a series of long notes going to no final point." Copeland managed to get into the book many of his favorite medical themes—that insanity can be caused by an infected colon, that "growing pains" are caused by "localized infection," that ignoring symptoms of tonsillitis can lead to "decreased mentality," that defective eyesight can "upset the digestion." He urged all students to undergo blood tests to help diagnose any "eccentricities and unconventional attitudes." He also proposed a plan by which all students would receive not only grades, but also critiques of their behavior and attitude.

On March 17, 1937, one of the vice presidents of Winston wrote Copeland that he would consider publishing the book if the senator would drop the school principal as his coauthor and have the book completely rewritten by another writer, someone the publisher had in mind, a writer of "considerable ability." Copeland declined, saying, "I am sick and tired of the whole subject anyhow, and I guess you are." The junior-high-school principal, however, wasn't, and because she considered the manuscript hers anyway, she told Copeland she was hoping to turn part of it into a series of magazine articles. Copeland answered her, "Let's not be discouraged. Everything new and unconventional always distresses the fossilized." It is not known if any magazine articles resulted from the aborted book.

That year, Frances Copeland also decided to write a book, which was published as *Mrs. Copeland's Guest Book.* It contained detailed recommendations for both hosts and guests—for example, to serve guests their breakfast tray on time so as not to give them time to smoke, "because it was bad for their health"; or to provide blankets in soft colors, and always to offer an extra quilt. In a discussion of parties, Mrs. Copeland wrote that one of her favorites was what she called "a kitchen party," at the end of dancing parties, where she served pancakes, eggs, and coffee.

She offered no medical advice, except this: "A great authority" (presumably the senator) says that "all pre-breakfast activities are a strain on the system, including, of course, getting up!" She offered a lot of practical advice, like "order, in a way, is a strength . . . a plea for everything in its place . . . 'order is Heaven's first law.' " Her husband found the time to edit the manuscript and made many subtle changes. In a discussion of table settings, he suggested changing "embarrassing" to "distressing," and even modified "guests" to "principals." In a paragraph mentioning their daughter-in-law, he substituted "charming girl" for "lovely girl." When Mrs. Copeland disclosed that she would refer to her husband throughout the text as "Doctor," because, she said, "I do not like the use of 'my husband' as a name," Copeland added the word "constant" before "use," so the sentence would read "I do not like the constant use of 'my husband' as a name."

That year, her husband accepted a challenge no one ever believed he would. After all, like many of his colleagues, he was stretched beyond endurance, and he had recently told the Senate that he "saw death written on the faces of some of his associates unless they rest soon." But he was drafted for a new office. He was asked by Republican leaders to run for mayor of New York City in both the Republican and Democratic primaries because the leaders didn't like the pro–New Deal inclinations of Fiorello LaGuardia. He accepted because the unconventional situation provided him with exactly the kind of circumstances he liked and excelled at: controversy and attention.

It was a hard and often ugly campaign. Copeland was frequently attacked as a "stuffed stethoscope." He called LaGuardia "the nominee of the Communists," and in retaliation was labeled "an ally of Adolf Hitler."

He lost in both primaries, partly because WPA workers were fearful of losing their jobs if they voted for him. As Copeland himself explained, "Unless I attacked the New Deal daily I could not attract Republican votes; if I did attack it I was sure to alienate men and women calling themselves Democrats, but who believed in things utterly foreign to Democratic traditions and ideals."

His supporters began to ask, Had Royal Copeland run his course?

In 1937, the Copeland bill received some unforeseen help. After 107 people, many of them children, died from a poisonous ingredient in "Elixir Sulfanilamide," Congress finally hurried the bill to passage. (A chemist, who later committed suicide, had added an untested solvent to the sulfa in order to create a liquid form of the drug.)

The bill now included a directive that labels must post all active ingredients and offer warnings about using the drugs under certain conditions, for instance, drugs intended for diagnosing certain illnesses or for weight reduction. For the first time ever, labels had to read "Use by instruction from physicians only." The bill, which levied fines and court injunctions, demanded "reasonable" sanitation in the production of all food, drugs, and cosmetics.

A new era of long-overdue improved consumer safety began when the Copeland bill—a revision of the Tugwell bill—was passed on June 2, 1938. It contained compromises, but it was still considered a good piece of legislation for Americans. In addition, the bill ushered in a renewed future for homeopathy, although most people didn't yet fully understand that aspect, and wouldn't for years to come.

As Copeland wrote of his bill, "The law has clearly been extended by supervision over cosmetics and devices. Careful provisions are present for the introduction of new drugs." Production could be stopped "where products become contaminated with micro-organisms injurious to health." The entrepreneur in Copeland, too, was pleased that "procedurally, the law is written so as not to harass business. Full notices and hearings are provided." He was unusually modest in saying, "We now have a law of which we can be proud. It marks a very great advance, probably beyond that of any other country in the world." It was, of

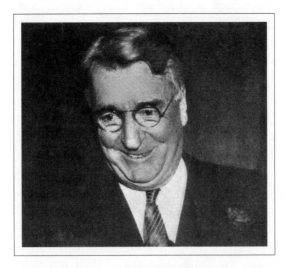

Copeland's smile shows that the long struggle to get his
historically important bill passed was worth the wait.

course, a massive achievement, a bold (but not yet flawless) safeguard for
American consumers.

Copeland was shrewd enough not to draw attention to the inclusion
of the *Homeopathic Pharmacopoeia,* and, in fact, in a speech delivered
before the bill was passed, he referred only to the *United States Pharmacopoeia.* But his message was clear when he said that the "pharmacopoeia
of the United States and similar publications have had a large part in the
promotion of health and the extension of life." It was, of course, the
"similar publications" that mattered the most to him: the *Homeopathic
Pharmacopoeia.* In another speech, he crossed out the word "sympathetic" in the line "In the course of my observations I have come to have
a sympathetic understanding of some of the difficulties enforcement officers are faced with in adapting to the needs of this modern generation a
statute framed to take care of the conditions of thirty years ago."
Unadorned understanding was good enough in this battle. Hyperbole
had its place, but not here, not at this moment.

ON THE morning of June 17, 1938, Copeland, who had been quietly
struggling with a serious kidney illness for many months, tried to get out
of bed. He said to his wife that he just couldn't open his eyes. "I'm so

tired," he told her, unable to get up. His colleagues had seen signs of strain in his face during the weeks preceding the passage of his bill, and a few hours before the 75th Congress was to adjourn the day before, he had, for just about the first time in his career, left the Senate floor early. At the urging of the Capitol physician, he had returned to his apartment at the Shoreham Hotel. In fact, his family doctor had wanted him to remain home that day and even several days before, but against medical advice Copeland had gotten dressed and gone to the Hill. Besides the new Food and Drug bill, there were other Senate matters he was involved with. He was in the midst of helping to get $325 million to improve the rivers and harbors in the country. He was trying to get an amendment to the Public Works Administration funds. He was seeking to improve subsidized ship construction in the nation. He had successfully introduced a bill to turn the Saratoga Battlefield in upstate New York into a national park. He was investigating airplane safety. He was helping to carve out an Equal Rights Amendment.

After he had left the Senate floor on June 16, he had worked the telephones from his bed at home, and helped ready a bill concerning firearms. He had telegrammed his son on June 13 that he was unable to attend a ceremony honoring Junior, or "Buster," as he was affectionately called in the family, because "Pop" is "still slaving in Senate Committee." On June 12, he had attended a meeting of the AIH, held in Philadelphia. The week before, the senator had visited Dexter to attend an alumni dinner for the high school (the new auditorium had been named after his father), and he was also present at the mortgage-burning ceremony for the Dexter Methodist Church.

Copeland's condition weakened during the day of June 17, and he slipped into a coma around 4 P.M. His wife, his son, his homeopathic physician, Dr. Harry M. Kaufman, and the Capitol physician, Dr. George W. Calver, were by his side when he died at 7:45 P.M. He was sixty-nine. The cause was classified as "circulatory collapse" at the time, although the *Evening Star* in Washington called it a heart attack. His doctor said he had been "a victim of the overwork and congressional strain against which he often had cautioned his colleagues."

An obituary in the *New York Tribune* mentioned that "he often told his colleagues to avoid excitement and shorten their working day. . . . Senator Copeland had not rested since 1937." Six years earlier, in a speech to the American Hospital Association, he had told his audience, "When the heart flags, then comes fatigue. A tired feeling and a weak heart are often associated." And, he had commented, "by the way, the general public regards the presence of a physician in political life as something unusual and even grotesque. I don't know why this should be the popular idea, because, after all, good government consists in the last analysis in the maintenance of good health on the part of the body politic."

He had maintained all his Senate business and had achieved his goal for homeopathy—"his crowning achievement," he told his colleague, junior New York Senator Robert F. Wagner.

But he forgot to take proper care of himself.

COPELAND'S DEATH shocked his friends and enemies alike, who telegrammed and phoned his widow messages of sympathy and support. President Roosevelt, Vice President John N. Garner, New York Governor Herbert Lehman, New York Mayor Fiorello LaGuardia, Postmaster General James A. Farley. Senator after senator. Congressman after congressman. Aide after aide. Worker after worker. Mrs. Copeland received more than 3,000 letters of condolence.

His death was marked by front-page notices, and editorial writers around the country wrote movingly of him. The *Grand Rapids Herald* mirrored what many others reluctantly concluded: "Senator Copeland's death is a restatement of that old adage 'Do as I say, Not as I do.' " Everyone seemed to understand that he had worked himself to death.

The whole of Dexter mourned its "worthy son" and "leading crusader-physician." At a local memorial service, the senior senator from Michigan, Arthur Vandenberg, spoke of his close friendship with "one of the great men of his time," who "died upon the battle-line of public service." And, he remarked to the packed auditorium, "never was he so happy and care-free as when he would cross over to my Senate desk and tell me, as he did repeatedly each year, that he was 'leaving for Dexter' in a few hours."

Even *JAMA* ran a polite obituary on June 25. It read like a curriculum vitae, containing not a single adjective, positive or negative. Copeland's last newspaper column ran on the same day as that obituary. It was titled "Skin Reveals Conditions of Body." Just two weeks before Copeland's death, the AMA had repeated to a correspondent a version of its line that "the homeopathy of Hahnemann is as dead as a last year's bird nest." If he could have, Copeland would have had a good laugh over that one.

But he also might have been a little concerned. Would homeopathy develop as a science and take advantage of what he called "the revelations of the laboratory?" Would homeopathy "not ignore the work of our friends of the other school?" Would homeopaths continue to obtain proper medical degrees? Would homeopathy, "a branch of positive philosophy," live up to the "crowning achievement" he had made?

For many people, it would seem that the AMA was right in stating that homeopathy was "as dead as a last year's bird nest." Certainly, even the remaining homeopaths would agree with another AMA statement, first made in 1934, that "homeopathy is rapidly dying out." After all, Hahnemann Hospital in Philadelphia closed in 1938, even though homeopathy as an elective continued to be offered at the medical school into the 1940s. (Copeland had been particularly proud of the honorary degree he had received from Hahnemann in 1921.) In New York, the Homeopathic Medical College and Flower Hospital merged with Fifth Avenue Hospital in 1938, and the college became known as New York Medical College. There was no longer anything homeopathic in its name. By the mid-forties, there were no strictly homeopathic colleges left in America. Had Copeland still been alive, he would have fought hard for homeopathy to become an intrinsic part of the curriculum at all medical schools in the country. Indeed, eight years after his death, the new leaders proposed such a plan at a meeting of the AIH. They also suggested changing the name of homeopathy to "homeotherapy." (Many homeopaths would not favor that route, and, not wanting to blend in with standard medicine, would continue to direct their attention to promoting postgraduate courses offered through the American Foundation for Homeopathy.) Still, the AIH prevailed, and in the late 1940s, the American Board of Homeotherapeutics was created, and its membership decided to seek recognition from the AMA for homeotherapeutics to become a subspecialty of internal medicine and for it to become an authorized course in medical schools. But the AMA would not consider such a proposal.

In fact, at the same time the AMA ran the obituary of Copeland, it also endorsed a harsh report from its Judicial Council on "association with cultists." The report stated that "some of our members are giving lectures in osteopathic and optometric schools and addresses before their societies. Some members are associated by a common waiting room in offices with them. Some members are by mutual agreement professional associates principally in the field of surgery. There are some instances of partnership in practice. All of these voluntarily associated activities are unethical." The report went on to say that relations with these cultists "do not 'uphold the dignity and honor of [our] vocation; or 'exalt its standards.' " The only time an association might be allowed was in an emergency, and even then, it was essential that the standard doctor let the cultist know that only the doctor of medicine had the necessary competence to solve the difficulty. Consultation with a cultist "was a futile gesture if the cultist is assumed to have the same high grade of knowledge, training, and experience as is possessed by the doctor of medicine." This was a charge that Copeland would have endorsed. Optometrists and the majority of osteopaths didn't have medical-school degrees, and until they did, the AMA rightfully, in his opinion, would consider their training "substandard, incorrect, and harmful to the people because of its deficiencies." Optometrists knew about vision-related concerns, but not much more. Osteopaths knew about bone-related issues, but little more.

Believing it had put homeopathy out to pasture, the AMA went to work in earnest on osteopathy. In 1942, it ruled that osteopathic interns should not be allowed to serve in army hospitals. The following year it decided to develop "suitable means to combat legislative recognition of cultists for participation in medicine and surgery." The targets of this campaign included homeopaths, chiropractors, naturopaths, and osteopaths, and was an attempt to make sure that licenses were given only to "graduates of approved schools." The AMA knew that its authority couldn't enforce such a law, although it wished it could "combat this evil of legislative recognition of cultists." When it came to license requirements, individual state governments legislated the ground rules. By 1931, thirty-nine states had given chiropractors some form of license or other form of recognition. By 1937, twenty-six states allowed osteopaths to practice on identical terms with MDs (although some of these states required further course work and training). Still, osteopaths didn't do well on required written tests because their course work had been less intense, compared with the regular medical-school curriculum. The same was true of chiropractors. In 1940, osteopathic schools began requiring that all entrants have two years of college work. Some states began to issue provisional licenses; still, the whole area of licensure would remain controversial for years.

During the winter of 1942, the AMA told a woman asking about naturopaths, osteopaths, and chiropractors that these practices were not considered to be in the field of medicine, saying, as it had done once before, that "the idea that all diseases can be cured through massage is ridiculous." The AMA's Bureau of Investigation then reminded the letter-writer that the AMA was the national organization only of doctors of medicine. "We would not have any confidence in the treatments proposed by a naturopath, and for one to claim that naturopathy is farther advanced than osteopathy or chiropractic is, in the opinion of this bureau, both ridiculous and meaningless." The bureau said that the only license it recognized was one issued by the state "to engage in the practice of medicine and surgery." Some "cult" practitioners, in order to obtain credentials, began to tell state governing boards that they used X-ray therapy "and other curative agents," but most were informed, nevertheless, that they were "encroaching upon the practice of medicine without being qualified so to do."

The early forties saw a rise in several other practices that the AMA was reluctant to embrace: dance therapy, once called "Medical Gymnastics," and "Rythmo-Specialty," which was first used on psychotic patients, and then on schizophrenics, as well as on war-scarred soldiers returning from World War II battlefields, and an electromagnetic touch therapy called polarity therapy. This therapy was developed by an American naturopath, chiropractor, and osteopath who used many ideas from ancient East Indian Ayurvedic medicine, a system of healing that includes diet—herbs and raw foods, especially honey, as well as properly cooked fruits and vegetables—cleansing of the body's toxins, massages, and yoga exercises. Polarity therapy involved energy flow, and its proponents believed that disease and pain were caused when the body's energy was unbalanced or blocked completely. (Reflexology, a form of total body healing involving the massaging of the feet, had been developed in the early 1930s, although the technique had ancient origins and connections to Chinese acupuncture, which used pressure points on the body to heal and relieve pain.) From the late 1800s into the 1940s, music therapy became an important healing tool, especially in hospitals.

Another pivotal piece of legislature—a signature of the New Deal—had been passed in 1935. The Social Security Act assured every American of an old-age pension. It did not include health insurance legislation, which had been considered. Most American doctors, and particularly the AMA, fearing what they called socialized medicine, opposed such insurance as being unfair to doctors and patients. The doctors dreaded government meddling in their affairs, although the American College of Surgeons at first supported mandatory health care insurance. But the AMA kept up a steady stream of protest to defeat the inclusion of health insurance under Social Security benefits. Since the end of World War II, health insurance, along with pensions, was offered to workers by some companies; in 1940 one in every ten persons was covered, and by 1945 one in five. The AMA finally agreed to noncompulsory group hospital insurance plans as long as the county medical societies monitored them. By the late forties, the private health insurance industry was thriving, and people were visiting their doctors more and more.

ONE OF the most crucial changes in American medicine occurred in 1941, when penicillin was finally purified and proved safe as an antibiotic for human use. This conclusive work was done by a German scientist and a group of English biologists, and further advances on the drug's production were accomplished in America during World War II. (By 1945, the year the war ended, American manufacturers were making 650 billion units of penicillin. Death from pneumonia occurred in less than 1 percent of the population during World War II, as opposed to 18 percent during World War I.) Diseases that had been plaguelike and were not helped by sulfa were eradicated in no time at all. Pneumococcal pneumonia. Syphilis. Gonorrhea. Meningitis. Gangrene. Rheumatic fever. Some staphylococcal and streptococcal infections. Even tonsillitis. Penicillin was called "the wonder drug," and to millions of Americans it was a miracle drug. It was effective, not poisonous, and was used in a dilute solution (almost like a homeopathic remedy).

In 1945, streptomycin became available. This antibiotic, produced by the bacillus streptomyces, effectively wiped out both tuberculosis and the plague. The world of germs would never be the same again. Cures were fast and lasting. Americans now besieged their doctors for antibiotics just the way they had once demanded homeopathic remedies. Surgery became even easier with advances in anesthesia and the emergence of muscle relaxers, and safer because of antibiotics. In gynecology, the Pap smear for the early detection of cancer was developed. Lifesaving kidney dialysis came into use. Cortisone, a steroid used for certain inflammatory and autoimmune illnesses, became available in the late forties, as did the first lens implants for cataracts. Psychiatric theories became more accepted in the country, especially Freud's theory of the unconscious, and the transference of the patient's underlying emotional difficulties to the analyst, which were then worked through in sessions often lasting years.

In 1947, the president of the American Naturopathic Association said his "separate school of healing" had "no use for sulfa, penicillin, and all that rubbish." He explained that these drugs "just prevent fever from doing its work. We *like* fever. When the body is healthy, it's a normal state, but when the body is diseased, that's a normal state, too—normal for a diseased body. See what I mean?" But now most people didn't see what he meant. He said that naturopaths "don't believe in vaccination, inoculation, contagion, infection, or drugs of any kind," and once again affirmed that germs do not cause disease. He added that only "a lot of crazy people" believe that they do.

But the tide seemed to be turning against these practitioners. People believed in antibiotics now. Naturopaths exhibited at one of their meetings a "spinalator," which was "a large, coffin-shaped apparatus" that allowed "spinal manipulation without manual labor." The public became confused and annoyed instead of intrigued. A memo written in 1944 by the AMA's Bureau of Legal Medicine and Legislation said that of the fifty naturopathic and chiropractic schools it knew of, "very few have even one adequately trained teacher on the faculty, and there are probably less than five expert all-time teachers in the entire lot of fifty institutions." The AMA also said that "not one of the schools actually enforces a matriculation requirement of even five minutes of high school study." It further reported that none of the schools was connected to "any worthy hospital," and, most important, "there is not one of these schools that does not ignore or even avowedly oppose the scientific point of view and the facts of medical science accepted by the authorities of the entire civilized world." These observations reflected the continuing clash between scientific methods and nonscientific methods. Well into the 1940s, the AMA documented such quackeries as a kidney disease cure said to be derived from the lymph glands of goats, an external cream for the cure of tuberculosis, a hypnotic cure for diabetes, and an "astro-bio-chemical" cure for asthma. The nonstandard practitioners claimed that as long as their patients got better, an investigation into how or why they got better shouldn't be a major concern.

CONTROLLED CLINICAL studies were established in the mid- to late forties as the "gold standard" for judging the validity of all medical treatment. This kind of study eliminated subjective conclusions based on the interpretations of the doctor or the patient. (Bad news for homeopathic provings—Copeland's "cloud of witnesses.")

In controlled studies, one group of patients received the drug under investigation and another received either a placebo (an inactive "pill"), another drug entirely, or sometimes no drug at all. The patients in the study, all with parallel symptoms, were randomly assigned to the groups. In the 1950s, the studies began to be "blinded"; in a single-blind test only the researchers knew who was receiving the real drug, and in a double-blind test no one knew—neither the patients nor the scientists doing the test and analysis.

Controlled studies had been used periodically since the turn of the century, although one involving the citrus treatment of a group of British sailors for scurvy, a once-fatal disease now known to be the result of a vitamin C deficiency, was first recorded in 1747. The AMA conducted a double-blind study in 1911, yet most of the studies were not blinded or randomized and didn't use placebos. (Recognition of the placebo as an effective control began in the 1930s, and the first actual trial of its effects was done in 1950.)

Copeland had lectured to his medical colleagues about homeopathic research, most of it originating in Europe. He had been particularly impressed with the 1908 high-potency work of the Spanish scientist M. Cahis, but this work with strychnine had never been duplicated. Copeland generally kept abreast of such research, even when he was in the Senate. He had heard of the work of the Egyptologist who conducted tests on extreme dilutions in 1928; the zoologists who conducted studies in 1923, 1925, 1927, and 1929; and the 1930s work by French, British, and American biochemists on enzymes.

In the 1940s, further clinical work on potencies was done by British bacteriologists and biochemists, as well as by two French botanists. German and French physicists did studies in the early and late 1940s. But this work wasn't being done by Americans, so it was hardly reported on or noticed at all by doctors of medicine in the United States. However, word about certain trials being performed in England and Scotland during World War II had gotten around; these tests involved the treatment of mustard-gas burns using not only mustard gas itself in a 30C potency, but also *Rhus tox.* and Potassium Dichromate, or *Kali bich.*, a remedy first proved in 1844 for the treatment of mucus discharge.

After the AMA rejected homeopathy as a subspecialty of internal medicine, the homeopaths were once again the outsiders, a status many homeopaths and other doctors would say they favored anyway. But Copeland had once told the AMA's Council on Public Health that "it is the outsider who feels that everything is wrong; take him in and he soon absorbs the spirit and the ideals of the majority." The remaining homeopaths didn't want any such absorption because they felt that their way was the only way.

Most medical doctors in America were in the process of becoming specialists of one kind or another—internists, pediatricians, obstetricians, and gynecologists. Those medical doctors who used homeopathy were scarcer than ever, and those who began studying it even scarcer— a few hundred out of the more than 5,000 medical-school graduates per year in the 1940s.

Several years before his death, Copeland had written about homeopathy: "It is an unfortunate fact that, in spite of a hundred years of practical use of this method, there is still much misunderstanding of its exact place in the practice of medicine." By including the *Homeopathic Pharmacopeia* in his final bill, he had left homeopathy an ideal legacy—not one just from the past, but one for the future. Now the leaders needed to take advantage of this gift and find homeopathy's "exact place" in modern medicine.

THIRTEEN

"Scientific Rule"

T HE WEATHER in the nation's capital was unusually cool for late June. Temperatures were in the low seventies; the sky was clear, almost cloudless. Inside a downtown Washington hotel that surrounded a fourteen-story glass atrium, thirty or so homeopaths crowded into a small conference room. Outside the room, in a moderate-sized lobby, a dozen tables were filled with books, pamphlets, catalogues, advertisements, software, and other items—including mugs and T-shirts—for sale or as giveaways. Also for sale were plenty of remedies—in pellet, liquid, spray, and cream form. One brochure from a laboratory advertised "Nosodes," or "potentized homeopathic remedies prepared from diseased tissue" that "contain no active organisms and are quite safe." Among the thirty available, sold in "various C potencies" were "Diphtherinum," "Influenzinum," "Mononucleosis," and "Morbillinum" (measles). This same lab also promoted over three hundred "Allergens," advertised as "derived from the antigens that induce an immune response in normal individuals who suffer from outdoor and other allergies." Allergens such as Bananas, Beef, Beer, Butter, Celery, American Cheese, Chocolate, Clam, House Dust, Mattress Dust, Ham, Honeydew, Lobster, Rice, Stinging Insects, Strawberry, Sunflower, and Wine were all available in 6X, 12X, or 30X dilutions. Also advertised were "Organotherapy Condition Protocols," which used "homeopathic forms of healthy organ tissues to treat dysfunctional organs"; there was "Colon Mucosa 4C" for constipation, "Pancreas 4C" for diabetes and prediabetes states, and "Veinous Wall 4C" for hemorrhoids. At another table, a demonstration of a small computerlike device was in progress; a brochure explained that the apparatus—"Meridian Stress Assessment (MSA)—used "electro-magnetic energy" that could "identify allergic substances and help choose the appropriate, optimal treatment dilution." The brochure said that "a low voltage electrical charge is introduced into the body, and the precise level of electric current conducted through the acupuncture points are measured." It further stated that "many double-blind studies have been done using this technology" and that the machine was primarily used in Europe.

Most standard doctors consider all such measuring instruments unscientific, having no diagnostic value at all because, as they see it, they are basically jazzed-up galvanometers that measure electrical resistance of the skin and are unable to identify allergic substances and remedies. Critics believe these machines should be confiscated by the government, and the practitioners prosecuted. (The FDA has been pushing for years to get some of the devices off the market—through warnings for false advertising, outright banning, and a few actual prosecutions.) The MSA brochure (and Web site) made no mention of FDA approval.

Inside "Plenary Room B," plastic chairs were lined up in neat rows. Small crystal lights embedded in mirrored disks crisscrossed a beige-colored ceiling. A young woman dressed in a long blue-and-white-checkered jumper with a short white puffy-sleeved blouse tucked inside, a white caplike scarf on her head, and white shoes worn with little white socks, checked badges and gave out booklets to everyone entering the room. She looked for all the world like Alice in Wonderland. But the participants were not going Down a Rabbit Hole or Seeking Advice from a Caterpillar. This was not a Mad-Hatter's Tea Party; this was the Fifth Scientific Symposium of the Homeopathic Research Network.

Copeland's decades-old observation that homeopaths "have a common cause and a common enemy" resonated in the room, as did his turn-of-the-century judgment that there needed to be a reproving of the remedies by expert diagnosticians, chemists, and pathologists. Overheard were comments like "We do not have a level playing field in homeopathy," or "There's a lot of politics, and politics is not science," or "We just have to keep pushing, and the truth will come out." All these remarks were similar to those that had been spoken about homeopathy, well, forever, even though the papers about to be delivered were new: "Homeopathic Research: A Challenge and an Opportunity"; "Statistical Analysis of Homeopathic Drug Proving"; "Homeopathic Treatment of Acute Otitis Media in Children—A Preliminary Randomized Placebo-Controlled Study"; "Using EEG and EKG Analyses to Detect Subtle Effects of Homeopathic Remedies"; "Homeopathy and Physics"; "The Placebo Response: Implications for Homeopathic Practice and Research."

Homeopathy appeared to be changing; it was becoming more proof-oriented.

The year was 2000.

THE HOMEOPATHIC Research Network was founded in 1993 by Jennifer Jacobs and Michael Carlston, two physicians who were attracted to homeopathy early in their careers.

Jacobs, a petite woman of fifty-five with short hair and glasses, is intense and focused, with a childlike voice that makes her seem more like a camp counselor or a children's librarian than the formidable scientist she is. Carlston, a bearded, sandy-haired man of fifty-one, has the demeanor of a stand-up comedian, although he is soft-spoken and often a mumbler; but he, too, is a passionate physician.

Sometime in the early 1990s, Jacobs had attended a medical meeting in Paris where homeopathic research was discussed; afterward she said she had a eureka moment. "I thought we should do the same thing in the United States." Carlston elaborated: "My idea in proposing the formation of the Homeopathic Research Network to Jennifer was to expand our nearly daily e-mail dialogue about homeopathic research along the lines of primary care research groups in which I had participated for years. Those groups are common in academic departments of family medicine throughout North America." He said that "the original motto was to prove and improve homeopathy (later borrowed by Peter Fisher of the *British Homeopathic Journal*) as we recognized the need to examine our work both for outsiders and insiders."

Jacobs was born and raised in Huntington, West Virginia, a residential and industrial hub on the Ohio River that borders Kentucky and Ohio. In 1842, Charles Dickens described the area that would become Huntington: "The Ohio is a fine broad river. . . . The banks are for the most part deep solitudes . . . unbroken by any sign of human life; nor is anything seen to move about them but the blue jay, whose colour is so bright, and yet so delicate, that it looks like a flying flower."

The only child of a clothing-store manager (he died when she was sixteen) and a clothing-store saleswoman (she died when Jacobs was thirty-five), Jacobs went to Ohio Wesleyan University, where she majored in biology, hoping one day to become a teacher. But, she says, "I saw people around me in premed and I thought, Why not? I was comparable to them," and so she decided to transfer to Wayne State University in Detroit. She graduated in 1972 with a BA in zoology and then went on to Wayne State's medical school, receiving her MD in 1976. While still in medical school, she coauthored a paper, "The Productivity of Women Physicians," that appeared in the October 25, 1976, issue of *JAMA,* and a follow-up paper, "Comparison of the Productivity of Women and Men Physicians," that appeared in the June 6, 1977, issue. She wrote in that journal that her first study "verified that productivity of women physicians is high" and that the second one showed that "despite major responsibilities for the home that most female physicians have, it is apparent that they take little time out from the work force compared to men physicians who do not have those added responsibilities."

After a year and a half of a residency in family practice at Bayfront Medical Center in St. Petersburg, Florida, Jacobs left in 1978 (the year the world's first test-tube baby was born) for Berkeley, California, to pursue an interest in midwifery and home births that she had developed during her residency. She said that Bayfront believed that home birthing was not practicing medicine "up to the standards of the community," and it threatened to take her license away. "It was a rude awakening, and when I first began thinking outside the envelope," she says, adding that "the environment of a community hospital made me realize medicine wasn't what I thought it was." She also began to see disturbing side effects from the various drugs she was prescribing to her patients for problems that were not getting solved, and she began to understand that the "problem was just covered over with all the medicines." She remembers being on call by herself at Bayfront when a man was brought in with his son. "He had had a heart attack," she says. "I gave him all the drugs. I went by the book. His condition became worse as he was given more and more medicine. Standard drugs. I watched him die before my eyes. He would have been better off if he had stayed at home." Jacobs is haunted by this experience.

In California, where home births were more accepted, she heard a lecture by Dr. Robert Schore, a prominent homeopathic physician who specializes in cranial osteopathy. "I had never heard of homeopathy before," Jacobs says, but "it clicked—it made sense, in terms of my worldview—symptoms being part of the body healing itself. . . . It was like a light bulb going on. . . . If you are just treating symptoms, it makes people get sicker. If there's an imbalance in the system, the illness will pop up some place else." She took a course at the International Foundation for Homeopathy (which was founded in 1978 by an MD named Bill Gray, who would later get in trouble with the FDA for allegedly selling a homeopathic product not listed in the *Homeopathic Pharmacopoeia*), and she says she "jumped in with both feet, and haven't done anything else since." She was influenced by other early teachers—George Vithoulkas, Dick Moskowitz, and Corey Weinstein—and finds that homeopathy is particularly effective for treating colds, ear infections, the flu, and fibromyalgia, as well as common allergies, premenstrual syndrome, chronic fatigue syndrome, and skin and gastric disorders. She often treats insomnia with a highly diluted extract of coffee, although she also uses "twenty other remedies, as well." She sometimes treats diaper rash with the highly diluted form of poison ivy—*Rhus tox.*

Michael Carlston grew up in Minneapolis, Minnesota, where his mother owned a sales and repair shop for radios, television sets, and stereophonic equipment. His father was in the navy, and was, Carlston says, "an alcoholic and an underachiever" who died of a heart attack at the age of forty-seven. His mother was "a real driving force," and, he quips, he himself is considered "the reincarnation of my great-grandma's husband," a gifted idealist. While still in high school, Carlston worked as an aide at an inner-city hospital and was disturbed at the sight of "people chained to their beds, like criminals." He received his BA, cum laude, from the University of Minnesota in 1977, where his honors thesis compared the Hippocratic and the Ayurvedic medical oaths. "Both oaths in their dependence on self-enforcement seem very much like religious moral teachings," he wrote. He received his MD from the University of Minnesota's medical school in 1980 and was introduced to homeopathy by Rudolph Ballentine, MD, a noted Ayurvedic practitioner, herbalist, homeopath, psychiatrist, and author, whom he met in a meditation group. From 1981 to 1984, he held a family practice residency at Bethesda Lutheran Medical Center in St. Paul, where he was twice a nominee for Outstanding Resident awards, and also took a one-year postgraduate course in homeopathy at the International Foundation in 1984.

As with Jacobs, an experience he had as a resident left a lasting impression: a patient dying of brain cancer was in great pain, and Carlston told her it was "okay to let go." He said that she then "died within a minute" after permitting her mind to pass that message to her body. He loves "the mystery" of medicine and even "loves that things don't make sense, that things are so rich and beyond our understanding." He says the " 'homeopathic community' is widely disparate—from the docs who use a little arnica without knowing *anything* about homeopathic principles to those who believe like one recently deceased M.D. homeopath that 'research in homeopathy is pointless because it is a spiritual science.' " But Jacobs and Carlston say that homeopathy is much more than spiritual, that it is also scientific, and they are determined to motivate homeopaths to acknowledge that their future depends on investigation, research, and innovation. Carlston admits, though, that "homeopaths tend to listen to patients so well, but to each other so poorly," illustrating once again how little those circumstances have changed in over a hundred years. Certain old battles remain, watched over, it seems, by ghosts of the purists, who do not want things to change from the way Hahnemann managed everything from symptoms to dilutions to shakings, and the moderates, who are willing to make concessions, as well as to incorporate standard medicine into their practices.

Many homeopaths now combine aspects of the purists (for instance, sometimes using only one remedy at a time per individual symptom) and the moderates (sometimes using more than one remedy at a time for a single symptom). But nothing is clear-cut. In 1992, the *Canadian Medical Association Journal* published the results of a clinical trial showing that three selected homeopathic remedies were not effective against plantar warts. In a letter to the editor, Jacobs protested the very approach they were describing, arguing that "the individualized aspect of homeopathy as well as its treatment of the total person rather than of specific symptoms has made it a particularly difficult subject for clinical trials." While she agrees that "individualization is the gold standard in homeopathic practice," she says it is "not practical on a research level." In other words, using three different remedies in the plantar warts trial proves nothing. The reply Jacobs received from the Canadian authors of the trial was more a lecture than an answer. "Homeopathic practice varies throughout the world, depending on the therapist's school of thought," they admonished her. "The 'unicists' advocate the use of a single medication for each patient. The 'pluralists' suggest several medications to be taken in a precise order. Finally, the 'complexists' prescribe several medications at the same time. There is no scientific evidence to show that one approach is better than another."

Unicists. Pluralists. Complexists. New descriptions for modern homeopathic researchers to consider. The *Homeopathic Pharmacopoeia of the United States* cites roughly 3,000 substances for use as medicines. Once, when asked how many remedies actually exist, Carlston, who was voted "Best General Physician in Sonoma County" (California), where he lives, joked that "it's like asking how many angels are on the head of a pin." Still, both Jacobs and Carlston know that sooner or later every single angel is going to have to be reexamined in a randomized, double-blind, placebo-controlled, peer-reviewed clinical trial, the gold standard of scientific medicine.

Jacobs and Carlston had achieved a great deal in their professions by the time they founded the Homeopathic Research Network. Each had experiences that helped mold the kind of researchers they would become. Carlston, certified by the American Board of Family Practice in 1984, and then recertified in 1991 and 1998, was also certified by the American Board of Homeotherapeutics in 1988; he considers himself a Kentian (James Tyler Kent) homeopath. "Kent believed that higher doses were more powerful and needed later in the treatment as disease is 'finer' or even spiritual in nature. As the patient improves, the treatment must be at a more fundamental level. In other words, a remedy that is more spiritual will work better," Carlston wrote in an article in the *American Homeopath.* He has served on the boards of the *American Journal of Homeopathic Medicine, Alternative Therapies in Health and Medicine,* and the *Journal of Alternative and Complementary Medicine,* and is also a peer reviewer for the standard journals, the *Archives of Family Medicine* and *JAMA.* He is not a member of the AMA (neither is Jacobs—both are members of the AIH). Carlston comments that "while the idea of subverting the AMA was always appealing, I haven't done it." He says that "homeopathy has a role as a dissident voice," adding that "oddly, I find myself in agreement with those editors of the *New England Journal of Medicine* who wrote that there is not alternative and conventional medicine, there is just good and bad medicine." He is on the faculty of the University of California at San Francisco Medical School and is an influential, as well as candid, advocate for the integration of alternative and complementary medicine into conventional medical education. "I respect experience and a critical mind, along with a caring heart," he says. "The pressures of medicine have killed hearts."

Carlston has sent patients for all sorts of treatments, including hypnosis and spiritual approaches, but says that "homeopathy comes more naturally." He told the *New York Times* for a magazine article about alternative medicine that he has "successfully treated schizophrenics, patients with Lyme Disease, AIDS, and other serious illnesses." He says that experience has shown him that contrary to what some people believe, herbs and homeopathy get along just fine together, and he sometimes uses full-strength herbs in his practice. "There is always a time and a place for different methods," he says. As for vaccinations, he says his recommendations are "clearly individualized," and that "most homeopaths view immunizations skeptically because of concern about ill effects in the short, and especially long term." Yet he says that he vaccinates in his office "routinely—tetanus and HepB most commonly; Diphtheria, HIB [flu], mumps, and DTaP [diphtheria, tetanus, and pertussis (whooping cough)] less often. I do not generally recommend polio, chicken pox, HepA, pneumoccocal vaccine."

He usually prescribes 12C for acute problems, and a one-time 200C for chronic problems, followed by 6C once a day; "but none of this is rigid," he says. He doesn't like giving people drugs; "it's difficult when I see a patient who wants to be on a prescribed medicine. I hate it. I see what it does to them in the long run." He says that "healing happens in all sorts of ways—the food we eat, the air we breathe, the interaction with the health care professional, the homeopathic remedy. . . . When a remedy doesn't work, I blame myself, but you do your best, that's all. I'll ask myself—'was it the water? the sugar pill? a life-style thing?' It all fits together. . . . Some people have psychological stuff—they get something out of being ill." Jennifer Jacobs says, "You're not going to get a good result if you're not prescribing the right remedy," although Carlston says that "sometimes you give the wrong remedy and the patient still gets better." Jacobs, who says, "I generally recommend that a person give homeopathy three to six months to see if it makes a difference," describes what is called "the homeopathic aggravation or healing crisis." She explains that "this occurs in my experience less than half the time, and is usually short-lived. Basically, it is part of the body getting rid of whatever imbalance there is in the system. This can occur with other types of healing as well, such as acupuncture," the 2000-year-old traditional Chinese therapy involving the piercing of the skin with hair-thin needles at special pressure points that are said to regulate the body's energy flow. (It became popular in America in the 1970s, and in 1996 the FDA counted acupuncture needles in the same category as hypodermic syringes and surgical scalpels.)

In 1978, Jacobs took a staff position at the Hering Family Health

Clinic in Berkeley, California, which she described as a "seventies idealis-
tic collective" where everyone "studied and learned about homeopathy
together." She also began apprenticing with a homeopath named Frederick Schmid. "He was a physician—German-trained in homeopathy—at
Marshall Hale Hospital (formerly Hahnemann Hospital) in San Francisco," Jacobs said, adding that she took a job at his hospital "as an
admitting physician for patients coming for surgery, to supplement my
income while learning homeopathy. It was one of those synchronistic
things where I found myself in this hospital with a full homeopathic
library and homeopathic medicines in the hospital pharmacy. Dr.
Schmid was using homeopathy in the hospital with his patients, and
when he found out about my interest, he took me under his wing and
invited me to observe at his practice. He died in 1980."

According to a 1979 letter from the legislative director of the AIH to
the AMA, such apprenticeships as Jacobs undertook with Schmid are a
reliable way for graduate MDs to study homeopathy. The letter went on
to say, "We estimate that between 15,000 and 20,000 MDs and
osteopaths practice homeopathy in the United States, although most of
them do not practice it exclusively," and added that "the licensing
requirements to become a homeopathic physician are the same as for any
other type of MD." In 1976, the year Jacobs received her MD, there were
a total of 13,561 graduates from American medical schools; by 1980, when
Carlston received his MD, there were 15,136 graduates. In the early 1980s,
Jacobs continued her training in America with George Vithoulkas, who
founded the Athenian School of Homeopathic Medicine in Greece. She
then opened a private practice in San Francisco, taught at the International Foundation for Homeopathy (she would be its president from
1984 to 1987), and then, in 1982, moved to Washington State and opened
the Evergreen Center for Homeopathic Medicine, informally known as
the Evergreen Clinic, in Edmonds, with her husband, Dean Crothers, a
doctor who also practices homeopathy. He received his MD from the
University of Washington and a diploma in homeopathy from the
Athenian School, and was president of the AIH from 1982 to 1984. Her
daughter, born in 1979, was never given antibiotics for any childhood illness, a custom even the august American Academy of Pediatrics encourages. (Only one of Carlston's three children ever needed an antibiotic
during childhood, and when two of them had pneumonia as teenagers,
he gave them antibiotics "because they were not getting better fast
enough.")

Jacobs, a moderate like Carlston, does not keep track of how many of her patients also go to standard doctors, and she will send patients to specialists if she feels they need treatment in addition to homeopathy. She keeps up with all the latest drugs. As for vaccinations, she says that "it is an entirely separate issue from homeopathy and there is no consensus in the field," adding that "my own position is that parents must educate themselves and make their own choice. I do not give advice on this to my patients." She says that, in general, conventional doctors are "suspicious" of her because "they confuse homeopathy with naturopathy and herbs." But, at the same time, she admits that they are grateful she can help their patients. Some of those patients who go to her remain on the standard medicines they used when they first came to her—anti-inflammatories, antidepressants, and medicines for lowering blood pressure—but her goal is "to get them off as much medicine as I can." She never immediately removes the drugs prescribed for high blood pressure, but with drugs for depression or heartburn, she says, "I try to get them off right away." She'll give her patients antibiotics "for backup, if they are not responding to homeopathy in a day or two"—especially for urinary tract infections.

She is determined to prove that homeopathy is "science-based." On October 14, 1993, she published a letter in the *New England Journal of Medicine* concerning a 1992 book review of *American Health Quackery* and the *Guide to the AMA Historical Health Fraud and Alternative Medicine Collection* that had appeared in the journal's pages. Jacobs objected to the reviewer equating all alternative medical practices "with those that are clearly fraudulent." The reviewer, Victor Herbert, MD, a former professor of medicine at Mt. Sinai School of Medicine in New York who died in 2002, was known for his discovery linking the lack of folic acid to anemia. Jacobs wrote that "in any field, be it business, industry, or medicine, there will always be those who are eager to take advantage of unsuspecting consumers for monetary gain. To dismiss the entire spectrum of alternative medicine with a blanket indictment ... is shortsighted, uninformed, and insulting to the integrity of the many dedicated practitioners who use these therapies." Herbert, in a reply, told Jacobs that she had "misrepresented" his book review and that he believed there were "three kinds of alternatives: genuine, questionable, and blatantly fraudulent." He placed homeopathy squarely in the third category because, he wrote her, "it is obviously fraudulent when bottles of homeopathic remedies 'potentized' by having been diluted past Avogadro's number—so that there is one molecule or less of active agent per ten bottles—are sold with representations of potency against dysfunction and disease."

Jacobs, who stands up for what she believes, knew that exchanging letters was not going to solve homeopathy's problems. She began to think about doing research after she read about the problems of childhood diarrhea in developing countries. She also wanted to help children with an illness that had no treatment beyond what the World Health Organization, a United Nations agency founded in 1948, recommended: namely, plenty of fluids (because most deaths are from dehydration and not from the diarrhea itself). Antibiotics were not recommended, and the illness had to run its course, in five or six days. Jacobs pursued an advanced public health degree and received an MPH (Master of Public Health) in epidemiology in 1990 from the University of Washington. For her master's thesis, she conducted a small pilot study in León, Nicaragua, using a variety of homeopathic remedies "in a unicist manner" on thirty-three infants and children with diarrhea. She tried, "individually," Aethusa, a flowering weed often used for convulsions and vomiting, as well as for diarrhea; Aloe, a remedy first proved by Constantine Hering in 1864 and often used for stomachaches; *Arsenicum album;* Belladonna; Bryonia; *Calcarea carbonica;* Chamomilla; China, from Peruvian bark; and Colchicum, or meadow saffron, often used for gout, bronchitis, and fevers. She also added *Croton tiglium,* from the oil of the seeds of the croton plant, which, when used full-strength, is a purgative or cathartic; Dulcamara, or woody nightshade (it is similar to Belladonna and is often used for cramps, asthma, and hives); Gambogia, from the fruit of the gambogia tree, often used for backaches as well as for diarrhea; *Mercurius vivus;* Nux Vomica; Podophyllum, or May apple, used for digestive complaints; Pulsatilla; Phosphorus; and Sulfur. "Adding the remedies to the standard oral rehydration treatment seemed ideal," she says, "especially since no recommended allopathic medication would have to be eliminated," and she could collect her data in a short time. Her results "were not conclusive, due to the small sample size, but did show a significant difference in the number of stools on the third day of treatment."

The following year, she returned to Nicaragua to conduct a larger study on eighty-one infants and children. Then, two years later, she replicated the study in Nepal. In 1994, her work won a prize, the Rafael Lopez Hinojosa Biennial International Award for Homeopathic Research, and her paper, "Treatment of Acute Childhood Diarrhea with

Homeopathic Medicine: A Randomized Clinical Trial in Nicaragua," was published in *Pediatrics*, the official journal of the American Academy of Pediatrics. Her research became the first modern homeopathic trial to be published in a standard peer-reviewed American medical journal. Jennifer Jacobs, and her colleagues in the study, made history. They included Margarita Jiménez, MD, MPH; Stephen S. Gloyd, MD, MPH; James L. Gale, MD; and Dean Crothers, MD, who had received the James Tyler Kent award for service to homeopathy in 1988. They had moved homeopathy to a new place, just as Royal Copeland had done fifty-six years earlier.

AMERICAN HOMEOPATHY'S new place in 1994 was hard-won and took years to achieve. Forty years earlier, its medical doctrines had been practically forgotten. Standard medicine made big advances in the America of the 1950s—the decade in which Jacobs and Carlston were born, she in 1950, he in 1954. Smoking was recognized as a cause of lung cancer. Hospitals established intensive care wards in 1952. A new antibiotic, Terramycin, was developed. The Salk polio vaccine came into use by 1955. Open-heart surgery progressed (the first pacemaker was implanted in 1958). CPR, or cardiopulmonary resuscitation, was first used in 1956. In 1953, James Watson and Francis Crick discovered DNA, the principal component of the chromosomes that transmit genes. This discovery marked a monumental advance in the study of molecular biology. The discovery is, in fact, considered by many scientists to be the true beginning of that science, because earlier, disease was only capable of being *described,* and now, disease could be *seen*—that is, scientists could actually get inside a cell to see what was happening.

Even though homeopathy was hardly on anyone's map in the 1950s, the AMA was still on the prowl for its remnants, and when it found one, as it did at the Cincinnati Centennial Medical Exhibit in 1957, it labeled it "obnoxious and subversive." Earlier, the organization had confiscated an anonymous pamphlet published on March 6, 1950, attacking the AMA for its "dictatorship" of public health. "Orthodox medicine is killing more people than war and disease combined," the pamphlet bellowed to a country in love with science. In 1956, the AMA answered a query about a homeopathic school in Mexico City as follows: "Graduates of these schools will tell you that they use homeopathic products only in those instances where others would use a placebo to give the patient relief. . . . Remedies are put up in such fantastic dilutions that chemists usually can find only the dilutant (usually milk sugar) in the tested product."

As for other "obnoxious" or "subversive" practices, the AMA "studied" (its word) osteopathy, saying (again) in 1952 that "all voluntary associations with osteopaths are unethical." This directive was "reaffirmed" (its word) by the AMA in 1955. Between 1953 and 1955, the group also decided that "the quality and content of chiropractic education does not belong within the field" of activities of the Council on Medical Education. Naturopathic schools were also included in these resolutions. The AMA contemptuously reported that some naturopaths objected to the Salk vaccine because it interfered with "the body's 'vibratory' rate.' "

Naturopaths fought back. They, too, wanted to be part of scientific medicine. In 1953, the National Association of Naturopathic Physicians (NANP) issued a new directive, hoping to raise standards and "obtain for the field that high type of graduate who will be a credit to the profession and of value to the public needs." Candidates for a doctor of naturopathy degree now needed at least "1080 clock-hours attendance time" in not less than three years (the work generally took four). In addition to naturopathic theories, the schools had to teach anatomy, pathology, chemistry, bacteriology, hygiene, and public health and sanitation. But even with more rigorous standards, naturopathy could not win over the standard doctors, especially after an official of the NANP told an inspector a decade later that "a good case of smallpox may rid the system of more scrofulous, tubercular, syphilitic and other poisons than could otherwise be eliminated in a lifetime. Therefore, smallpox is certainly to be preferred to vaccination."

The homeopaths who were still around also fought for their profession. An article in the AIH's journal of November 1955, titled "Modern Medicine Rediscovers Homeopathy," had urged members "to investigate modern medicine," even "various anti-biotics," which most homeopaths avoided. "Indiscriminate use" was a concern, and the author, Dr. Henry W. Eisfelder, told his readers that he had often used highly diluted antibiotics to "combat" the overdosage generated by standard doctors. (In 1951, an amendment to the Food, Drug, and Cosmetic Act had said that prescription drugs were unsafe for self-medication and were to be used only under a doctor's supervision.) Homeopaths maintained that ignoring "like cures like" and treating acute illnesses with antibiotics encouraged chronic illnesses. Dr. Eisfelder revealed in his AIH article that Dr. Garth Boericke, a prominent homeopath, had "failed to get the credit for work he did" when it was discussed in the October 1955 issue of *Better Homes and Gardens,* "wherein thousands of Floridians 'chewed or sucked, but did not swallow' a certain pill and thereby went free of mosquito bites even though the insects did light on their skin." The "secret remedy," Eisfelder said, "proves to be our well-known Staphysagria, which Dr. Boericke has been testing together with our armed forces during the years following W.W. II. . . . The dose is the 6X tablet Triturate." *Delphinium staphysagria* is a plant remedy that dates back to the ancient Greeks and Romans, who used the seeds as a purgative as well as an antidote for insect bites.

Some homeopaths began to realize that they needed scientific proof to back up their theories. Indeed, chemical testing of a handful of homeopathic remedies such as mercuric chloride and quinine—as well as testing of the microdilution principle itself—went on sporadically in the 1950s, mostly in England, France, and Russia, although in one case an American homeopath by the name of James Stephenson took part in a microdilution study. In 1953, two Frenchmen, Alphonse Gay and Jean Boiron, said they were able to differentiate between a container consisting of sodium chloride that had been diluted beyond Avogadro's number and six other containers that held only distilled water by using a galvanometer, which was said to be capable of detecting the strength and direction of electrical currents in the magnetic field.

By 1953, the AMA, in its battle for preeminence, had become so conscious of its public image that it even got in touch with the National Association of Radio and Television Broadcasters "in an effort to eliminate, or at least curtail, the improper portrayal of physicians in television and radio." As part of its campaign, it also wanted unequivocally to rid the profession of homeopathy. In 1955, *JAMA* published a placebo study involving more than a thousand patients, and the following year, the journal told a correspondent that homeopathic remedies are only placebos used "to give the patient relief from fancied or self-limiting conditions." It told another correspondent that "there just isn't much" to homeopathy and called the AIH "meager," adding that "one or two" names on a list of AIH officers published in 1941 "have their place in our quackery files." In 1957, the IHA—the International Hahnemannian Association—disbanded, and its membership merged with the American Institute of Homeopathy. Membership was not robust, but also not "meager," as the AMA maintained.

That same year, the AMA, stressing science for a world that now understood DNA, revised its Principles of Medical Ethics to include this sentence: "A physician should practice a method of healing founded on a scientific basis; and he should not voluntarily associate professionally with anyone who violates this principle." By 1958, the American Osteopathic Association wanted to become more scientific, too, and began emphasizing high standards as well as scientific research. And the following year, the AMA (which now called its Bureau of Investigation the *Department* of Investigation) began gradually to shift its position on osteopathic training and agree that AMA members "could now ethically take part in the education of osteopathic students." Naturopaths, chiropractors, and homeopaths were not to be included.

DESPITE THE AMA's disapproval, homeopathy (and other practices the AMA labeled "obnoxious and subversive") would fare slightly better in certain ways during the next decade. The psychedelic, frenetic, frantic era of the sixties—with its civil rights movement and expansion of the war in Vietnam—saw every sort of boundary challenged. In the spirit of the times, offbeat, unconventional medical care became increasingly faddish. The rush for such care was similar to the rush for homeopathic remedies in the mid-1800s. Yet despite the renewed interest in homeopathy, fewer homeopaths than ever were practicing in America. And despite the nonconformity of the decade, standard medicine was seeing such extraordinary scientific gains as the development of the CAT, or computerized axial tomography, scan of the human body, the Sabin oral measles vaccine, oral contraception, kidney transplantation, coronary bypass surgery, and the first heart transplant.

Confident that it could prevail against unconventional medicine, the AMA redoubled its efforts, and enlisted the federal government. In 1961, the AMA sponsored jointly with the FDA a National Congress on Medical Quackery, which discussed continued ways to educate the public, as well as ways to regulate such obvious quackeries as a magnetic hearing aid advertised as a cure for blindness and rheumatism, or Jolly's Dutchess Pills (ingredients unknown), or a hypnotic cure for diabetes, or scented coal as a treatment for bronchitis, or several so-called antibiotics that were simply not. The following year, in 1962, Congress passed the Kefauver-Harris Amendments to the Food, Drug, and Cosmetic Act, which required that drugs be proved effective before distribution to the public. Although Copeland's legacy to homeopathy was basically kept intact (the *Homeopathic Pharmacopoeia* was still part of the act), some remedies were marginalized by the new amendments. For instance, remedies for common illnesses like colds or stomachaches were still permitted to be sold over the counter, but those for more serious illnesses (heart problems) now required prescriptions. In addition, some remedies below 6X were now judged to be toxicity risks. But no one in the FDA kept a sharp eye out for delinquents, beyond occasional warning letters to homeopathic drug companies.

Standard doctors soon received quite a jolt. In 1965, the year the AIH issued a new edition of the *Homeopathic Pharmacopoeia,* a leading homeopathic doctor by the name of Wyrth Post Baker obtained confidential reports that showed that close to 2 billion homeopathic pills or tablets were sold in the United States that year, and that an estimated 12 million persons used homeopathic remedies without the advice of a physician (this despite the fact that the FDA reported that by 1970 there were fewer than two hundred homeopathic practitioners in the country).

The AMA decided that it clearly needed a new approach to nonstandard medicines. With its attempt at disparaging homeopathic remedies by dismissing them as placebos seemingly going nowhere, the organization now fixed its attention on a new category it called "useless drugs." Not necessarily only unconventional drugs were troubling the group, but also "unneeded aspirin, vitamins, and habit-forming laxatives." The medical establishment was concerned about the overuse of such commercial products as Anacin, Midol, Alka-Seltzer, Tums, Rolaids, Ex-Lax, and Murine. In 1965, the AMA also decided that a stronger bureaucracy might aid its war on nonstandard treatments, and the organization formed a brand-new Committee on Quackery (the same year Medicare and Medicaid were established, which the organization opposed, believing they would eventually lead to socialized medicine). The AMA also created a Committee on Medical Practice, a Committee on Human Reproduction, a Committee on Exercise and Physical Fitness, and a Subcommittee on Classification of Sports Injuries. But new committees wouldn't mitigate the fact that the influence of the AMA was now decidedly waning. According to one of its own internal reports, this decline was occurring because of "outdated procedures," "widespread uncoordination," "over-staffing," and "unclear authority." The changing attitudes among Americans, as well as the growing influence of medical specialty societies, also had an impact. The spirit of the sixties had infiltrated the AMA's center of power.

In 1968, trying to be less rigid and more realistic, the AMA decided, to the astonishment of most people, that osteopaths were eligible for membership in the association. Twenty years later, there would be close to 25,000 licensed osteopathic doctors and surgeons and fifteen fully accredited osteopathic schools in the country.

AT THE beginning of the next decade, technological advances in standard medicine inspired many nonstandard practitioners, especially after a British pharmacologist by the name of John R. Vane figured out in 1971 exactly how aspirin works. He won a Nobel Prize for discovering that the drug suppresses the body's production of prostaglandins, or hormonelike messengers involved in inflammatory responses that are found in most cells. Aspirin might often be "unneeded," as the AMA had said in the sixties, but it was no longer unexplained. But what about homeopathic remedies? Would their effects be explained?

Meanwhile, chiropractors, too, wanted to be a part of new scientific advances. In 1974, the year that MRI, magnetic resonance imaging, was introduced (the spine was now revealed in all its details) and the year after DNA cloning was originated, the Council on Chiropractic Education was formed and finally began to revamp the curriculum and admission procedures at chiropractic schools. Some chiropractors would drop the name because of its controversial history and instead call themselves spinal manipulative therapists, which they thought had a more moderate sound. But opposition would linger, and chiropractic schools would continue to be censured for their lack of a strong scientific foundation, as well as for their lack of postgraduate residency programs.

But chiropractors carried on. In 1976, a group of them sued the AMA for conspiracy against their procedure and won a historic court judgment in their favor. Years later, some chiropractors, weary of continuing ridicule but still not willing to attend standard medical schools, began calling themselves orthopractors. The name didn't stick, and the country didn't care, even though it would take twenty years for all chiropractic colleges to obtain acceptance from both the Council on Chiropractic Education and federal authorities. Chiropractic would then defy all AMA forecasts, despite practitioners' lack of an MD, and become one of the most widely used alternative procedures. Americans trusted chiropractic. Many standard doctors would remain critical of its claims and applications (especially on young children), its overuse of X-rays, and various odd techniques that seemed to serve no purpose, such as "nasal specifics—inserting a balloon in the nose and inflating."

The 1970s also saw the development of angioplasty, the procedure in which a balloon that standard doctors approved of is inserted and then inflated to clear clogged coronary arteries. The decade also saw the creation of a more accurate and dependable dose of the standard heart medication, digitalis, for congestive heart failure. Of course homeopaths, too, used digitalis—in the form of its source, *Digitalis purpurea*, or foxglove—as an important remedy for various heart ailments ranging from an irregular pulse to heart failure. But only in small doses. (Thirty years later, an alternative-medicine clinic on the East Coast inexplicably experimented with full-strength foxglove, only to stop their testing following the death of a patient. Cardiologists said that medicine sometimes needs to leave progress alone. Many homeopaths would agree.)

AFTER THE scramble for unconventional medicines that increased in the 1960s, the words "complementary" and "alternative," along with the term "holistic" (which first came into use in the 1920s), began to be widely adopted in the 1970s for unconventional medical treatments like acupuncture, chiropractic, and homeopathy.

Jennifer Jacobs does not consider homeopathy "complementary," because, she says, it competes on equal terms with conventional medicine, which, she argues, "should be threatened" by it. Michael Carlston, by contrast, says that "homeopathy may be the ideal form of complementary medicine." The word "complementary" had actually first been used in 1889 by a homeopath when Dr. E. B. Nash wrote in the *Transactions of the International Hahnemannian Association* that "in regard to complementaries we often see the reports of cases in our journals, when some marvelous results with some particular remedy have been accomplished, that this remedy had to be followed by some other remedy to finish the cure."

The AMA, more worried about its own problems than about any complementaries, turned to brightening its own faded image. In 1975, the group folded its Department of Investigation and then, three years later, its Committee on Quackery. It eventually formed still another committee, this one called the Council on Scientific Affairs, which "provided analyses of current medical and technical subjects with the help of recognized experts in the field." (The Association of American Physicians [AAP] had always remained involved in academic, scientific, and clinical research. "We . . . want a society in which we learn something," its first president had said in 1896, adding that the AAP would not become involved in medical politics or ethics.)

With the AMA's withdrawal from the field, in general, after 1975, the pursuit of quackery was taken up by individuals and consumer groups. In 1984, the year the *Helicobacter pylori* bacterium was established as the cause of ulcers, and three years after AIDS was first described in the United States, three separate California groups joined to form the National Council Against Health Fraud. The NCAHF is a nonprofit consumer group whose concept was originated by Stephen Barrett, MD, a psychiatrist and author who leads his own organization, Quackwatch, which started in 1969 as the Lehigh Valley Committee Against Health Fraud. Barrett, a 1957 graduate of Columbia University's College of Physicians and Surgeons, interned at Highland Park General Hospital in Michigan and did his residency in psychiatry at Temple University in Philadelphia. In 1984, he received the FDA Commissioner's Special Award for Fighting Nutrition Quackery. Other organizations taking up the fight against quackery include the Committee for the Scientific Investigation of Claims of the Paranormal, founded in 1976, and the American Council on Science and Health (1978), as well as numerous state and regional associations that publish antiquackery newsletters and magazines. None of these groups has any connection to the AMA.

Barrett says that the word "alternative" is "tricky," because "it is a marketing term and not a definable group of methods." Wallace Sampson, MD, a professor emeritus of medicine at Stanford University and the editor in chief of the *Scientific Review of Alternative Medicine,* agrees, saying that the term "is an intentional invention of sectarian medicine advocates to place a more acceptable, benign face on the problem of anomalous, aberrant, and misrepresented claims." Both men have taken up the gauntlet against what they consider medical fraud. Homeopathy, especially, would have new problems—coming from the outside, as well as from the inside.

In 1980, conflicts involving the direction of homeopathy once again erupted when the officers of the newly organized National Center for Homeopathy, founded six years earlier, resolved that "homeopathy is a postgraduate specialty of medicine practiced by licensed health care workers." Lay members—those without medical degrees, licenses, certificates, or any other educational credentials—were angered by this

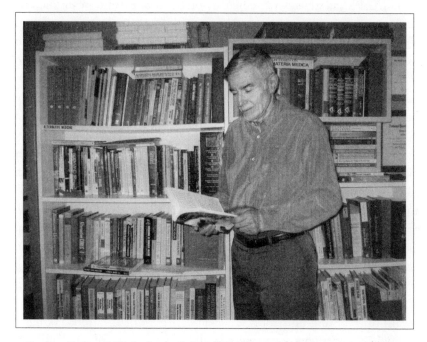

Stephen Barrett, MD, in front of part of his 5,000-volume Alternative Medicine
Collection, which he refers to as "quackery-related books"

directive, which they thought smacked of elitism. These disgruntled
members formed a new group to train homeopaths (no MDs or cumber-
some certificates required) called the American Center for Homeopathy.
Now, instead of the purists opposing the moderates, the fully trained
were being resisted by those they considered the dilettantes. The more
authoritative International Foundation for Homeopathy (IFH) still
offered approved courses (as would the National Center), but these organizations now had to compete with educational programs many homeopaths considered less serious.

New opponents appeared outside the fold of homeopathy as well. In
the early 1980s, the Federal Bureau of Investigation looked into a fake
"HMD" (homeopathic medical degree) that could be bought by mail
order or at a brief summer-school session. Even though authorities in the
individual states could take legal action against such abuses—as they did
with all medical fraud, including impostors and writers of fake prescriptions—homeopathy had still another blemish to deal with, one that
would add to its troubles.

Homeopaths tried to cope by emphasizing certification. In 1982, the Homeopathic Academy of Naturopathic Physicians was organized, with the goal of advancing homeopathy at naturopathic schools, as well as encouraging board certification. That year, under the guidance of the American Association of Homeopathic Pharmacists (AAHP), a revision of the *Homeopathic Pharmacopoeia* was begun, employing what Martin Kaufman, a professor of history and a writer on homeopathy, called a "testing by modern drug provings." This not only served as a defense against critics, but represented real scientific progress. Kaufman explained that the AAHP also "sent 'regulatory letters' to manufacturers who advertised 'homeopathic' drugs which had not been tested or approved by the AAHP, and submitted questionable advertisements to the federal authorities for FDA action." But homeopathy still needed a great deal more of what Copeland once referred to in a speech when he said that "so long as men live they will differ on all questions not actually proved by scientific rule." And "scientific rule" now meant controlled clinical studies. Such applied science could go a long way toward erasing homeopathy's remaining scars and blemishes.

In 1980, several doctors from Glasgow, Scotland, conducted a significant clinical trial involving the use of homeopathic remedies versus standard anti-inflammatory drugs in rheumatoid arthritis. The results, while not overwhelming, showed that the homeopathic treatment was what they pronounced "effective." Many more European trials followed, studies involving the flu, allergic rhinitis (hay fever), gall bladder problems, and fibrositis, among others. Most of these trials showed that homeopathic remedies worked to some extent—indicating in the case of fibrositis, according to the report, that there was "a significant reduction in tender spots by 25%," or in the case of hay fever that "patients using homeopathy showed greater improvement in symptoms than a placebo" and that "no evidence emerged to support the idea that placebo action fully explains the clinical response to homeopathic drugs," or in the case of flulike symptoms that "the effect [of homeopathy] was modest, but nevertheless, of interest." None of these trials was received without severe criticism by standard doctors, who faulted their design, size, management, evaluation, and, most important, their inability to be duplicated, an essential scientific rule. Some homeopaths said that the bar was set higher (as always) in the case of homeopathic trials, while standard researchers said that this was simply not the case. Science was science.

The most disputed clinical trial was one undertaken at a French government research institute in 1985, when a scientist by the name of Jacques Benveniste announced that he had proved that high dilutions of substances left a "memory" in water. The high dilutions, made from white blood cells—basophils—were said to have changed the very structure of the water. The experiment, supposedly replicated at four or five other laboratories (both numbers are given in summaries), was written up in the prestigious science journal *Nature,* even though an editorial in the very same issue called the findings unbelievable. After much debate, a team of investigators from an embarrassed *Nature* went to the original laboratory and couldn't duplicate the results. This team included the editor of the journal, an investigator of scientific frauds, as well as a magician—a real-life, professional wizard. Leading homeopaths said that duplication wasn't successful because of the team's unfamiliarity with homeopathic principles, the protocols of the experiment, and a built-in bias against homeopathy. But standard doctors countered that not only did the experiment defy the known laws of chemistry and physics, but the work had been inappropriately performed in the first place.

According to Wallace Sampson, "careful analysis of the study revealed that had the results been authentic, homeopathy would be more likely to worsen a patient's condition than to heal, and it would be impossible to predict the effect of the same dose from time to time." Sampson, a 1955 graduate of the University of California at San Francisco Medical School, later wrote that if water molecules could "somehow become rearranged and 'remember' the solute's essence and mimic its action," then "the 'solution' should retain every action of every molecule that was in the preparation at the beginning of the 'potentization.' " He went on, "That would amount to a nearly infinite number of actions (including that of any alcohol present) but homeopaths do not explain why the claimed actions are only those of the material on which they focus." He concluded that "one might just as well ascribe the 'effects' of homeopathic 'solutions' to that of a religious miracle as opposed to rearranged water molecules." Robert Park, the former chairman of the Department of Physics at the University of Maryland, has written that "in due course a well-respected group at University College London reported in *Nature* that they had repeated Benveniste's experiment as precisely as possible and found that no aspect of the data is consistent with previously published claims."

The whole episode amounted to a minor scandal and seemed to leave the homeopathic community with a permanent sense of shame. At the 2000 Homeopathic Research Network symposium, a former government health official sighed and then remarked, "You're not going to get far talking about the memory of water to government agencies." In an essay published in the British journal *The Lancet* in 2000, a standard doctor, doubtful that solvents have memory, asked, "How could one confidently cause a solvent to develop amnesia so it could be used in homeopathic solutions? When we are drinking water, what memories are we consuming and what is their effect on us?"

Yet despite the absence of scientific proof, Americans continued to be infatuated with alternative treatments, contraptions, and diets. In 1982, the AMA, which claimed it had "a membership population of 250,821 out of a total doctor population of 250,821," wrote in a newsletter that "wellness" was the new catchword, and that "although 'health' and 'wellness' might seem to be synonymous, the wellness educators seek to go beyond traditional definitions of health." There was no further explanation. In 1983, the World Health Organization listed some prevalent "unorthodox therapies." These included such practices as kinesiology, which entails muscle-testing as a whole-body evaluation tool; Kirilian photography, which was said to gauge by high-voltage imaging the body's so-called aura in an effort to discover problems before symptoms emerge; impact therapy, which underscores core aspects of problems and avoids what it believes are unneeded details in the healing process; Rolfing, which employs soft-tissue manipulation and movement; cymatics, the investigation of the structure of waves and vibrations; radiesthesia, which uses a pendulum to detect healthy or sick vibrations in the body; radionics, which traces energy patterns; orgone therapy, which uses individual blankets and chambers to charge the body's faulty electrical system; pyramid therapy, which uses pyramid-shaped constructions to replenish cosmic energy to cells; and Dianetics, a semispiritual practice involving long-buried traumas.

Homeopaths continued to defend their beliefs. In 1984, the Homeopathic Nurses' Association was created to promote homeopathy in nursing schools, and in 1986, HomeoNet, the first online network, was built. While helping to advance homeopathy, these groups didn't foster scientific investigation. But it hardly mattered. Americans wanted "health" and "wellness," and would do just about anything to attain them.

FOURTEEN

"Another Tool in the Bag"

D URING THE 1990s, consumer groups kept finding fault with alternative medicine. Steven Novella, MD, an assistant professor of neurology at Yale, a founder of the Connecticut Skeptical Society, and a board member of Quackwatch, wrote in the *Connecticut Skeptic* that arguments like those Jennifer Jacobs and others cite concerning the "individualized" aspect of homeopathy place it solidly "in the halls of pseudoscience." He said that homeopathy is basically "untestable," and even though homeopaths are making an effort to use clinical trials, he wondered why they "do not alter their treatments based on the results of such research." Michael Carlston, trying to defend homeopathy's position, wrote that "one hundred highly publicized negative trials would not end a system of medicine so well established by tradition and familiar to hundreds of millions worldwide. Some homeopaths therefore argue that research has nothing to offer those who would continue to use homeopathy." He realized all too well that the tide of science might be running against homeopathy, although he added, diplomatically, "However, research can still play a role in this independent-minded community."

Yet to many people, homeopaths seemed to be a "community" that lived in another century. After all, the hard science that made homeopathy seem outdated continued to advance. It became possible in the mid-nineties to map the very structure of bacteria, viruses, neurotransmitters, and cell receptors in the brain. The Human Genome Project was launched with the intent of identifying all the approximately 30,000 genes in human DNA. (It was completed in 2003.) Science was zeroing in on the biochemical and neurobiological meanings of living and dying. Standard drugs, previously obtained only from natural sources, could now routinely be synthesized in the laboratory—among them, Atropine, used to dilate the pupils, which was once extracted from Belladonna, and monoclonal antibodies (proteins that the body's immune system uses to inhibit cancer cells), which were developed in a laboratory and served to revolutionize some cancer treatments. (There were earlier examples: Salvarsan, a synthetic compound made from arsenic created in 1911, and certain amphetamines synthesized in the 1930s.)

After Jacobs's famous childhood diarrhea study was published in *Pediatrics* in 1992, criticism of it had poured in, along with occasional praise. The AMA's Council on Scientific Affairs condemned it in its "Report 12" for "inconsistent/incorrect data analysis; use of different diagnostic and treatment categories but combining them in the conclusions of efficacy; and lack of chemical analysis of different treatments." In other words, for being somewhat of a procedural mess. Joe M. Sanders, Jr., MD, the executive director of the American Academy of Pediatrics at the time of Jacobs's study, told a spokesperson for the FDA that "just because an article appears in a scientific journal does not mean that it's absolute fact and should be immediately incorporated into therapeutic regimens. It just means that the study is [published] for critique and review and hopefully people will use that as a stepping stone for further research." (Jacobs later divulged that she heard rumors that the editor of *Pediatrics* had almost been fired for publishing her study.)

The Letters to the Editor section of *Pediatrics* published many diverse reactions to the study. Some said Jacobs's work was "helpful," "practical," and "generally well-designed," while others chided it "for having no definition of study failure," for not checking "for double-blinding," and "for not providing data on toxic risk." Later, an American doctor writing in the English medical journal *The Lancet,* called the study "methodologically sound" but also described "an additional obstacle to the ready acceptance of homeopathic medications—the complexity of the prescribing process." This doctor pointed out that most parents would find it next to impossible to figure out whether their child had " 'one cheek red, other pale,' or 'blue circle under eyes' " and thus could not be reliable historians during the process of figuring out exactly which homeopathic remedy was the correct one. Copeland had once written that homeopathy's "one and only demand for recognition was its peculiar way of determining the remedy for the removal of symptoms of disease."

But most standard doctors argue that going through a long list of very specific but pertinent symptoms in order to help a crying child to feel better might be considered by some parents not just "an additional obstacle," or even "peculiar," but a totally unmanageable—and abnormal—barricade.

Jacobs and her team replied that the letters raised important points and reminded the correspondents that the study was "preliminary." Addressing the letter in *Pediatrics* that complained of a toxicity risk in the use of *Arsenicum album,* Jacobs agreed that "extremely low homeopathic potencies of toxic substances like arsenic can be dangerous," adding that "it is our understanding that these have been voluntarily withdrawn from the over-the-counter market by homeopathic manufacturers." (In 1986, Drs. Harry D. Kerr and L. A. Saryan conducted a trial, the results of which were published in the journal *Clinical Toxicology,* showing that low-potency [3X] Arsenicum tablets posed a threat if taken as directed on the label.)

One critique in particular had nothing kind to say. Wallace Sampson, along with an educator, William London of the American Council on Science and Health, said in a "Special Article" in *Pediatrics* that Jacobs's study "not only included no safeguard against product adulteration," but also offered no clinical or even public health significance whatsoever simply because the only remedy needed for mild childhood diarrhea is adequate fluid intake. (Sampson later wrote that there was only one less bowel movement with the remedies and such a result was hardly significant. But *Resonance,* the magazine of the International Foundation for Homeopathy, challenged Sampson's dismissal by reporting that the study, and its presentation at a meeting, "was much acclaimed for its combination of enthusiasm, rigor and humility." The article explained that "Dr. Jacobs won the audience at the expense of a journalist who was observing that the reduction of diarrhea by one day was nothing to brag about. 'If you are a mother and have to change a diaper five or six times a day, it does mean a lot,' replied Jacobs!")

Notwithstanding, the four-page "Special Article" was considered by many standard doctors as meticulous in its detailing of the errors found in Jacobs's study. Sampson and London argued that because of "the extraordinary concepts and claims of homeopathy, the method of study should be nearly faultless and results should be reported cautiously." Jacobs rejoined that Sampson and London's article was published without informing her in advance and giving her an opportunity to respond.

"It was quite disturbing the way it was handled," she said, and she concluded that it was done "to placate people." She means, of course, the community of standard doctors. (The article was a source for the criticism in the AMA's Council on Scientific Affairs's "Report 12.")

Some homeopaths nearly went on the warpath in response to the article. Dr. Edward H. Chapman, the president of the AIH at the time, wrote *Pediatrics* that Sampson and London were on "a mission to debunk complementary medicine," and that "homeopathy represents a challenge to the conventional bio-medical model." He reminded the editors that "research into homeopathy is in its infancy." Trials had shown that homeopathy worked, at least to some extent, and others had to be developed that would show *how* it worked.

But the criticism was almost relentless. In an article called "Homeopathy: The Ultimate Fake," Stephen Barrett wrote that "a 30X dilution means that the original substance has been diluted 1,000,000,000,000, 000,000,000,000,000,000 times. Assuming that a cubic centimeter of water contains 15 drops, this number is greater than the number of drops of water that would fill a container more than 50 times the size of the earth." He went on, "Imagine placing a drop of red dye into such a container so that it disperses evenly. Homeopathy's 'law of infinitesimals' is the equivalent of saying that any drop of water subsequently removed from that container will possess an essence of redness. Robert L. Park . . . has noted that since the least amount of a substance in a solution is one molecule, a 30C solution would have to have at least one molecule of the original substance dissolved in a minimum of 1,000,000,000,000,000, 000,000,000,000,000,000,000,000,000,000,000,000,000,000,000 molecules of water. This would require a container more than 30 billion times the size of earth." (In his book *Voodoo Science,* published in 2000, Dr. Park said that Hahnemann's "anecdotal evidence" would never be taken seriously today and that he was "presumably unaware that he was exceeding the dilution limit in his preparations because he published his major work . . . in 1810, one year before Avogadro advanced his famous hypothesis.")

But homeopaths remained undaunted by such arguments. Dr. David J. Tulbert, of the Center for Classical Homeopathy in Toronto, presented a paper before the Fourth Scientific Symposium of the Homeopathic Research Network, which was held at the Renaissance Hotel in Washington, D.C.; its title was "Hypothesis for the Structure and Action of Sub-Avogadro Homeopathic Dilutions." Tulbert discussed the "unusual storage properties of sub-Avogadro dilutions, including their indefinite shelf life, sensitivity to chemicals, sensitivity to environmental influences, and the revival of potency by succussion."

Some criticism of Jacobs came from homeopaths themselves. Michael Carlston wrote *Pediatrics* that some of the data in "the interesting and potentially important trial" was incorrect and didn't add up. He later said, "I criticized the use of the diarrhea index score because the WHO [World Health Organization] criteria were not weighted heavily enough." Jacobs defended herself by pointing out that in one case a "table was added late in the publication process and was not adequately proofread," and that in another case she "is unclear how this 8 became a 7 in the final version." But the current was clearly moving in favor of establishing a scientific basis for homeopathy. Edward Chapman, who praised Jacobs's study (which had been partly funded by the Boiron Research Foundation, a division of Boiron, a leading manufacturer of homeopathic remedies, and the Standard Homeopathic Company, another manufacturer), conceded that medicines in future homeopathic studies must be routinely tested to prevent criticism of adulteration. Homeopathy needed to become more legitimate in science's eyes.

Many other homeopathic studies, some that made standard doctors want to avert their eyes, were completed in the early nineties. One, in 1990, and another in 1992, used nuclear-magnetic-resonance-imaging technology in an attempt to present evidence of submolecular activity in the remedies. In 1994, a meta-analysis of 105 toxicological tests showed, according to the report, that "homeopathic remedies may be useful in treating toxic exposures." Still other studies attempted to use quantum physics to illustrate that on some level electromagnetic energy in the remedies interacts with the chemistry of the body. Some of these studies had negative results, and received little or no publicity—a meta-analysis in England, and one involving veterinary medicine in France. (The use of homeopathy among veterinarians across America and abroad was increasing, and the British completed a study that showed that remedies reduced birth difficulties in cattle and were also helpful in certain horse diseases. A 1997 survey by the American Animal Hospital Association reported that 21 percent of all pet owners used some form of alternative medicine on their pets, especially for skin diseases, concussions, breathing difficulties, teeth problems, and diarrhea.)

In 1996, a study conducted in France claimed to show evidence of beta radiation (that is, of the nucleus of an electron) emanating from homeopathic remedies. In fact, in 1999, Jacques Benveniste, whose study about water having a memory caused a stir fourteen years earlier, now insisted that the water had an "electro-magnetic signature" that "can be captured by a copper coil, digitized, and transmitted by a wire . . . over the internet . . . to a container of ordinary water." This caused outright revulsion among standard doctors.

Homeopaths also read with interest a report in 1997 by a well-known homeopathic educator, Dana Ullman (he holds a master's degree in public health but is not an MD), that scientists at the American Technologies Group, a controversial research and development company with an interest in products for the environment, "discovered, identified, and characterized a unique type of (non-melting) ice crystals that maintain an electrical field." Ullman, once arrested decades ago—in 1976—for practicing medicine without a license, wrote that the discovery would have significant applications in combustion enhancement, cleansing agents, and "medicine and pharmacy." Homeopaths wondered if this particular discovery could open the door to homeopathic "proof," showing that their remedies are a type of liquid crystal. In fact, one of the scientists Ullman referred to, Shui-Yin Lo, had presented a paper— "Molecular Basis of Homeopathic Preparation"—before the Third Scientific Symposium of the Homeopathic Research Network held in San Francisco during the winter of 1995. But Lo's credentials had been criticized by Quackwatch, which noted that his findings were never published in a first-rate scientific journal. In addition, American Technologies Group, his employer, was later accused of fraud for a product that was said to increase gas mileage and engine performance in cars but did not.

If standard doctors remained unconvinced of homeopathy's scientific efficacy, so did some homeopaths. In 1999, the editor of the *British Homeopathic Journal* wrote that "we are still far from a comprehensive grasp of what is going on in ultra-molecular dilutions, and how they act. For instance, what happens to them when they get into the body? How are they received by the biosystems?" Jennifer Jacobs herself told an interviewer for OneBody.com, an Internet health site, that "my guess is that science has not advanced enough yet to explain how homeopathy works," an argument that Barrett and other critics say is the major hallmark of a quack. Yet Jacobs believes that, in time, research will show how homeopathy works on a molecular level.

Dr. Iris R. Bell, a homeopathic researcher at the University of Arizona, says that biomarkers, or physiological factors like chromosome abnormalities, basal metabolic rate, and body temperature, will have to be factored into future clinical studies. A project she undertook in 2000 discussed "measures such as electroencephalography [electrical activity of the brain], electrocardiography [electrical activity of the heart], blood volume plethysmography [the use of an instrument called a plethysmograph to measure blood flow in an arm or leg], skin temperature, physical activity monitors, and electromyography [the use of an instrument that records electrical activity in muscles]," which, she said, "can offer, over real-time, dynamical, non-invasive indicators of subtle remedy effects." A researcher at a Homeopathic Research Network symposium suggested to the audience that understanding sound might provide some answers as to why the remedies work. Michael Carlston himself writes that "no single theory adequately accounts for both of the essential homeopathic principles, similia and potentization. We remain a long way from understanding how these extreme dilutions can directly create clinical effects."

But there are those who will never be persuaded: Dr. Frank Wilczek, of the Massachusetts Institute of Technology, and one of the world's most eminent theoretical physicists (he shared the 2004 Nobel Prize in Physics), was asked in an interview about the role certain subatomic molecules called muons could play in homeopathic remedies, especially in light of evidence found in 2001 by the Brookhaven (N.Y.) National Laboratory that these rare particles have unknown properties outside the standard model of particle physics. "I find it extremely difficult to imagine a connection," Wilczek said. "There are several potential explanations for the [Brookhaven] result that are well within the framework of conventional physics. If there were something really weird going on, involving small interactions among many particles, I don't think this is necessarily the first place we'd bump into it."

Dr. Murray Gell-Mann, who won the Nobel Prize in 1969 for his discovery of elementary particles he named "quarks," says that for homeopaths to say that there is a memory of a substance when there are no molecules left is, quite simply, "garbage physics."

IN 1992, the United States Congress granted $2 million to create the Office of Alternative Medicine at the National Institutes of Medicines. With that act, alternative medicine officially became of interest to the American government. Dr. Daniel Moerman, a medical anthropologist at the University of Michigan, observed that creating the division "was like setting up an office of deviltry within the Catholic church."

It happened because of bee pollen, which is said to strengthen respiration because of its concentrated enzymes, although Stephen Barrett has written that "no scientific study supports any claim that bee pollen is effective against any human disease." Indeed, in 1990, 1992, and 1994, even the Federal Trade Commission weighed in against pollen, and barred four companies from making unreliable statements about the substance; the FTC was also concerned about contaminants and the potential for allergic reactions to some of the products. But it took an advocate of bee pollen therapy for allergies, Tom Harkin, the Democratic senator from Iowa, to successfully place a clause for the creation of the new office into a National Institutes of Health provision.

Opponents of the government's involvement in alternative medicine protested and said that such an office could offer legitimacy to all sorts of quackeries; they even suggested that the government wanted to become involved in alternative medicine only because it detected potential financial gain for the health industry. In the past, critics had also faulted private funding of alternative-medicine research. Most doctors—both those who use alternative medicine and those who don't—pay little attention to such criticisms and are grateful for the underwriting of any scientific research, a great deal of it coming from private foundations; without it, or the support of drug companies, much research, standard as well as alternative, might not progress at all.

Jennifer Jacobs, now a leader in homeopathic research, was asked to serve on the advisory board of the Office of Alternative Medicine, which she did from 1992 to 1996. From 1993 to 1997, the office funded eighty-eight grants for research involving acupuncture, music therapy, massage therapy, hypnosis, yoga, transcranial electrostimulation, herbalism, and homeopathy.

Despite the government's interest, the criticism of homeopathy continued. In 1994, the National Council Against Health Fraud wrote in one of several position papers that it had issued since 1984 that "the marketing of homeopathic products and services fits the definition of quackery established [in 1984] by the United States House of Representatives committee which investigated the problem (i.e. the promotions of 'medical schemes or remedies known to be false, which are unproven, for a profit')." The position paper went on, "The United States Food, Drug, and Cosmetic Act lists the *Homeopathic Pharmacopoeia of the United*

States as a recognized compendium, but this status was due to political influence, not scientific merit," a reference that was a direct blow to Royal Copeland's legacy. Later, Barrett would write in Quackwatch that "if the FDA required homeopathic remedies to be proved effective in order to remain on the market, homeopathy would face extinction in the United States." (In 1994, he petitioned the FDA on behalf of forty-two doctors, medical researchers, educators, and lawyers, to regulate homeopathic remedies more carefully, and "in the interim . . . issue a public warning that although the FDA has permitted homeopathic remedies to be sold, it does not recognize them as effective." Such a warning has yet to materialize.) In 1998, Dr. David Kessler, who served as FDA commissioner from 1990 to 1997, and had opposed the 1994 Dietary Supplement Health and Education Act, which liberalized the marketing of supplements and herbs, told a *Good Housekeeping* magazine panel that homeopathic remedies don't work. Stephen Barrett, who also served on the panel, had asked the question that elicited this response, and, according to Barrett, Kessler, now the dean of the University of California–San Francisco School of Medicine, said he did not attempt to ban homeopathic remedies because he felt that Congress would not go along with it.

Homeopaths knew that regulations were on their side. The Dietary Supplement Health and Education Act of 1994 had defined herbs and supplements as "orally ingested foods," thereby making proof of effectiveness no longer a requirement. Manufacturers of vitamins, minerals, enzymes, glandulars, and even ginseng and garlic, were responsible for the safety of the substances they sold (all considered foods, and not drugs), and the FDA could step in only if there was a problem after the item (the "food") reached the marketplace. Many people felt that the act was a step back into another era; indeed, an "observational study" in *The Lancet* suggested that "research into hazards and risks of dietary supplements should be a priority" because they "are associated with adverse events that include all levels of severity, organ systems and age groups."

But homeopaths also had faith that their remedies were safe, and didn't worry, even after the National Association of Boards of Pharmacy (NABP) voted favorably in 1994 on a resolution that acknowledged that some homeopathic products sold are not approved by the *Homeopathic Pharmacopoeia of the United States.* This resolution said all homeopathic products had to meet not only the standards of this pharmacopoeia, but also those set by the FDA. The resolution brought trouble to Jennifer Jacobs's former teacher, Bill Gray, who sold Dr. Gray's Small Pox Shield, a homeopathic preparation that the FDA told him was not listed in the *Homeopathic Pharmacopoeia.* In a "warning" letter dated April 2, 2003, the FDA decreed that the concoction was, in fact, a biologic that needed a special license. The FDA noted as well that Gray's Web site stated that his remedy was "available only by prescription, and that this prescription is provided through [the] website for a fee." The FDA threatened that "failure to promptly correct these violations may result in regulatory action such as seizure and/or injunction without further notice."

Even though homeopathy was no longer of direct interest to the AMA, the organization still had some surprises in store for it. Even some pleasant surprises. In 1995, the AMA dropped the word "quackery" from its vocabulary and began using the words "alternative medicine" and "unconventional medicine" after its House of Delegates passed a resolution saying that the AMA "encourages its members to become better informed regarding the practices and techniques of alternative or unconventional medicine." Still, two years later, the first paragraph of the twenty-three-page report of the AMA's Council on Scientific Affairs quoted from a *New England Journal of Medicine* editorial calling many alternative treatments "well known," many "exotic and mysterious," and still others "dangerous." The use of the word "dangerous" did not surprise homeopaths, who were used to hearing it from standard doctors. Later, putting danger aside, the AMA reported that alternative medicine was "ranked among the top three subjects for their journals to address in 1998," even though it also called it "perhaps the most controversial arena in medicine—an arena that purports to be a circus, where fantasy and illusion regularly mingle with reality."

Inadvertently, the AMA contributed to the controversy over homeopathy's effectiveness. Almost unaware that it was contradicting itself, the organization made a stunning appraisal that same year. For the very first time, one of its journals used words to the effect that homeopathy actually works. This surprise appeared in a year-long double-blind, randomized, controlled homeopathic study performed at fifteen clinics throughout Germany from 1995 to 1996, the results of which were published in the AMA's *Archives of Otolaryngology—Head and Neck Surgery.* The study, which received very little publicity, concerned a prescribed remedy called Vertigoheel, and an investigation found it to be as safe and effective as its standard counterpart, Betahistine, in a treatment of the symptoms of vertigo, dizziness, and motion sickness. Betahistine hydrochloride, known as SERC, is a histaminelike drug first reported in

JAMA in 1966. Vertigoheel is not "ultra-highly diluted," according to its manufacturer; it contains five ingredients in 3X to 6X dilutions. These are *Conium maculatum* 3X, the poison hemlock; *Cocculus indicus* 4X, another poison from the fruit of the levant nut tree, or Indian cockel; *Ambra grisea* 6X, made from the intestines of sperm whales; Mineral Oil 8X; and inactive Magnesium Stearate, a mineral salt used as a cohesive agent. The study might have been neglected, but it was science-based, and good news for homeopaths.

By 1997, most of the AMA's specialty journals—including the *Archives of Pediatric and Adolescent Medicine,* the *Archives of Internal Medicine,* the *Archives of Family Medicine,* the *Archives of Dermatology,* the *Archives of Neurology,* and the *Archives of General Psychiatry*—had published trials, studies, and surveys on alternative medicine. The AMA now said that its specialty journals "deliver through the rigors of science, a cogent and well-constructed survey of the evidence-based understanding of alternative medicine." In 1998, *JAMA* published a defining study called "Trends in Alternative Medicine Use in the United States, 1990–1997," by a team comprising David Eisenberg, MD; Roger B. Davis, ScD; Susan L. Ettner, PhD; Scott Appel, MS; Sonja Wilkey; Maria Van Rompay; and Ronald C. Kessler, PhD. The study reported not only a high use of complementary and alternative medicine, but also an increase in its use from 1990 to 1997. According to the study, which had a total of 3,594 participants, "the therapies increasing the most included herbal medicine, massage, megavitamins, self-help groups, energy healing, and homeopathy." Another study published in *JAMA* that same year, "Why Patients Use Alternative Medicine," conducted by John A. Astin, PhD, indicated that "along with being more educated and reporting poorer health status, the majority of alternative medicine users appear to be doing so not so much as a result of being dissatisfied with conventional medicine but largely because they find these health care alternatives to be more congruent with their own values, beliefs, and philosophical orientations toward health and life." That year, *JAMA* also picked Barrett's Quackwatch as one of the nine Web sites "that provide reliable information and resources."

Nineteen ninety-eight proved to be a favorable year for homeopathy. In addition to the Vertigoheel study, Jennifer Jacobs, along with her colleague and husband, Dean Crothers, MD, and Edward H. Chapman, MD, published "Patient Characteristics and Practice Patterns of Physicians Using Homeopathy" in the AMA's *Archives of Family Medicine.* The authors wrote that "patients seen by the homeopathic physicians were younger, more affluent, and more likely to present with long-term complaints. Physicians using homeopathic medicine surveyed spent more time with their patients, ordered fewer tests, and prescribed fewer pharmaceutical medications than physicians practicing conventional medicine." (The authors cited statistics showing that in 1997 the worldwide sales of homeopathic remedies added up to approximately $1.15 billion.) The following year, in 1999, the *Journal of Head Trauma Rehabilitation* published a Harvard Medical School study (Dr. Chapman was one of its authors) that showed there could be a place for homeopathy in the treatment of mild traumatic brain injury. A larger study was recommended.

But not everything was favorable for homeopathy. Faring less well was a medical book published by Jacobs in hardback in 1996, and in paperback in 1998, cowritten with Dr. Wayne B. Jonas, the director of the Office of Alternative Medicine from 1995 to 1999 and a homeopath who describes himself as a "99% conventional doctor." *Healing with Homeopathy: The Doctors' Guide* promptly found a place on Quackwatch's list of "unreliable" books because, Dr. Barrett said, such books "promote misinformation, espouse unscientific theories and/or contain unsubstantiated advice." Dr. Robert L. Park wrote in a review of the book: "The danger is that it reinforces a sort of upside-down view of how the universe works, like trying to find your way around San Francisco with a map of New York. That could be dangerous for someone who is really sick—or really lost."

In 2000, the AMA published its own book on what it now called CAM (complementary and alternative medicine). *Alternative Medicine: An Objective Assessment* included seventy-five articles that had appeared in its journals, covering such subjects as acupuncture, chiropractic, herbal medicine, naturopathy (called "Diet, Nutrition, and Lifestyle"), aromatherapy, yoga, and homeopathy (including the 1998 study of patient characteristics and practice patterns by Jacobs, Crothers, and Chapman). The book was far from entirely approving. One article concluded that CAM "is largely a political term" because "the types of interventions considered to be alternative are likely to change over time and vary from region to region." Included was an article called "A Close Look at Therapeutic Touch," which had been coauthored by a nurse, an educator, Stephen Barrett, and a sixth-grade student who thought up the whole idea for her fourth-grade science project. The study, which Barrett shepherded to publication in *JAMA*, received a lot of publicity because it was done so professionally by someone so young. It determined that the claims of therapeutic touch are "groundless and that further professional use is unjustified."

Medical professionals agree that the critics' hearts are in the right place with their concerns, and that Quackwatch, particularly, provides an essential service tracking fraudulent and worthless services. Barrett's consumer safeguard instructions are especially applauded. He says that "the first thing is to maintain an adequate level of caution with respect to claims. Second, identify reliable sources of information and follow what they say." But some homeopaths insist that he often appears as unyielding, insular, and full of zealotry as he thinks some of them appear when it comes to proving their procedures work. They say that certain practices are intolerable to Barrett, as well as to Sampson, and that homeopathy is among these because it has yet to be proven scientifically. (Barrett says it is because "homeopathy clashes with reality," although in 1986 he offered a possible protocol—"an idea"—for testing homeopathic remedies to Dana Ullman, who headed a homeopathic foundation at the time and had approached Barrett. Nothing ever came of the matter.)

Homeopaths welcomed a decision made on December 3, 2001, when a California Supreme Court judge ruled in favor of a homeopathic manufacturer in a case involving charges of false and misleading advertising of homeopathic products. Barrett and colleagues made an effort to persuade the court that many homeopathic claims were false, but the judge, according to Barrett, "refused to permit testimony about the scientific impossibility that ultradilute products can work."

Stephen Barrett conscientiously tries to elevate himself above squabbling. In an effort to make sense out of the many complementaries and alternatives, he has suggested that "to avoid confusion, they should be classified as genuine, experimental, or questionable." John Renner, MD, a board member of the National Council Against Health Fraud, furthered Barrett's ideas by suggesting five categories of alternative medicine to the AMA's Council on Scientific Affairs. These are: Proven, or scientifically tested; Experimental, or in the process of undergoing controlled trials at reputable places like academic medical centers, the NIH, or the FDA; Untested, or having never been subjected to rigorous testing (herbals and homeopathy are in this category); Folklore, or "passed down through cultural tradition and oral history," like chicken soup for colds; and finally, Quackery, or the commercial marketing of products and therapies that can cause harm and where "anecdotal testimonials are the main basis for the 'success' for these modalities." Homeopathy was elevated out of the Quackery category for the first time by at least one consumer group, and though it was categorized as Untested, it wasn't considered harmful. That was progress, especially when coupled with the AMA's remarkable acknowledgment in 1998.

Although officially no longer part of anti-quackery, the AMA did still take an interest in water. Yes, water. As a study in its *Archives of Family Medicine* stated, "Bottled water has become a status symbol and is frequently used in place of tap water." It pointed out that both bottled and tap waters "are considered safe to drink," but went on to ask, "Is either more beneficial in preventing tooth decay and is there a difference in purity?" The answer, based on the testing of fifty-seven samples of five categories of bottled waters, was that some bottled water has *more* bacteria and *less* fluoride than tap water. The International Bottled Water Association called these findings "sensationalized," because it was "not clearly reported that these bacteria are not harmful in any way to human health and do not have the potential to cause disease or illness." (By 2002, water was a very big business, with sales of $35 billion worldwide, and with 65 percent of Americans drinking it in bottled form.) Water is a big concern for Quackwatch, too, which posts ten articles on "Water-related Frauds and Quackery" and provides access to a Canadian Web site called Aquascams. It's not just plain and flavored waters that people are purchasing in bottles; it's so-called structure-altered waters, waters that can "heal," waters that can "reverse or delay ageing," waters that contain "electrical energy," and waters that can deliver "vibrations."

DESPITE STANDARD acceptance, if not outright approval, of homeopathy, the disparagement kept up. In the fall of 1998, representatives from twenty-three countries met in Heidelberg, Germany, for the Second World Skeptics Congress. As Matt Nisbet, the public relations director of the Committee for the Scientific Investigation of Claims of the Paranormal, wrote at the time, "North American and European medical experts emphasized a serious problem: the public is not getting scientifically valid information on alternative therapies." He quoted Barry Beyerstein, an English psychologist, who said that "alternative medicine's enduring popularity stems from widespread public scientific illiteracy, aggressive alternative medicine industry marketing, New Age faddishness, inadequate media criticism, a growing distrust of authority that includes the scientific and medical establishment, and an anti-doctor backlash." Nisbet reported that Beyerstein told the audience at the Skeptics conference that "natural is considered safe. Though I like to remind people that tobacco is a naturally occurring substance."

"Patients seldom ask their regular physicians how the drugs they have been prescribed actually work," Michael Carlston has written in an article about allergies. "Instead, they merely trust that the drug will [work], and that their physicians are careful enough not to poison them." He adds, "Physicians become homeopaths because homeopathy works better for most health problems than the techniques we learn in medical school." But, Stephen Barrett told a magazine interviewer, "most homeopathy is simply buying products off the shelf," adding, "How long does it take to become a homeopath? Two seconds. You just call yourself a homeopath, and you are one. You could study it a lot, but so what? You can study astrology for a hundred years, but it's not going to make it work." Barrett, who was chided at a homeopathic research meeting for not being "an active, working scientist," agrees with what Arnold S. Relman, MD, the former editor of the *New England Journal of Medicine*, wrote in an essay published in 1998 about the celebrated alternative doctor Andrew Weil: that his theories are a forsaking of common sense, are the result of "stoned thinking," and follow the rule that there is not one scientific truth but many truths. (Relman included the popular holistic endocrinologist Deepak Chopra in his discussion.)

In *Healing with Homeopathy,* Jacobs and Jonas include statements that Royal Copeland might have written: "Homeopathic medicine is not a complete system of medicine in itself and should be used along with conventional medical knowledge." But, Barrett says, echoing the AMA's words uttered over the course of the nineteenth and twentieth centuries, homeopathy is "a masquerade fakery" and "pseudo-science." He and other critics are particularly disturbed by homeopathic encouragement of self-medication, although Jacobs told an interviewer that "people have to be careful about not trying to treat themselves for chronic conditions." Still, she also said, "I do think there's a place for over-the-counter use of homeopathy, but for chronic problems I recommend they seek a trained homeopathic practitioner." This explanation is not satisfactory to those who are not convinced the remedies are completely safe or to those who worry that medical problems will be overlooked. Michael Carlston reports that 82 percent of homeopathic use is self-care. "People are buying it on their own," he says. " 'Mom and Dad' have the biggest practices," he commented during a conference presentation. Many homeopaths treat themselves for chronic problems, but Carlston doesn't. "It's like doing a self-portrait without a mirror," he says.

Jacobs and Jonas write in their book that "just as the discovery of infectious agents revolutionized our ability to care for many diseases at the turn of the century, the discovery of what happens when a homeo-pathic preparation is made and how it impacts the body might revolu-tionize our understanding of chemistry, biology, and medicine. If it turns out to be only a placebo response, it will still provide important infor-mation on how our minds and bodies operate."

In 1995, a three-day conference called "Placebo: Probing the Self-Healing Brain" was held at Harvard University. Arguments about the meaning of "placebo" ranged from stating that "placebos do not help dis-ease, only the way patients perceive disease," expressed by Howard Spiro, MD, the founding editor of the *Yale Journal for Humanities in Medicine,* to asking, "Why is the placebo regarded as pejorative? Is it threatening to medicine?" voiced by Arthur Kleinman, MD, the chairman of Harvard's Department of Social Medicine and director of the World Mental Health Project. A year later, the Office of Alternative Medicine hosted a placebo and nocebo (negative effect) conference. Herbert Bensen, MD, an associate professor at Harvard and the president of the Mind/Body Medical Institute in Boston, said that "there were three components that drive placebo and nocebo: beliefs and expectations of patients, their health care providers' beliefs and expectations, and the interaction between the two."

Michael Carlston says that the most important question to ask about patients is "Did they get better?" He adds, "I care that they get better." He does not care necessarily by what means. And, he told the Homeo-pathic Research Network symposium in 2000, "it doesn't make any dif-ference if homeopathy is a placebo or not. All clinicians use placebos unwittingly. It's the part of the healing process we don't understand."

THE GOVERNMENT continued to be interested in alternative medicine, now sometimes called integrative medicine. In July 2000, President Bill Clinton assembled the first White House Commission on Complemen-tary and Alternative Medicine to help advise Americans on "the great potential and possible perils associated with the use of CAM." The commission was headed by Dr. James Gordon, a psychiatrist who runs the Center for Mind-Body Medicine in Washington, D.C., and is on the faculty of the Georgetown University School of Medicine, as well as the Uniformed Services University of Health Sciences in Bethesda, Maryland. Quackwatch was extremely critical of Gordon, not only because he "volunteered for one year at the Haight-Ashbury Free Clinic in San Francisco, helping ease young seekers through their experimentation with drugs," and apparently favored a dancing technique involving whirling and spinning called dynamic meditation, but also because he seemed to have a special interest in UFOs. Quackwatch also said that Gordon held that his White House Commission's report "has the potential to be, for medicine in the 21st century, as important as the Flexner Report was to medicine in the 20th century."

Gordon told the AMA's *American Medical News* that CAM opponents have a "McCarthyite mind set—the inquisitor's mind, not the scientific mind. There's a lack of thoughtfulness in that approach—knee jerk is the right word," he said.

In 2000, the AMA seemed to switch directions again, issuing a statement on CAM that was, as the *New York Times* put it, "tepid at best." The AMA said at this time "there is little evidence to confirm the safety and efficacy of most alternative medicines." Still, during the summer of 2001, the *Annals of Internal Medicine* published a study that indicated that CAM is not going to go away anytime soon. Even so, Dr. Robert S. Baratz, president of the National Council Against Health Fraud, said, "The notion of alternative medicine is like a magic carpet. It will get you nowhere."

By 2001, the office of Alternative Medicine, now called the National Center for Complementary and Alternative Medicine (NCCAM), already had a budget of $90 million for research, with $113 million projected for 2003. Nearly thirty health insurers and HMOs covered various CAM procedures, but still not homeopathy. (According to the *Archives of Internal Medicine,* chiropractic is covered in all fifty states, acupuncture in seven, naturopathy in two.) But, in general, most Americans are willing to pay out of pocket.

Quackwatch reported that in 1997 a London health authority "decided to stop paying for homeopathic treatment after concluding that there was not enough evidence to support its use." At a Homeopathic Research Network symposium, a doctor was overheard saying that whenever it came to homeopathy, "politics at the highest level" was always involved in opposing it, and "powerful people can crush you."

Nonetheless, Gordon's White House Commission report, issued in 2002, after testimony from seven hundred witnesses, recommended many positive steps, including an increase in CAM educational opportunities, better and more consistent manufacturing practices to ensure the safety of all CAM products, improved product information, the formation of a central government office within the Department of Health and Human Services to coordinate CAM activities, more research money, and more coverage of CAM therapies by insurance companies and Medicare.

Jennifer Jacobs, who became president of the AIH in 2000, had testified that homeopathy "deserves careful, unbiased evaluation." She also spoke of placebos, but as a research component, saying that "once the efficacy of homeopathy is established firmly, the use of placebo can be eliminated by randomizing subjects to receive either conventional medical care or homeopathy." She said that this "would give a more accurate representation of what homeopathy has to offer in actual clinical practice. Longitudinal studies of homeopathic patients over several years should document the preventive as well as curative aspects of this modality as well as cost analysis."

Opponents of homeopathy rose up and delivered a vigorous cry of protest. On March 25, 2002, the National Council Against Health Fraud urged President George W. Bush and members of Congress to ignore the White House Commission "because its recommendations go far beyond any data or findings of the Commission and also go beyond reason and rationality." The group's statement went on, "Widespread adoption of unproven, disproven, and irrational methods would cost the American public billions of dollars and thousands of human lives."

Two new private groups had been trying to help the public sort out the "unproven" and "disproven." In 1999, an independent company, ConsumerLab.com, began testing herbs, vitamins, and supplements; the results are offered to the public on a subscription basis. The company is not planning to test homeopathic remedies; it did not give a reason for this decision. Some products tested by ConsumerLab were shown to contain not only less than the label indicated, but also entirely different ingredients, and some contained high levels of pesticides. Natural Standard (at naturalstandard.com), begun in 2000 by a Harvard-trained doctor with an advanced literature degree from Oxford, also provides, for a fee, impartial, evidence-based CAM information that undergoes "blinded editorial and peer-review prior to inclusion." They test "selected herbs used in homeopathy," such as Belladonna or arnica.

But the protests got louder. Further "reason and rationality" was needed. In 2002, the World Health Organization (WHO) took on what the *New York Times* called "a Herculean task," to become "a global watchdog over unconventional medicine." Jonathan D. Quick, MD, director of the Department of Essential Drugs and Medicines Policy at WHO, said there are "uninformed skeptics who don't believe in anything, and uncritical enthusiasts who don't care about the data. We want to convince the skeptics that some things work, and make the enthusiasts more cautious because it can kill them."

The AMA, never really able to let go of homeopathy as a scapegoat, even after allowing that it might work, now decided that the persistent popularity of the treatment might "be due to [its] patient-centered view of illness, where the key to resolving health issues lies in understanding and treating all symptoms, not just those that fit the text book description of a specific disease." And, once again to the amazement of most standard doctors, a personal essay by a medical student published in *MS JAMA* (Medical student *JAMA*) said that "if used within its limits, homeopathy will complement modern medicine as another tool in the bag." Copeland would have found it hard to believe he was reading these words in an AMA journal.

"We homeopaths are like monkeys that know how to drive a car," Michael Carlston wrote humorously in an essay on allergies that seemed to respond to the *MS JAMA* essay. "We can fill up the car with gas and take you to all kinds of wonderful places but we didn't design the car. Other physicians are still monkeys but instead of hopping in and going for a ride, they would rather investigate the car by banging on the tires and twisting off the antenna." He is saying what has always been said about homeopathy, that homeopaths use the tools in their bag to bring gentle relief to the whole body, while conventional doctors use their tools to tinker and tinker with its parts.

FIFTEEN

"A Long-Felt Want"

J ENNIFER JACOBS works out of offices in a residential area of Edmonds, Washington, fifteen miles north of Seattle. The town of 40,000 people overlooks Puget Sound, whose shores were once filled with so many trees that at the turn of the century the area supported eleven shingle mills. Blue herons, double-crested cormorants, and Canada geese are among the dozens of visitors to its beaches, marshes, mudflats, and treetops. Rhododendrons, wisteria, and evergreens grow along the sides of the two-story angular wood building that houses the homeopathic clinic Jacobs runs with her husband, Dean Crothers. Inside is a lobby with a skylight, a reception area, a conference room, two examination rooms, two bathrooms, and a tiny kitchen. A small room is set aside for Jacobs's research assistant, whom she describes as "a detail-oriented person who does data processing" for her clinical studies.

A lot of new research is being conducted in homeopathy, and Jacobs is focused in her strong-minded belief that over time homeopathy will be proved scientifically. She is also "very interested in using homeopathy in epidemics," where she thinks it can play a significant role. Meanwhile, she also now wants to try "to make homeopathy simpler—not as taught in classical homeopathy."

Yet, despite her determination, she remains controversial. After her expanded diarrhea study of 126 infants and children was published in the *Journal of Alternative and Complementary Medicine* in 2000, questions about her work persisted. She was unable to find a standard medical journal to publish the work, which had been carried out in a "private,

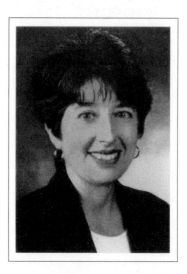

Jennifer Jacobs, MD

charitable health clinic" in Kathmandu, Nepal, where Jacobs was joined by six other health practitioners, including Crothers. The study, actually completed in 1993, produced the same results as the previous ones, showing that "individualized homeopathic treatment decreases the duration of diarrhea and number of stools."

But skeptics continued to take a dim view. Standard doctors maintained that the small variations in duration and number of stools are common and hardly worth noting. They would agree with what Wallace Sampson wrote years earlier: "We are left wondering how, nearly into the 21st century, well trained physicians and scientists can cling to absurd viewpoints, and misinterpret the natural world and how it really works."

Critics even began to whisper that doctors who became homeopaths in the first place were usually malcontents who were never in the forefront of their respective classes and thought they could distinguish themselves only by becoming outsiders. They were merely restless and rebellious, the critics said. Sampson wrote in 1998, in fact, that although he was "on dangerous ground because of lack of data," still, "good doctors know who the other good doctors are." He went on, "One of the darkest, most secret, and little-mentioned factors in the Alternative Medicine controversy is that AM advocates are not in the higher ranks of good doctors. Many or most are probably in the lowest rank of quality." Critics also became increasingly suspicious of homeopathy's more and more frequent tendency to appear to blame patients for their illnesses, and to assume that an invisible weakness was contributing even to the illnesses of infants.

Some skeptics also began to say that "randomized trials aren't everything." Even some homeopaths agreed. In 2000, Dr. Marianne Heger, a doctor at the Research Center Homint, in Karlsruhe, Germany, told an audience of homeopaths listening to a reading of her paper "Outcomes Research" that all the answers "are not to be found in clinical trials." She favored a "multi-disciplinary approach that emphasizes the benefits to the patient." At this same gathering, a Scottish homeopath agreed that clinical trials "might not be the gold standard" after all, adding that "the patient knows if he is getting better so maybe we should be looking at patient-centered trials." These debates seemed to put homeopathy right back into its dark ages before "scientific rule."

It was not alone in its retreat. In March of 2000, a poll conducted by the People for the American Way Foundation showed that 79 percent of Americans believed that creationism, the belief that God created humans and controlled their growth, should be taught in public schools along with Darwin's theory of evolution, which was thought "far from being proved scientifically." One of the pollsters said, "The poll's results might reflect a postmodern feeling that no single view can provide complete understanding of most issues." Perhaps reflecting a similar attitude, Sampson has written that homeopathy is based not only on ideology, "but is a reaction to the complexities of modern medical thought."

Whatever the roots of a belief in homeopathy, Jacobs pressed ahead with her research. In 2001, she published a preliminary pilot study on the use of homeopathic remedies in acute Otitis media, or ear infection, in the *Pediatric Infectious Disease Journal,* the official publication of the Pediatric Infectious Diseases Society and the European Society for Paediatric Infectious Diseases. After analyzing seventy-five children, eighteen months to six years old, she concluded that "a positive treatment effect of homeopathy when compared with placebo cannot be excluded and that a larger study is justified." (Standard medicine treats ear infections with pain medication and antibiotics, although a study in 2002 done by researchers from the Children's Hospital Medical Center in Cincinnati, Ohio, showed that in some cases parents are willing to forgo antibiotics and use only pain medication because of concern that antibiotics will contribute to the emergence of antibiotic-resistant bacteria.)

While discussing her work with ear infections at the 2000 Homeopathic Research Network symposium, Jacobs said that the parents of the children were very motivated to use homeopathy. She also disclosed to the audience that an American standard journal she wouldn't name had requested two revisions of her paper, which she completed, but then the journal ended up rejecting her study anyway.

Jacobs's pilot study was dismissed by some standard doctors for not only being unimpressive, but also insignificant. Even a fellow colleague grumbled. Wayne Jonas said the study "does not convince me Otitis media should be treated by homeopathy," although he also remarked that a larger study could conceivably change his mind. An earlier pilot study to assess "appropriate study design" for trials "comparing homeopathy with allopathic treatment of acute Otitis media" had been published in the *Pediatric Infectious Disease Journal* in 2000, but one of the authors confessed that publication "was made a little easier" because of the "clout" of one member of the team. This survey suggested that one of the difficulties with studies like Jacobs's was that "conceivably a given case of acute Otitis media could require any one of the medicines in the homeopathic pharmacopeia" and because of this problem, randomizing patients to specific medications would be difficult. The study concluded that "failure of therapy may be difficult to define."

The audience of the Homeopathic Research Network had groaned at Jacobs's revelations about her frustrated efforts with the unnamed standard journal. Groaning is not an uncommon reaction whenever standard medicine enters the dialogue. "It's not necessary to be a good homeopath and learn a new remedy every week—this is typical of allopathic medicine, to start with one [drug] and suddenly have a new medicine," a homeopath said to much whistling and applause, responses that were also heard a great deal. Chortling is another familiar sound that greets what homeopaths call "the allopathic party line." Loud versions of that sound greeted a homeopath talking about the use of steroid inhalers in the treatment of asthma. "They make the disease massively worse," the speaker told his laughing audience.

The reactions to her Otitis media work were mixed. When a doctor asked Jacobs which remedies worked and which did not in her study, she replied that she hadn't considered the issue "because the study was so small." Another homeopath suggested that the studies "shouldn't allow more than one remedy." Still another argued no, there needed to be combination studies, because consumers were now buying mixed remedies. It was also suggested that the standard-medicine model of sequential analysis, or one step at a time, be used. Another homeopath thought a study should be prepared comparing standard medicine to homeopathic remedies with respect to ear-infection relapses within one or two years. Someone else said "replications are urgently needed." Jacobs agreed with this latter assessment, understanding that replications are key in all scientific investigations. Still, an audience member reminded the group that the success of homeopathy during the nineteenth-century cholera outbreak had "lots of data, but doubts still exist." This person asked, "How can we be sure modern replication will be easy to achieve?" Another homeopath tried to explain that scientists were close to showing an energy transfer between single cells.

Many scientific strategies and terms were being tossed around, as the pressure to enter a more modern age was felt by almost everyone assembled in the room. But it was not clear which ones mattered to homeopathy. Wayne Jonas had told the gathering that, in general, "research is daunting to people." It is daunting to both scientists and the lay public. Most theoretical and scientific jargon is also daunting, and it is often difficult for a layperson to distinguish genuine scientific terms from less than genuine ones that are used improperly or inappropriately as a means either to impress an audience or to keep it at bay. (For example: Is the "Casimir effect," which describes the appearance and disappearance of light, a real facet of quantum mechanics? Yes. It was predicted in 1948, and verified forty-eight years later, in 1996. On the other hand: Is there a "psychotronic amplification system"? No. Quackwatch calls this term "gibberish" and says it is used because it "sounds scientific and technical.")

Some homeopaths decided simply to abandon scientific terminology. "We need to throw away labels. We are studying medicine," a homeopath told the 2000 symposium. Still another reminded the audience how difficult it was—if not impossible—to merge science and homeopathy, and said that performing experiments on their remedies is often "like listening to a bird's chirp during a jet airplane take-off."

But Jennifer Jacobs is not overwhelmed by the task. In the fall of 2001, she went to Tegucigalpa, Honduras, to perform a new pilot study, this time on the homeopathic treatment of dengue fever, a mosquito-born infectious disease, which, like malaria, is generally found in tropical places. Dengue, which the World Health Organization says affects 50 to 100 million people annually, causes joint pain, headaches, rashes, and fever, which usually lasts around ten days. A vaccine has been developed and is expected to reach the market for the general public by 2005. (The U.S. Army has had a vaccine since 1995.)

With the cooperation of the Honduran Ministry of Health (which even provided cars and drivers paid for out of the grant's budget), Jacobs and her associates in the study worked in two clinics in the poorest, most crowded areas of the city. Most of their patients lived in wooden shacks with electricity but no plumbing or sanitation. Jacobs wrote in an e-mail to her colleagues in the United States that "we have found the people to be warm and friendly and they have accepted us well. We have enrolled 13 patients into the study, out of the 60 that we need. It is a bit behind but we got a slow start. The lab technicians and health workers are on strike here. We have had to hire a private lab to do our lab tests, and some of the health workers are helping us outside of their strike. It is crazy! We start work at 7 A.M. every day as people start going to the clinics at 6:30. It is hard to sleep late because the streets are full of noise very early. By 10 P.M. we are ready to crash!"

The pilot study used six different homeopathic remedies: Belladonna, Euphrasia (made from a wildflower; used for eye difficulties), Aconite, Bryonia, Gelsemium (from a climbing plant with poisonous flowers; used for fever), and *Rhus tox.* Jacobs told the 2002 Homeopathic Research Network symposium that she "didn't feel comfortable giving just one remedy," and so it was decided to do the study with multiple ones. However, "technical troubles" (Jacobs's phrase) forced the study to be abandoned a few months later. These troubles included blood tests that revealed that "a large number of people had other illnesses," and, more important, that they didn't actually have dengue fever. All was not lost, however; Jacobs says she built a strong connection with the Health Ministry, and she conducted a new, very large placebo-controlled, double-blind clinical trial of childhood diarrhea in Honduras in 2004. She first explained that this trial would have three "arms": the use of individual remedies, combination remedies (several medications "combined together in one pill"), and placebos, but later said that "the cost for carrying out an individualized study of this magnitude would have been $750,000, and funds were not available, either privately or from NCCAM." Three hundred children were enrolled in two groups. "The 2-arms, without individualized treatment, is a third of the cost," she says, adding that "the kids are in homeopathic combination or placebo." She will analyze all the criticisms of her earlier diarrhea studies, especially the one by Wallace Sampson that appeared in *Pediatrics.* She hopes her new study will be "airtight." In 2003, the *Pediatric Infectious Disease Journal* published a meta-analysis of all of Jacobs's previous diarrhea studies, which showed that her combined data indicated a positive response with the use of remedies

Jacobs is planning another pilot study, codesigned with Christine Girard, a naturopath connected with the Yale-Griffin Prevention Research Center in Derby, Connecticut. This one will investigate the safety and efficacy of homeopathic remedies in the treatment of ADHD, or attention deficit hyperactivity disorder, in children aged six to twelve years. According to her research plan, "it often takes three to four months to see the full results of homeopathy; therefore, the duration of this pilot is eighteen weeks. Following baseline measurements, subjects will be randomized into two groups of equal size and will receive one of two treatments: the individualized treatment prescribed by the homeopathic provider, or placebo. Individualized homeopathic prescribing will be done by board-certified naturopathic physicians. Potency selection will be individualized, based largely on whether or not the subject is taking allopathic medication for ADHD." (The leading standard drug used in ADHD is the stimulant Ritalin, or methylphenidate; other drugs sometimes used include anticonvulsants, antidepressants, antihypertensives, and antianxiety medications.)

Jacobs says that "the prescribers are free to use whatever remedies they want, so there are at least a thousand possibilities," adding that "we need to be clever in our design, and also true to the homeopathic spirit." She says that some remedies "more likely to be used for ADHD are Stramonium, Calcarea phosphorica, Tarentula, and Tuberculinum." Stramonium, made from the poisonous plant also known as Devil's Apple, brings on delusions—as well as sedation—if given full-strength. *Calcarea phosphorica (Calc. phos.)* is a Schussler tissue salt, often used for toothaches as well as for certain psychological problems. Tarentula, or Tarentula Cub, is a remedy that uses the entire *live* spider of the same name for toxic infections of the body. Tuberculinum is a remedy often used for coughs and immune system problems, and is produced from dead tuberculosis bacterium.

Jacobs says that the naturopathic doctors working in the study will also be homeopaths with certification from the Homeopathic Academy of Naturopathic Physicians. "It's a long-term process," she says, "and with a one-time study you can't answer all the questions. The idea is to look and see if there is a possible trend—see what's going on—and if it looks good, we'll do a bigger study." (At the 2002 symposium, Christine Girard spoke about the study and was asked by Michael Carlston "if how well kids are liked" will be a criteria of success in the study. "Maybe further down the road this will be done as an outcome," Girard answered; "this is a pilot at this point.")

Jacobs is conducting another pilot study in Seattle, this one treating hot flashes in seventy-five breast cancer survivors. The trial, conceived in 1998, is being underwritten by the United States Army, which has had a breast cancer research program since 1992. (The army has given more than 1,800 grants to more than 830 institutions.) Jacobs writes that "our goal is to determine whether homeopathy is an effective treatment to improve the quality of life in breast cancer survivors," and that the pilot will use "the classical approach and a combination of homeopathic medicines." She goes on to explain that "homeopathic medicines have been used to treat hot flashes and other menopausal symptoms for more than 100 years. . . . Because homeopathy is a system that treats the physical, emotional, and mental symptoms of a patient, it might be of value to women suffering from the myriad symptoms associated with estrogen withdrawal." She concludes, "There have been two previous studies done to evaluate the use of homeopathy for menopausal symptoms. Both found an improvement with homeopathy, but the number of patients was small and the methodological quality was poor."

ASIDE FROM working hard to incorporate science into homeopathy, many practitioners want to stress that their form of healing has to be as professional and exacting as any other medical practice. Alan Trachtenberg, MD, the acting director of the Office of Alternative Medicine in 1994, told the 2000 Homeopathic Research Network symposium that there is now "a big move to get practitioners without licensing out of the field." A year earlier, Dana Ullman, the homeopathic educator, had published an article in the *Journal of Alternative and Complementary Medicine* about homeopathy and managed care. The article, which Ullman later posted on his Homeopathic Educational Services Web site, quoted some 1998 statistics from the National Center for Homeopathy showing that 44 percent of all homeopaths in America are "medical doctors or osteopaths," 16 percent are naturopaths, 15 percent are chiropractors, 12 percent are veterinarians, 7 percent are nurses, 4 percent are dentists, and

2 percent are acupuncturists. Ullman explained that there are four recognized naturopathic colleges, but "less than 100 naturopaths have sought certification from the Homeopathic Academy of Naturopathic Physicians." (The colleges, in Oregon, Washington, Arizona, and Canada, have a four-year program, and require premedical course work in biology and chemistry.) He also referred to the Council on Homeopathic Certification, "a new certifying body" that allows "unlicensed and licensed individuals to apply for certification." He writes that "as of 1998, they have certified almost 200 homeopaths, granting them a Certification in Classical Homeopathy." He says that managed care will cover homeopathy "within the next ten years," especially if certification matters are cleared up.

Although certification doesn't guarantee excellence, nearly forty states now have laws allowing CAM to be practiced, although chiropractic is licensed in all states. Acupuncture is licensed in thirty-eight states. Homeopaths with an MD don't need a special license (except in Arizona, Connecticut, and Nevada). Naturopathy is licensed in approximately thirteen states, and is trying for more. Three states—Illinois, Kentucky, and Texas—have consumer guidelines. Illinois and Kentucky allow homeopathy as well as acupuncture, art therapy, biofeedback, bodywork/manual therapy, herbals, hypnosis, light therapy, magnetic stimulation, massage, music therapy, reflexology, traditional Chinese medicine, and yoga.

Education is another controversial subject. The AMA says, "We believe the way to become trained is by education, not legislation." Medical doctors and skeptics of homeopathy agree. The issue of whether or not to have an MD still divides homeopaths, almost more than the ancient quarrels about dilutions and single or multiple remedies. Michael Carlston says he doesn't mind working with "non-doctors," and that what bothers him is "people who think they know more than they know. If you think you know everything, you can't learn anything." Yet he also says that one of his teachers (as well as Jacobs's), George Vithoulkas, now head of the International Academy of Classical Homeopathy in Alonissos, Greece, "went to a homeopathic medical school in India, but quit because he said, 'What am I going to learn?' So he read and he saw patients." According to Carlston, Vithoulkas's only training was as a civil engineer. He didn't have an MD. This does not matter one bit to Carlston because he thinks that Vithoulkas is a great teacher and practitioner. The National Center for Homeopathy lists twenty-two "educational programs" that have either been approved, or are under review. (Two are correspondence courses.)

Carlston wanted to contribute to homeopathic education. He is the editor and principal author of what he calls the first contemporary textbook on homeopathy for conventional medical students. *Classical Homeopathy* is a slim 181-page book, published in 2002 as part of a series on CAM produced by Churchill Livingstone, an imprint of Elsevier Science, one of the world's oldest and best-known health and science publishers. The company publishes 400 books and 1,200 journals a year. Carlston, who writes that "classical homeopathy is often considered the holy grail of clinical homeopathy," says that the book is actually intended for all interested students, practitioners, and teachers, "as well as academically inclined and interested lay readers." The publisher calls it "a thorough introduction to homeopathy," so it doesn't yet fulfill Copeland's dream of a comprehensive medical-school textbook "intended to satisfy a long-felt want."

Carlston writes that "the greatest challenge to homeopathy today is to produce skilled practitioners." Notwithstanding, Jennifer Jacobs says that she believes that the mandatory teaching of homeopathy in medical school "won't happen in my lifetime, but maybe in my grandchildren's."

All the same, as Wayne Jonas had reported in 1997, 80 percent of medical students want some form of CAM training, and, according to a 1998 survey that appeared in the *Archives of Pediatrics and Adolescent Medicine,* many primary care doctors, especially pediatricians, are interested in taking alternative medicine course work "within the context of biomedicine," or standard medicine. The *Archives of Family Medicine* published a report in 1997 by Carlston, Jonas, and Marian R. Stuart, which showed that alternative medicine "has begun to establish a presence in United States medical schools and Family Practice Residency programs." Jonas says that homeopathy "is a CAM system that few professionals know about and fewer still understand," and he calls Carlston's book on classical homeopathy "one of our best guides."

Jacobs and Jonas report in their book *Healing with Homeopathy* that "many 'physician-extenders,' such as physician's assistants (PAs) and nurse practitioners (NPs), are becoming interested in homeopathy, and work independently under the supervision of a physician." Osteopaths who use homeopathy generally receive a doctorate in homeotherapeutics from the American Board of Homeotherapeutics, while naturopaths can

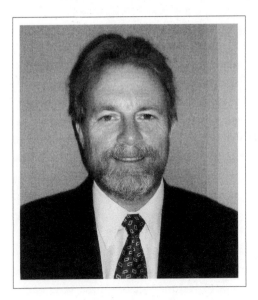

Michael Carlston, MD

receive a doctorate in homeopathy through the Homeopathic Academy of Naturopathic Physicians. The National Board of Homeopathic Examiners, which was started by chiropractors, offers a diploma for homeopathy on various levels of expertise—not only to chiropractors, but to acupuncturists, osteopaths, PAs, NPs, nurses, dentists, and medical doctors.

Jacobs prefers that homeopaths have medical training and worries about strictly laypeople using homeopathy. "The biggest fear is that something serious will be overlooked, that someone will come in with a headache who has a brain tumor," she told *New York Newsday* in 2000, adding, "That's less likely when you've had the training to be suspicious."

More and more homeopaths seem to be donning caps and gowns. By 2001, seventy-five U.S. and Canadian medical schools, including those at the University of Arizona, Columbia, Harvard, UCLA, Yale, and Johns Hopkins, had CAM courses in their curriculums. Seventy-one schools discuss homeopathy. But Harvard Medical School, for one, does not relish doing so, saying in a letter of query in 2001 that it found that "American audiences were resolutely uninterested in this tradition of medicine." It went on to say that "this is partly because the D. Hom (doctors of homeopathy) in this country are not well organized and have little 'presence' in American healthcare institutions." The letter said further that "we have discussed this problem at great length with the directors of Homeopathic professional associations, but the leadership seems to lack the vision and determination to make homeopathy an acceptable alternative as, for example, acupuncture." It concluded, "Part of the problem, of course, is that the mechanism of action of the medicines is controversial, and the evidence for homeopathy has not been controlled for time spent with the doctor." (Michael Carlston has written about a discussion he once had with an unnamed "European researcher" to conduct "a homeopathic trial" with American patients whose only treatment would be the homeopathic interview.)

Dean Crothers, Jennifer Jacobs's husband and partner in running the Evergreen clinic, received the Samuel Hahnemann Award for Teaching in 1997. He says that one should be a physician first and a homeopath second, adding that he is "ambivalent about homeopathy being taught in medical schools as a specialty." After the AMA turned down a request in the 1940s that it become a subspecialty of internal medicine, the subject hasn't been broached to the organization again. Meanwhile, other subspecialties have been created—cardiovascular disease, gastroenterology, hematology, and, in 1972, medical oncology.

Crothers says that "on the one hand, having homeopathy taught in medical schools at all would greatly enhance the credibility and accessibility of homeopathy in the eyes of the public and the medical profession. On the other, there would be a tendency to reduce the scope of the subject in order to fit it into the already full curriculum. If homeopathy were presented in one or two required courses as an introduction to homeopathic medicine, and in such a way that it was clear that postgraduate study and certification were necessary in order to practice the specialty, we would be moving in the right direction." Carlston says that "every physician should know some homeopathy," and he would like it to become a specialty. Jacobs disagrees, arguing that in many ways it is actually a "ludicrous" idea to make homeopathy a specialty, because it "has an entire philosophy of its own, and is the opposite of internal medicine, where mostly drugs are given." She would like ideally to see homeotherapeutics someday become "a separate specialty board within the AMA."

IN THE spring of 2002, the Homeopathic Research Network held its Sixth Scientific Symposium at the Rittenhouse Square Sheraton Hotel in downtown Philadelphia. This occurred several blocks from the site of the constitutional convention of 1787 and during the same week that the FDA approved a surgical instrument that uses radio-frequency waves to correct vision, a less invasive approach than laser surgery.

The meeting included presentations about the use of homeopathy in pediatric care, in brain injuries, for the incision pain of surgery, and in epidemics. Speakers got very technical. They talked about a patient's "global health rating," "the need to be cautious of low level ambient electrical, magnetic, or radiation noise," "the use of psycho-physical measures," and the "toxidation" of the environment. But along with all the scientific and scientific-sounding language (there is no such word as "toxidation"), other concepts were heard in the conference room, some of them sounding as if they belonged in Wonderland: "There's something in the water, it's not just the mother tincture." Or, "The water could have effects from something nearby." Or, "A lot of stray things turn up." Or, "The death of a friend could have caused the illness." (Psychological and emotional symptoms were discussed almost more than physical symptoms at the meeting.) Many participants held computers on their laps—some with games of solitaire running on them. Others talked on their cell phones. One researcher said, "There are no clear leads on what is causing homeopathic relief," while another remarked that "despite the high dilutions, the safety of remedies needs to be studied." Another doctor repeated the often-heard remark to the effect that "a large number of conventional drugs have no known mechanism of action, so why do we have to prove homeopathy?"

But despite the continued intrusion of Wonderland, hardheaded science seemed to be prevailing. Shortly after the symposium, Dr. Rebecca Elmaleh, a homeopath who practices in New York City, spoke to the Biennial Case Conference of the AIH, held at the same hotel in Philadelphia, about her treatment of molluscum contagiosum, a viral skin disease. Right before her presentation, Dr. Elmaleh was proudly introduced as the instructor of the first-ever Category 1 AMA course in homeopathy, which meant that the AMA's Accreditation Council for Continuing Medical Education, or ACCME, had given Beth Israel Medical Center, where the two-year course was given, the right to award credits to students.

More than a century ago, Copeland's colleague at the University of Michigan, W. A. Dewey, said that all MDs should be taught homeopathy by "masters of the art." Such masters were surfacing everywhere. The

American Academy of Family Physicians accredits one hundred CAM courses a year, and the ACCME evaluates hospitals, colleges, and universities as to their suitability to offer qualified courses to physicians. According to ACCME's mandate, these courses must not advocate "unscientific modalities of diagnosis or therapy." Dr. Murray Kopelow, the chief executive of ACCME, says that alternative medicine is "an important topic" for his organization but that there has to be "valid evidence" to the practice. In any case, ACCME approves the institutions that provide the courses, not their content.

The AMA's newspaper, *American Medical News,* reported Dr. John Nelson, the secretary-treasurer of the AMA, as saying that "the fact that medical schools and residencies are teaching it does not mean they are endorsing using alternative medicine therapy." (He also said that "not all CAMs are scams—acupuncture and chiropractic care have been proven.") Homeopathy was not singled out.

Elmaleh, who did her residency in family medicine, said that her course was sponsored by the Boiron Institute. According to the AMA, more than 40 percent of funding for continuing medical education comes from such commercial sponsors, which, it said, is an increase from only 17 percent in 1994. Elmaleh was vague about the details of Boiron's underwriting of her course, and in fact couldn't recall the exact year her course was given, other than "some time in the last three or four years." Beth Israel Medical Center has no record of it, or of Elmaleh. The Boiron Institute didn't respond to inquiries about its sponsorship, nor did two other homeopaths who also work at Beth Israel. Like homeopathy itself, some matters, even educational ones, often remain enigmatic.

But at the case conference, Elmaleh was completely straightforward and professional as she discussed a seven-year-old girl who had previously received standard steroid cream for her condition, which consisted of soft, shiny warts, along with eczema. After a lengthy interview, Elmaleh had prescribed five remedies to the child: Sulfur (30C); Thuja (15C), from the conifer tree, which is also used in aromatherapy for acne and hair loss; *Nitric acidum* (5C), made from the corrosives sodium nitrate and sulfuric acid; Causticum (5C), from potassium hydrate, a remedy created and proved by Hahnemann, and often used for bladder, larynx, and eyelid problems; and Staphysagria (5C), or larkspur, used for insect stings and bites. Elmaleh said that her patient took these remedies once a day on weekdays and alternated them on Sundays, and that after the child told her that she had recently become more tidy in her room, but not obsessively so, she decided to add *Arsenicum album,* 30C, to her regimen. She said that eight months after the *Arsen. alb.* was included her patient's skin disorder disappeared. Most people in the audience seemed to accept the cure as proof of the eternal mystery of science.

When Wallace Sampson was asked in the winter of 2003 if scientific evidence might change his mind about homeopathy (and if he believed that such evidence was achievable), he gave a long and detailed answer. He said that "there are several problems. One is the nature of therapeutic trials, another is the nature of statistics, and another is in the question. . . . As for trials, no trial completely proves or disproves. No matter how well randomized and blinded, the variables of human populations, responses, and variability of observations all reduce the likelihood of one study proving a hypothesis. Clinical trial statistics assume equal populations in experimental and control groups, which are not attainable. This makes all results from individual trials approximations."

When asked to comment about Jacobs's early plans for her newest diarrhea trial, Sampson, who knows a great deal about clinical trials because of his former position as the associate chief of the Oncology Division at Santa Clara Valley Medical Center, gave a scientifically precise if intellectually demanding reply. He said that "even if the trial had no defect, even with a power of 90%, having the three arms increases the possible subgroupings, thus the chances for a chance hit—especially if the multiple end points remain the same, thus further lessening the chance for the result to reflect reality." He went on, "Homeopathy trials such as for diarrhea are even more fraught with error potential because measurements are not objective. They usually measure symptoms (like diarrhea). . . . Even 'systemic reviews' and meta-analyses of multiple trials are fraught with potential and real error. We have reviewed all such reviews for homeopathy and for acupuncture. They do not all come up with the same results. That means that the methods are not reliable enough to be generally applicable. (We think we know how to do a good one.)" And he says, "With homeopathy, prior probability—plausibility—of the null hypothesis being negated is near zero, thus making any positive result less probable of representing reality. Prior probability in this case reflects effects of basic science laws and prior data from trials and other sources. Next, for a false proposition, the more trials, the more likely the chances of a false positive result (though at the beginning of each trial the chances are the same as the previous time). In a way, it is like quantum mechanics. It is the nature of mathematics that if previous trials were negative or uninterpretable, the more one tries to determine if the hypothesis is true, the more elusive the truth becomes—the less likely a positive trial gives certainty that the result or the hypothesis is true. If most previous trials are positive, the likelihood of true representation increases with each success." In conclusion, Sampson says, "do not blame me for this, the problem is in the nature of statistics. There are ways to approach truth and reality more accurately than by carrying out a large trial, but they [Jacobs et al.] use the plausibility principles above, and all work to the disadvantage of the homeopathic proposition." About approving Jacobs's new protocol, Sampson says that "for all of the above, I would have to assign only a 'likely to be true or false' value to it. I would also have reasons to disbelieve the accuracy of how the data would be presented, in view of Dr. J's previous errors and misstatements in her publications, and partially because of Dr. J's high advocacy profile. (It seems that high advocacy serves to subtract from credibility, but that principle does not work in the other direction. In other words, skeptics are more often correct than advocates.) But even independent of that, stating the case just a bit inaccurately, but for illustration, the 'cards' are 'stacked' against Dr. Jacobs, even though the deck has been shuffled, and the cards are in random order."

Still, Sampson says that if Jacobs "were to send the proposed protocol, I would try my best to comment on it with help from experts in the performance of trials and statisticians." Jacobs has no plans to show Sampson her proposal. In fact, she believes that his answer to the question of whether or not scientific evidence might change his opinion of homeopathy is "self-evident." In short, nothing will change his mind. "I have no further comments nor interest in the views of Wallace Simpson," she says, calling his reply "double-talk."

At the Homeopathic Research Network symposium in 2002, Jacobs had commented that "there's a backlash against homeopathy now—it's under the radar." She went so far as to say that her study in *Pediatrics* "would not have been published in this climate." Another homeopath said that he "was more disheartened today than ever before." Even so, Jacobs also acknowledges that "slowly but surely as the research piles up, it will count, and some people will believe it, and others will not." Iris Bell, MD, PhD, says, "It's not going to be simple."

In an article entitled "A Critical Overview of Homeopathy," which appeared in the March 4, 2003, issue of *Annals of Internal Medicine,* Drs. Wayne Jonas, Ted Kaptchuk, and Klaus Linde wrote that although homeopathy "has recently undergone a worldwide revival, there is a lack of conclusive evidence on the effectiveness of homeopathy for most conditions." They also said, "Homeopathy deserves an open-minded opportunity to demonstrate its value by using evidence-based principles, but it should not be substituted for proven therapies."

Michael Carlston writes in *Classical Homeopathy* that "in some ways, research has made homeopathy more mysterious. A decade ago, very few physicians would have predicted that any good study would produce a result favorable to homeopathy. . . . At the same time, many good studies do not support homeopathy. That homeopathy has not simply shriveled up under the bright light of scientific examination is surprising and intriguing. Research has given us a sense of what needs to be done. We have much yet to learn."

The National Library of Medicine in Washington, D.C., has nearly 2,000 articles on homeopathic trials completed, homeopathic research in progress, homeopathic databases, surveys, discussions, and instruction in medical schools. Even though homeopathic trials have been making inroads, they are still crawling along in their infancy, so homeopathy is unable to satisfy Copeland's hope that it be "properly understood" and eventually become so routine that it is "nothing more than a method of therapeutic application." It *is* a "therapeutic application"—the fact that an estimated 15 million Americans use it is proof enough of that definition. But it is not yet routine or understood. Many people seem to think that it might never be fully understood, and most standard doctors say there is nothing there to be understood.

Jacobs says that these days homeopathy "is just lumped together with everything else in complementary medicine. Over the past ten years, some medicines have been more accepted than others—e.g., herbs and vitamins—and more allopaths are now using herbs instead of drugs. Homeopathy is often scoffed at because of the infinitesimal dose."

There is one particular homeopathic remedy that is rarely "lumped together with everything else." Oscillococcinum, made from the heart and liver of ducks, is considered the most popular and most widely used remedy in the world for cold and flu symptoms. (It has been the subject of a few clinical studies that reported a decrease in symptoms.) Stephen Barrett writes in "Homeopathy: The Ultimate Fake," that the remedy's

" 'active ingredient' is prepared by incubating small amounts of freshly killed duck's liver and heart for 40 days. The resultant solution is then filtered, freeze-dried, rehydrated, repeatedly diluted, and impregnated into sugar granules. If a single molecule of the duck's heart or liver were to survive the dilution, its concentration would be 1 in 100 (200 times). This huge number, which has 400 zeroes, is vastly greater than the estimated number of molecules in the universe (about one googol, which is 1 followed by 100 zeroes). In its February 17, 1997, issue, *U.S. News & World Report* noted that only one duck per year is needed to manufacture the product, which had a total sales of $20 million in 1996. The magazine dubbed it 'the $20-million duck.' "

A "Point/Counterpoint" debate between Jacobs and Sampson published in *Alternative Therapies in Health and Medicine* journal in September 1995 remains pertinent today. Jacobs's essay is titled "Homeopathy Should Be Integrated into Mainstream Medicine," and Sampson's is titled "Homeopathy Does Not Work." Jacobs insists that "nothing in homeopathy is inconsistent with contemporary physics, even though there is not a universally accepted scientific explanation for the mechanism of action." She reminds her readers "that the mechanism of action of aspirin was unknown until the early 1970s, and no one today understands how Ritalin, a stimulant in adults, helps hyperactivity in children." She asks, could it be homeopathic? Sampson argues that "homeopathy has cured no disease, has not extended life, and has not deepened our understanding of biology, health, or illness. The concept conflicts with the entire body of knowledge of pharmacology, chemistry, physics, and every other field of science. . . . No research has been done to show homeopathy to be equal to its rival—allopathic, rational biomedicine." He asks why homeopathy cannot explain "why the small amount of alcohol in an original tincture is not also made more potent by such dilutions, thus curing or causing drunkenness."

Eight years later, in 2003, Jacobs answered Sampson's question this way: "The alcohol in the original tincture is mixed with 87% alcohol at each stage of dilution and succession so you are mixing alcohol in alcohol. The alcohol, itself, is not undergoing any dilution." However, Michael Carlston said that the alcohol in an original tincture "might" become more potent, although he acknowledged that he has "never seen such a study." He said that "as etoh [ethanol, or grain alcohol] is a toxin which creates an 'intoxicated' state, a homeopathic preparation of etoh should help clear it from the system. As individuals vary, simply giving 'the hair of the dog' would not be as good as specifically administering the remedy which most precisely suits the specific patient's state. Nux Vomica is commonly recommended for hangovers."

These very different answers to Sampson's question might seem confusing, but Carlston, who said he "doesn't like to theorize so much," claimed that Jacobs's "reply is correct—as is mine." Then he said that "dilutions can be made many ways—not only in alcohol," and that "you could dilute alcohol in water, not just alcohol. Homeopathic remedies can be prepared with many dilutants."

But Jacobs countered that "Michael is incorrect. I do not think he considered that the 87 percent alcohol is used at all stages of dilution." Carlston agreed that she "has a good point," but that "alcohol is not the sole possible medium of dilution so this becomes a different matter." Jacobs replied that "it is very uncommon for dilutions to be made in something other than water/alcohol. Theoretically, it is possible to make a potency of alcohol by dissolving it in something else, but I have not heard of this."

Two modern homeopaths. Two medical doctors in the twenty-first century. Two contrasting views. Jacobs said that her answer "is the practical one," and Carlston's is "theoretical." Doctors of all specialties have been debating one another for centuries. In 1925, Copeland wrote, "I well remember the early days of the general acceptance of the germ theory. There was never a medical society meeting but two or three, or the whole group of doctors engaged in a verbal combat over the idea that diseases can be produced by plants or animals of microscopic size."

Epilogue

From 1960 to the early 1990s, scientific advances were perceived by many American homeopaths as more and more of a threat. These practitioners became afraid of (and angry at) the future and seemed more content to stay in a familiar past. They became unwilling even to integrate this past they so treasured into the present. They forgot what Copeland had so often lectured his students about, that Hahnemann saw all medical advances "in one symphony of perfect harmony." They even turned away from conventional medical degrees. Personal provings and anecdotal evidence once again became for them proof enough.

And then in 1993 came the Homeopathic Research Network, a group of homeopaths with medical degrees who wanted to apply the gold standard of clinical trials to their chosen specialty. It was almost as if homeopathy decided to join science in time for the twenty-first century.

Indeed, in 2000, one prominent spokesperson for alternative medicine laid out a road map for the appropriate testing of CAM. Stephen E. Straus, the first permanent director of the National Center for Complementary and Alternative Medicine, testified before the House Appropriations Subcommittee on Labor about his budget for 2001, saying that "credible, not anecdotal data must be provided to the public." He added that "advances in neurobiology will reveal more about ancient practices such as acupuncture and meditation, as well as the phenomenon of 'the placebo effect' as we tap the healing power of the mind."

His mention of the placebo effect was significant. Standard doctors believe that if homeopathy works at all it is because of this effect, or perhaps due to spontaneous recovery—the body healing itself over time. There are myriad descriptive phrases for the placebo effect, ranging from "a powerful therapeutic agent" to "a therapeutic maneuver," to "make-believe medicine," and one particularly evocative definition by Dr. Anne Harrington, a historian of science at Harvard—namely, "lies that heal." Some modern homeopaths are even ready to believe that if science can't explain why their remedies work, the placebo effect could turn out to be what is responsible for their cures. But mainstream homeopaths are not ready to give in so easily. In 2001, the National Center for Homeopathy said that attributing homeopathy's successes to the placebo effect was, in effect, dismissing homeopathy. The center urged scientists to focus not only on submolecular "transfers," but also on "the areas of energy transfer." (It even invoked cell phone transmissions as an area of possible study—that these magnetic fields might possibly hold some clue to a remedy's source of power.) An article on alternative medicine and the laws of physics by Robert Park in the *Skeptical Inquirer* discussed the idea from a book called *Conjuring Science,* by C. P. Tourney, that alternative-medicine practitioners' "nostalgia for a time when things seemed simpler and more natural is mixed with respect for the power of science." The members of the Homeopathic Research Network appear to fit this particular model.

Still, there remain skeptics who will never be convinced that homeopathy could one day be science-based, a part of biomedicine. The most they will concede is the placebo effect, going along with the Mayo Clinic's definition of a placebo as something that "may work on the power of suggestion," and concerning which "scientists speculate that a person's confidence in a certain treatment may activate chemical impulses in the brain that diminish symptoms." Indeed, these skeptics wonder if another mind-body synergy might be involved. Could it be that the psychotherapeutic aspect of homeopathic prescribing—that is, the connection between patient and doctor, as well as the long and detailed process of history-taking—is involved in the success of remedies on people? It is in this vein that Michael Carlston pronounces that "the most potent placebo is the physician." Granted, many homeopaths prefer to think of this healing connection between the doctor and patient in a spiritual light. For instance, at one homeopathic conference, an audience member asked a speaker if his teenage patient's "spiritual journey, of going into the darkness of illness and coming out of it, had helped her." (The girl, who had an autoimmune disease, had also been a victim of sexual abuse, and had talked about it with her doctor for the first time.) "Yes," the speaker replied. During a question-and-answer session at the 2002 Homeopathic Research Network Symposium, a member of the audience told the group that "when a homeopath goes 'Aha, this is the remedy!' that's a big energy going out in the world, and the patient is sitting there. Thoughts are energy."

Thoughts are energy? Was the speaker waxing mystical? Not really, as far as modern scientific thinking goes. This is not science fiction, but a possible actuality. It is also part of the "advances in neurobiology" theme that the first director of the National Center for CAM talked about at the turn of the twenty-first century.

In a laboratory experiment, Eric Kandel, the Nobel Prize–winning psychiatrist and neuroscientist, has demonstrated through his work with the nervous system of sea slugs that learning can actually alter brain cells. Newly created proteins can remake neurons in the brain. In his medical-school textbook, *Essentials of Neural Science and Behavior,* edited along with James H. Schwartz and Thomas M. Jessell of the Center for Neuro-biology and Behavior at the College of Physicians and Surgeons of Columbia University and the Howard Hughes Medical Institute, Kandel states in one of the chapters he has written that "we no longer think that certain diseases (organic diseases) affect mentation by producing biolog-ical changes in the brain while other diseases (functional diseases) do not. The basis of contemporary neural science is that all mental processes are biological and any alteration in those processes is organic." He goes go on to write, "Insofar as social intervention works, whether through psychotherapy, counseling, or the support of family or friends, it must work by acting on the brain and, quite likely, on the strength of connec-tions between nerve cells. Moreover, the absence of demonstrable struc-tural change does not rule out the possibility that important biological changes are nevertheless occurring. They may simply be undetectable with the techniques available to us."

So one has to ask if it is remotely possible that homeopathic remedies could somehow affect the connections between nerve cells. Or if the remedies might act in the same way that psychotherapy does, even to the extent of altering the physiology of the brain. Or if the patient is being affected by some combination of the intense relationship with the ho-meopathic doctor and the remedies. In an e-mail exchange with this author, Kandel remarked that "homeopathic medicine may work in many vague ways, as a placebo, as a mechanism of interaction between patient and physician, as a spiritual relief of an ailing patient. The point is it does not act specifically against the disease to which it is directed."

Jennifer Jacobs writes in *Healing with Homeopathy* that in a certain sense homeopathy "captures the hope of the magic bullet: to embody the complex process of healing in a simple and safe procedure. Ultimately all healing is a personal journey. . . . Sometimes it seems to come from with-out, sometimes from within—sometimes it does not come at all. In any case, healing comes when illness motivates a person to seek change.

Though the process may seem long and chaotic at times, it always begins with this intention toward a more satisfying life."

The simple reality remains that despite most people's tendency and desire to embrace scientific medicine, homeopathy is still sought-after all around the world. Millions and millions of Americans pursue "change" and "a more satisfying life" through the use of homeopathic remedies.

A somewhat elliptical but heartfelt letter in the May 13, 2000, *Lancet* by Dr. V. S. Rambihar hints at just why. He writes that "a post-modern science has developed since the 1980s, of deconstructionism, responding to the collapse of normal science. Normal science (before 2000) refers to a puzzle solving approach, with uncertainty managed and values unspoken. A post-normal (not post-modern) science has since appeared, emerging from the new science of nonlinear dynamics, which recognizes irregularity, subjectivity, and uncertainty as intrinsic and fundamental. This new science is variously also called chaos, complexity, or nonlinear dynamics." Rambihar goes on to assert that "science or evidence lies in the eye of the beholder, changing with time, place, and circumstance. Science may mean absolute truth and validity to some, with a relentless pursuit of certainty, whereas others may accept the inevitability of uncertainty, and the contextual and thus subjective nature of reality."

Most standard doctors are more than willing to admit that if homeopathy—as a "personal journey" in Jacobs's sense, or not—is to have a place in twenty-first-century medicine, its only real future lies in the outcome of replicable clinical studies of its entire repertoire of remedies. Even Stephen Barrett, who believes scientific proof will never happen, nonetheless says that "proponents interested in research should consult with homeopathy's critics to see whether they can agree on the type of research needed to test homeopathy's theories and methods and to determine *in advance* what various experimental outcomes would mean—pro or con."

In addition, all homeopaths need to have medical degrees from reputable medical schools, and be fully licensed. During much of Copeland's life, homeopaths were, of course, practically indistinguishable from allopathic doctors. Their training was identical. Still, Copeland's cures, while always popular, were firmly ridiculed, even though scientific advances were often integrated into homeopathy.

Two critical questions remain. Will homeopathy step into the future with facts and scientific confidence, hand in hand with standard medicine? Or will it remain the distinct alternative it has always been, one that may or may not be "proved" someday?

Sources

An explanation concerning sources: The Royal Samuel Copeland Collection at the Bentley Historical Library of the University of Michigan in Ann Arbor was my primary and most important research tool in the writing of this book. Not only is the collection superb, but the library is a welcoming and peaceful place for a writer to work. In the spring and summer, the large desks in the reading room face a flowering sculpture garden. In the winter, the snow-covered garden remains restful and soothing. I am grateful to the entire staff (listed separately in my acknowledgments) for their knowledge, help, and patience. Chapter notes use the identification "RSC Collection/Bentley," and then list the box numbers where the material was found and the titles of the documents.

Another important research tool was the American Medical Association's Historical Health Fraud and Alternative Medicine Collection, housed in the AMA's headquarters in Chicago. The published guide to this impressive collection was instrumental in leading me to the documents I studied during the time I spent in the archives room. Archivist Robert Tenuta was very helpful and courteous to me, although he was sometimes handicapped by restrictions that prevented me from consulting certain reference books that were right next to the table where I worked. (Nonmembers of the AMA—like me!—are only allowed to look at the Health Fraud Collection.) Still, often with begging and pleading, I got to look through some of those wonderful, age-old reference books shelved tantalizingly nearby. Finally, I am grateful to the AMA for waiving the fees pertaining to the photo of the advertisement of Copeland and Pluto Water.

Many books—all detailed in the Selected Bibliography—provided background material, descriptions, and facts that informed my account. All books will be identified by their author and title in the chapter notes, and complete information about them can be found in the Selected Bibliography. Seven books in particular provided essential information—they were my "lodestars"—and also acted as important catalysts for certain insights and opinions expressed by the author. Direct quotations from any of them (as well as from all the other books) will be noted.

The essential books include: Fontanarosa, ed., *Alternative Medicine,* a collection of articles from *JAMA* (*Journal of the American Medical Association* and the *Archives* Journals); Coulter, *Divided Legacy: The Conflict Between Homeopathy and the American Medical Association;* Jacobs, ed., *The Encyclopedia of Alternative Medicine;* Porter, ed., *Medicine: A History of Healing;* Hahnemann, *Organon of the Medical Art;* Lockie and Geddes, *The Complete Guide to Homeopathy: The Principles and Practice of Treatment;* and Starr, *The Social Transformation of American Medicine: The Rise of a Sovereign Profession and the Making of a Vast Industry.*

An eighth book also deserves to be on this list. It is an unpublished PhD dissertation by Raymond J. Potter, Western Reserve University, June 1967. This work, "Royal Samuel Copeland, 1868–1938: A Physician in Politics," served as a useful guidebook and provided me with chronological as well as some biographical material. I will identify it in the chapter notes as "Potter dissertation" and will record page numbers when I quote directly from it.

The Web addresses listed have been checked as carefully as possible for accuracy and reliability. Please contact the author c/o Knopf if access is denied or if the site has "disappeared," as can happen with such sites.

AUTHOR'S NOTE

The phrase "no medicine medicine" comes from Robert L. Park, "Alternate Medicine and the Laws of Physics," *Skeptical Inquirer,* Sept. 10, 1997; the Jennifer Jacobs quote comes from Jonas and Jacobs, *Healing with Homeopathy,* p. xvii; the Michael Carlston quote is from Carlston, ed., *Classical Homeopathy,* p. 1.

PROLOGUE

My description of bloodletting is drawn from various sources, most especially from John Upshaw, MD, and John O'Leary, MD, "The Medicinal Leech: Past and Present," in *The American Surgeon,* Mar. 2000, published by Southeastern Surgical Congress, Atlanta, Georgia; Kansas State Historical Society, "Bloodletting Tools," www.ksha. org/cool/coolmed.htm; Geoffrey Mock, "The Long Respected History of Bloodletting," www.dukenews.duke.edu/news/diologue_newsrelease30ab.html; Museum of Questionable Medical Devices, "Phlebotomy and the Ancient Art of Bloodletting," by Graham Ford, www.mth.org/quack/devices/phlebo.htm. **RSC Collection/Bentley:** Box 21: RSC, *What Is Homeopathy?* **Books:** Porter, ed., *Medicine;* Wilbur, *Revolutionary Medicine.*

ONE: "Like a Pleasant Dream"

The following were consulted for information about medicine in the eighteenth and nineteenth centuries, Samuel Hahnemann, and homeopathy: Morris Fishbein, MD, "The Rise and Fall of Homeopathy," in *Fads and Fallacies in Healing* (New York: Blue Ribbon Books, 1932), posted at www.homeowatch.org/history/Fishbein; "Sappington Cemetery State Historic Site," www.mostateparks.com/cemeteries; *Scientific American* 4, no. 37 (June 2, 1849). **RSC Collection/Bentley:** Box 21: RSC, *What Is Homeopathy?* **Books:** Lockie and Geddes, *Complete Guide to Homeopathy;* Coulter, *Divided Legacy;* McCabe, *Let Like Cure Like;* Porter, ed., *Medicine;* Shapiro and Shapiro, *Powerful Placebo;* Hahnemann, *Organon;* Starr, *Social Transformation.*

Many of the facts about Dexter, Michigan, Roscoe and Frances Copeland, and young Royal and Cornelia Copeland were drawn from Roscoe P. Copeland, "A Letter to His Children, Royal and Cornelia, March 6, 1926," in the Dexter Area Museum (I am extremely grateful to Nancy Van Blarcum for unearthing this and other documents during my visit to the local museum; Nancy even gave me a tour of Dexter, pointing out places she knew would be of interest to me); and Norma McAllister, "Residents Serve Village over Long Period of Time," *Chelsea Standard/Dexter Leader,* July 15, 1999; **RSC Collection/Bentley:** Box 20: RSC, selected speeches, 1925. Box 21: RSC, selected speeches re health, 1925. **Books:** McAllister, *Judge Samuel William Dexter; History of Washtenaw County*, vol. 2.

Many of the facts about the American Medical Association, the American Institute of Homeopathy, and the University of Michigan Medical School were drawn from "Minutes of the First Annual Meeting of the AMA," *Digest of Official Actions, 1846–1958* (courtesy of the American Medical Association Archives); and Howard Markel, MD, PhD, "The University of Michigan Medical School, 1850–2000: An Example Worthy of Imitation," *JAMA,* Feb. 16, 2000. Information about Avogadro's number is from www.gemini.tntech.edu/~tfurtsch/scihist/avogadro. **RSC Collection/Bentley:** Box 8: assorted letters, 1914–15. Box 9: assorted letters, 1916–17. Box 113G: "RSC's Testimony to University of Michigan Medical School—1921." Michigan University Homeopathic Medical School Collection/Bentley: Box A13: "Obetz, Henry—An Explanation: A Communication to the Honorable Board of Regents of the University of Michigan." **Books:** My knowledge of the early years owes much to Coulter's *Divided Legacy* (especially chap. 2, "The Sectarian Attack on Allopathy," pp. 87–137, and chap. 3, "The Allopathic Counterattack," pp. 140–237); *The Proceedings of the American Institute of Homeopathy, 1846* (quoted from p. 125). Coulter, *Homeopathic Science;* Davenport, *Not Just Any Medical School;* Cramp, *Nostrums and Quackeries;* Hahnemann, *Organon.*

TWO: "As Fixed as the Law of Gravitation"

Information in this chapter was drawn from the following: "Circumcision Information Resources," www.cirp.org/; Roscoe Copeland, "A Letter to His Children," Dexter Area Museum; W. B. Hinsdale, MD, "Nux Vomica," notes on a lecture, Homeopathic Medical College Collection, Bentley Historical Library; also Hinsdale, "Private Scrapbook of Collected Articles by Wilbert B. Hinsdale, MD"; and further from this collection, RSC, "Reference Handbook of the Medical Sciences," entry on homeopathy; "Homeopathy Special Data, Articles and Clippings," *Digest of Official Actions, 1846–1958,* AMA Archives; Howard Markel, PhD, "The University of Michigan Medical School, 1850–2000: An Example Worthy of Imitation," *JAMA,* Feb. 16, 2000; Oliver Wendell Holmes, "Homeopathy and Its Kindred Delusions," www.quackwatch.org; "Medicine in the Civil War," University of Toledo Libraries, www.cl.utoledo.edu/canady/quackery/quack8.html; "Past and Present of Washtenaw County," Dexter Area Museum; Dana Ullman, "A Homeopathic Perspective on Health and Healing in the 21st Century," www.homeopathic.com/new/understandingnature.htm. **RSC Collection/ Bentley:** Box 1: assorted correspondence, some undated; RSC letter, "Dear Doctor Doran," 1906. Box 9: "My Dear Doctor," letter to RSC from Joseph Pettee Cobb, Dean of Hahnemann Medical College in Chicago, Mar. 11, 1916, re "militant and at the same time diplomatic" phrase; RSC letter, "Dear Mr. Williams," Oct. 30, 1907. Box 17: "Letter RSC, Jr., to RSC," Mar. 31, 1930. Box 21: RSC, "Emergencies in Ophthalmology"; RSC, "Homeopathy's Appeal to the Practitioners of the Old School." Box 23: Dr. Cyrus Bump, "The Teaching of Materia Medica." Box 25: "Response of Dean Copeland to the Congratulatory Address"; RSC, "Hahnemann's Place in the Medical World"; W. A. Dewey, MD, "Homeopathy and Its Place in Medicine"; RSC, "Emergencies in Ophthalmology"; RSC, "Belladonna"; RSC, "Blood Pressure as a Factor in Eye Disease"; RSC, "Address to Nurses," Bureau of Homeopathy. Box 26: RSC, "Jamaica Real Estate

Board Address"; RSC, "Address to Class of 1901." Box 32: "Response of Dean Copeland to the Congratulatory Addresses." Box 33: RSC, "Address to Class of 1901"; RSC, "The Value of an Opportunity"; RSC letter to his sister. Box 34: RSC, assorted obituaries. Boxes 133–36: RSC's notebooks (oversized). **Books:** Lockie and Geddes, *Complete Guide to Homeopathy* (the quotation re the *Kali iod.* type is from p. 132); Coulter, *Divided Legacy* (p. 227 re *Boston Medical and Surgical Journal,* 1854–55); Coulter, *Homeopathic Science;* Jacobs, *Encyclopedia of Alternative Medicine;* Schaller, *Health, Quackery, and the Consumer;* William Boericke, MD, *Homeopathic Materia Medica* (www.homeoint. org/books/boericmm/index.htm, pp. 104, 206, 209); Porter, ed., *Medicine;* Hahnemann, *Organon;* Potter dissertation ("His first operation . . ." is quoted from p. 32); Starr, *Social Transformation.*

THREE: "We Shall Deserve to Win and We Will Win"

Information in this chapter was drawn from the following: www.baycitymi.org; www.multimag.com/city/mi/baycity. I'd like to thank Phil Adair, in the Bay City City Hall Engineering Department for taking the time to help me identify street names during the time RSC lived in his city. Also consulted: *History of Bay County, Michigan* (Chicago: H. R. Page & Co., 1883); "Brochure on Naturopathy," AMA Archives; "Naturopathic Doctors," *Digest of Official Actions,* AMA Archives; "Pluto Water Ad with Royal Copeland Remarks," AMA Archives; P. P. Wells, MD, "A Revolution in Old Physic!" *IHA Transactions, 1889,* p. 32, www.julianwinston.com/archives/periodicals/ iha/php. **RSC Collection/Bentley:** Box 1: RSC letter, "Dear Mr. Runyan," Aug. 11, 1907. Box 21: RSC, "Annual Address to American Hospital Association"; RSC, "The Part the Physician Should Play in Public Life"; RSC, "What Should Be the Provisions of a Model Medical Practice Act." Box 23: RSC, "Hahnemann's Place in the Medical World"; RSC, "Autobiography"; RSC, "Homeopathy and Polology." Box 34: "Senator Royal S. Copeland," *America Forward.* Box 113G: assorted news clippings. (Note re Mary DePriest Ryan Copeland: There are no letters, official documents, or substantial references to her in the entire RSC Collection. It would appear that she has been excised, even though she was married to RSC for seventeen years.) Information about RSC's surgery on the blind Civil War veteran is from "Copeland's Life Upset Traditions," New York *Daily News,* June 18, 1938. **Books:** Coulter, *Divided Legacy* (information on George Simmons, MD, and AIH membership is largely taken from this book; information about Mark Twain is quoted from pp. 288–89); Lockie and Geddes, *Complete Guide to Homeopathy;* Porter, *Medicine;* Davenport, *Not Just Any Medical School;* Starr, *Social Transformation.*

FOUR: "Much Missionary Labor Yet to Perform"

Information in this chapter was drawn from the following: Charles Woodhull Eaton, MD, "The Facts About Variolinum," *Transactions of the American Institute of Homeopathy,* 1907, pp. 547–67, www.whale.to/v/eaton.html. **RSC Collection/Bentley:** Box 1: W. B. Hinsdale, MD, "Mercurius Corrosivus Poisoning," *Medical Century,* Dec. 1900 (I am grateful to Dean Crothers, MD, for helping me identify the remedy Strychinium sulphuricum, mentioned in Hinsdale's essay. Dr. Crothers found it in *The American Homeopathic Pharmacopoeia,* by J. O'Conner, published in the late nineteenth century); "Report by E. D. Campbell," *Chemical Engineering and Analytical Chemistry,* May 16, 1904; unsigned biographical sketch of RSC. Box 20: "Letter to 'Mr. Copeland' from Dr. Copeland," Feb. 12, 1938. Box 21: RSC, "The Operation for Cataract"; RSC, "Therapeutics of the Eye"; RSC, "Is There But One School of Medicine?" (re Osler quote); RSC, "Address to Nurses"; RSC, "Homeopathy in the 20th Century"; RSC, "The Propagandism of Homeopathy"; *Scientific American* entry on homeopathy by Dr. Pemberton Dudley, professor of Institutes of Medicine, Hahnemann Medical College, Philadelphia; W. A. Dewey, MD, "Homeopathy and Its Place in Medicine." Box 23: RSC, brief autobiography. Box 34: Alva Johnson, "Master Hinter," *New Yorker* profile, Aug. 18, 1928; selected news articles about RSC as mayor of Ann Arbor, Mich., 1901–3. **Books:** Potter dissertation (additional information about RSC as mayor, and material on the separation of Mary and Royal Copeland); Coulter, *Divided Legacy* (the information about membership in the IHA in 1892 is from n. 216, p. 399); Lockie and Geddes, *Complete Guide to Homeopathy;* Vithoulkos, *Science of Homeopathy.*

FIVE: "The Sacred Fire of a Wise Ambition"

Information in this chapter was drawn from the following: The characterization of homeopaths using "figurative language" is from the *Minutes of the National Medical Convention, 1846,* p. 89, AMA Archives; "Brochure on Naturopathy," AMA Archives; the term "pseudo-homeopaths," used by Samuel Hahnemann, is from Dana Ullman, "A Condensed History of Homeopathy," Homeopathic Educational Services, www.homeopathic.com; "From Quackery to Bacteriology"/"Women's Health Care," Document 4, www.cl.utoledo.edu/canady/quackery/quack4.html (also same address but at end "quack3b.html"); James Harvey Young, "The Long Struggle for the 1906 Law," *FDA Consumer,* June 1981; National Library of Medicine, Pure Food and Drugs, "Images from the History of the Public Health Service"; information on AMA membership in 1904 from Robert Tenuta, AMA reference archivist; "Proving of X-Ray," *IHA Transactions,* 1897, pp. 47–76, www.julianwinston.com/archives/periodicals/iha/php. **RSC Collection/Bentley:** Box 1: RSC letter, "Dear Dr. Brown," Oct. 5, 1906. Box 2: letter, "Dear Doctor," Jan. 20, 1910; RSC letter, "My Dear Sister," Dec. 15, 1908; letter from Committee on Pharmacopoeia, AIH, Feb. 15, 1907. Box 21: "Homeopathy and Its Place in Medicine," by W. A. Dewey, circa 1910; RSC, *What Is Homeopathy?;* RSC, "Bureau of Homeopathy"; RSC, "Definite Medications"; RSC, "The College Alliance"; RSC, "Member of the Class of 1901"; RSC, "The Scientific Resemblance of Homeopathy"; RSC, "Address to Nurses"; RSC, "Annual Address to American Hospital Association," Aug. 14, 1932. Box 23: RSC, "Hahnemann's Place in the Medical World"; document re cause of disease, in report for Single Board of Medicine for All Schools, 1906. Box 34: Alva Johnson, "Master Hinter," *New Yorker* profile, Aug. 18, 1928; RSC, "Food Fads"; Memorial Address by Senator Arthur Vandenberg. **Books:** Coulter, *Divided Legacy*—statistics on homeopathic medical schools and some information on the AMA is largely taken from this source, as well as from Starr, *Social Transformation;* some additional statistics and information on the AMA and patent medicines is from Burrow, *AMA,* and Cramp, *Nostrums and Quackery;* Gevitz, ed., *Other Healers.*

SIX: "Eventually Those Who Came to Scoff Will Remain to Learn"

Information in this chapter was drawn from the following: **RSC Collection/Bentley:** Box 1: assorted letters of May 17, 1907. Box 2: RSC, "Letter to President and Board of Regents, University of Michigan," Sept. 7, 1908; letter, "Dear Doctor," Sept. 7, 1908; RSC letter to student, "My Dear Sir," n.d.; letter, "My Dear Doctor," Oct. 22, 1908; letter, "My Dear Doctor," Oct. 21, 1908; letter, "Dear Friend," Feb. 4, 1909. Box 3: RSC letter, "Dear Doctor Myers," Sept. 8, 1909; RSC letter, "Dear Dr. Butler," Mar. 12, 1910; letter, "Dear Doctor," Jan. 10, 1910. Box 6: RSC letter, "To Parke-Davis & Co.," Oct. 8, 1910; letters, Parke-Davis & Co. to RSC, Oct. 8 and Oct. 18, 1910. Box 8: RSC letter, "Dear Dr. Brooks," Dec. 1, 1915; RSC letter re J. D. Rockefeller, Jr., using allopathic doctor and not a homeopath. Box 20: letter, "Dear Doctor," Jan. 20, 1910; RSC letter, "Dear Joe," May 5, 1910. Box 21: RSC, "Definite Medication"; RSC, "The Elimination of Sectarian Dogma from Scientific Medicine"; RSC, "Emergencies in Ophthalmology"; RSC, "Homeopathy and the New Thought in Science" (Note: The English scientist RSC mentions is "Strutt of Trinity College," and his book is *The Bequerel Rays;* the French scientist is Dr. Alfred Robin); RSC, "Saving the Babies in a Great City." Box 23: RSC, "Short Autobiography"; New York Homeopathic Medical College Board of Trustees reports and minutes. Box 34: "Joint Annual Homeopathic Convention." Box 35: scrapbooks, 1908–11; "To the Alumni of the New York Homeopathic Medical College and Flower Hospital," 1908, re Dr. Biggar on homeopathy; also *Utica Daily Press,* Dec. 10, 1910. Additional information on Flower Hospital is from www.nymc.edu/today/today/asp.; "A Brief History of New York Medical College," www.homeoint.org/cazalet/histo/newyork.htm; also Potter dissertation, and "Research in Homeopathy," www.lyghtforce.com/king_bio/research.htm. Some information about Abraham Flexner is drawn from Coulter, *Divided Legacy,* and Starr, *Social Transformation.*

SEVEN: "Masters of the Situation"

Information in this chapter was drawn from the following: "Flexner Report," www.carnegiefoundation.org/elibrary/index.htm#prof. "Summary of John D. Rockefeller's Charities, 1863–1903, Rockefeller Family Archives; National Eye Institute, www.nei.nih.gov/; James Harvey Young, PhD, "The New Muckrakers," chap. 7 of *The Medical Messiahs: A Social History of Health Quackery in 20th Century America,* www.quackwatch.org. **AMA Archives:** *Digest of Official Actions;* AMA Department of Investigation file on RSC; "Homeopathy: What Is It?"; J. H. Hohnstedt, MD, "Self-Medication," *Kentucky Medical Journal,* Dec. 15, 1912. **RSC Collection/Bentley:** Box 1: RSC letter, "Dear Mrs. Knight," Oct. 8, 1906. Box 2: letter, "My Dear Doctor," Oct. 10, 1908; letter, "Dear Dr. Copeland," June 11, 1908. Box 3: letter, "My Dear Doctor," Mar. 11, 1910; letter, "Dear Sir," Jan. 16, 1910. Box 4: RSC letter, "My Dear Parents," Sept. 13, 1910. Box 6: letter, "Dear Doctor," Jan. 17, 1913; RSC letter to editor of *Medical Times,* "Dear Sir," Feb. 21, 1931. Box 7: RSC letters, "Dear Dr. Downing," Oct. 8, 1913, and Mar. 30, 1914; letter, "My Dear Doctor," Sept. 1, 1913. Box 21: RSC, "Definite Medication"; RSC, "The Present Status of Scientific Medicine"; RSC, "The Future of Homeopathy"; RSC, "Transplantation of the Cornea: The Preliminary Report of a Single Case"; W. A. Dewey, MD, "Aspirin: A Dangerous Drug"; State Board of Charities reports. Box 23: RSC, "Outline of Talk to Interns"; RSC, "If Medical Colleges Were Under State Supervision, Could the Medical Profession Be More Uniformly and Efficiently Trained Than the Present System?"; RSC letter to Board of Trustees, New York Homeopathic College, n.d.; Flower Hospital's Operation Books, 1914. Box 34: news article, "Lengthen Medical Course: Homeopathic College Now Requires Five Years' Study," n.d.; "Flower Hospital's New Private Hotel for Sick Is Open," *New York Globe,* Jan. 28, 1914; W. A. Dewey, MD, "Aspirin: A Dangerous Quack Nostrum," *Homeopathic* (a newspaper published in Perkasie, Pa.), June 19, 1913; Alva Johnson, "Master Hinter," *New Yorker* profile, Aug. 18, 1928. Box 35: re AMA wanting a Department of Health, *New York Herald,* May 22, 1910; re calorimeter, *New York Tribune,* Jan. 27, 1911. **Books:** Burrow, *AMA;* Shapiro and Shapiro, *Powerful Placebo;* Fishbein, *History of the American Medical Association;* Gevitz, ed., *Other Healers;* Starr, *Social Transformation;* Potter dissertation ("After a while, however, he discovered . . . ," paraphrased from p. 114).

EIGHT: "Losing at the Edges"

Information in this chapter was drawn from the following: **AMA Archives:** *Kentucky Medical Journal,* Dec. 14, 1912; Cramp, *Nostrums and Quackeries;* Martin I. Wilbert, *The Limitations to Self-Medication: Uses and Abuses of Proprietary Preparations and Household Remedies* (Washington, D.C.: Government Printing Office, 1915); 1914 AMA statistics from Robert Tenuta, AMA reference archivist; "Naturopathic Doctors"; "Homeopathic Prophylaxis," www.homeopathic.org/crtoddh.htm. **RSC Collection/Bentley:** Box 6: Horace Porter Gillingham, MD; RSC letter, "Dear Sir," Feb. 21, 1913. Box 7: RSC letter, "My Dear Parents," Apr. 28, 1914. Box 8: RSC letter, "Dear Dr. Burrett," Jan. 24, 1916; letter from George Starr White to RSC, Dec. 23, 1915. Box 9: "1914 Inspection Report"; letter from George Starr White to RSC, Feb. 12, 1916; RSC letter, "Dear Dr. Laidlow," Mar. 9, 1916; RSC letter, "Dear Mr. MacKay," Jan. 21, 1916. Box 20: RSC, "I regard the bottler as just as important . . . ," n.d. Box 21: RSC, "What Is Homeopathy?"; letter from George Starr White to RSC, Feb. 22, 1916; RSC, "The Proof of Homeopathy"; RSC, "Attrition and Homeopathy"; RSC, "Members of the Class of 1901"; "Minutes of College Commission," Dec. 20, 1913; RSC, "Bureau of Homeopathy"; RSC, "The College Alliance of the AIH." Box 23: RSC, "The Teaching of the Materia Medica"; Flower documents pertaining to polio epidemic in 1916. **Books:** Fontanarosa, *Alternative Medicine* (Ted Kaptchuk, MD, and David Eisenberg, MD, "Chiropractic," pp. 508–20); *Chronicles of the Twentieth Century* ("First Cancer Virus Discovered by Rous," Jan. 21, 1911); Copeland, *Dr. Copeland's Home Medical Book* (p. 249 re cancer); Hahnemann, *Organon;* Gevitz, ed., *Other Healers;* Starr, *Social Transformation.*

NINE: "But One of Many Methods of Treating Sickness"

Information in this chapter was drawn from the following: Frederick M. Dearborn, MD, *American Homeopathy in the World War* (Chicago: American Institute of Homeopathy, 1923); RSC, "Hospital Unit 'N,' " www.homeoint.org/books2/wwi; Jim Middleton, "The One Dollar Miracles of Battle Creek," the Animating Apothecary, jimmiddleton@juno.com or www.animatingapothecary.com/; "History of Cereals Time Line," www.Kelloggs.com. **AMA Archives:** "Obesity Cures," in *Nostrums and Quack-*

ery; "Letter to the AMA from Acting Commissioner of Health, City of Cleveland," Jan. 9, 1919; letter, "Dear Sir," May 24, 1927; letter, "Dear Dr. Leithauser," Apr. 9, 1928; AMA letter, "Dear Dr. Smith," Feb. 7, 1931; Naturopathy Correspondence, 1914–1939; "Naturopathic Doctors"; AMA Law Department, "Naturopathy"; "Epidemic Lessons Against Next Time," *New York Times,* Nov. 17, 1918. **RSC Collection/Bentley:** Box 1: William J. Murray, "The Gift of Public Service" (published in *Circulation*); letter from the Battle Creek Sanitarium, "Dear Doctor," Oct. 24, 1906. Box 9: RSC letter, "Dear Dr. Kellogg," Jan. 25, 1917. Box 20: RSC medical advice column questions, 1920–21. Box 21: RSC, "Dr. Copeland Tells How to Trade Overweight for Pep"; RSC, "Modern Chemists and Nature"; RSC, "The Policeman and the Public Health"; RSC, "Colonic Cleanliness"; RSC, "Saving the Babies in a Great City"; RSC, "What Is Homeopathy?"; RSC, "Homeopathy," in *Reference Handbook of the Medical Sciences,* p. 284; RSC, "The Propagandism of Homeopathy"; RSC letter to deans of homeopathic colleges, begins "The old Jewish religious life . . ."; "Is There But One School of Homeopathy?" prepared by a committee of the faculty of the Homeopathic Medical School of the University of Michigan; W. A. Dewey, MD, "Aspirin: A Dangerous Quack Nostrum." Box 22: RSC letter, "My Dear Dr. Dunlevy," May 9, 1918; RSC, "Typhus Fever"; RSC, "Plague"; RSC, "Every Great War . . ."; RSC, "Vaccination"; RSC, "What You Should Know About Influenza"; influenza document dated Sept. 19, 1919; influenza bulletin issued by the Trust Fund for Homeopathic Research and the Materia Medica Department, New York Homeopathic Medical College; RSC, statement about whiskey, Jan. 26, 1920. Box 25: RSC, "The Health of a Nation"; RSC undated speech: "To the Jews of Buffalo." Box 26: "I found that movies kept the minds of the people . . . ," from Laurence Reid, "Senator Copeland Has the Floor," n.d.; scrapbooks of health articles; re polio epidemic, *New York Times,* Oct. 3, 1920. Box 34: RSC, "How Daylight Savings Aids in Fighting Epidemics"; "Politics Interfere, Says Copeland," *Brooklyn Eagle,* Oct. 20, 1921; "Immigration Evils Shown by Copeland," *Standard Union* (Brooklyn), 1921; "Health Expert Club Speaker," *Jackson* (Michigan) *News,* Feb. 2, 1921. Box 113G: "To the Board of Trustees of the AIH, Report of Inspection Made October 24, 1919"; "Commissioner Copeland," n.d.; RSC letter to president of University of Michigan, "My Dear Doctor," Dec. 15, 1921; James W. Ward, MD, "Homeopathic Activities." **Books:** Hahnemann, *Organon* (quote from p. 123); Lockie and Geddes, *Complete Guide to Homeopathy;* Potter dissertation (p. 214, letter to Raymond Potter from Col. Royal S. Copeland, Aug. 15, 1965).

TEN: "Hitch Your Cart to a Star"

Information in this chapter was drawn from the following: "Dexter Area Sesquicentennial"; "Western Washtenaw Bicentennial Celebration"; "Letter to Royal and Cornelia Copeland from Roscoe P. Copeland"—all in the Dexter Area Museum. **AMA Archives:** AMA Department of Investigation file on RSC; "Senate Investigation of Diploma Mills," *JAMA,* Dec. 22, 1923; "Bid for Medical Research Bureau in Interior Department," *JAMA,* May 17, 1924; "North Carolina State College of Agriculture and Engineering Commencement Speech by Royal S. Copeland," 1923; Chuck-Muck-La Water information from "Mineral Waters" file; "Buffalo Litho Water" file: letters, Nov. 10, 21, 24, and 31, 1921, and Jan. 3, 1922; letter to the *Journal of the Indiana State Medical Association,* "Dear Dr. Bulson," Dec. 5, 1924; "Dear Dr. Cramp," Dec. 6, 1924; "Dear Dr. Bulson," Dec. 9, 1924; United States Department of Agriculture, Circular No. 78, Mar. 20,

1914; "Bill for Medical Research Bureau," *JAMA,* May, 17, 1924; "Peril of Fake Serums Told," *Chicago Herald and Examiner,* Feb. 22, 1924; "Dear Sirs, Questions and Answers," *Hygeia,* May 5, 1927; AMA Department of Investigation file on Bernarr Macfadden. Additional information on Macfadden is from www.riverflow.com/macfadden. **RSC Collection/Bentley:** Box 1: William J. Murray, "The Gift of Public Service"; miscellaneous Senate biographical material; RSC appointment calendars. Box 15: RSC letter, "Dear Father," July 13, 1923. Box 16: RSC letter to members of the Dexter Women's Study Club, "Dear Friends," Aug. 30, 1928. Box 20: RSC letter, "My Dear Jurney," Sept. 2, 1925; letter from solicitor general, "My Dear Senator Copeland," Sept. 3, 1925; assorted documents and letters pertaining to "Camp Copeland"; assorted documents and letters pertaining to Copeland Restaurants, Inc.; assorted documents and letters pertaining to Copeland Services; night letter to Mr. Burns re Key West, May 14, 1925. Box 21: RSC, annual address to American Hospital Association, Sept. 14, 1932; letter from Macfadden Publications, "Dear Senator Copeland," Jan. 22, 1925; letter to RSC from Advertising Record Corporation, "Dear Sir," Feb. 17, 1925; RSC, "Without Silica and Lithium, Potash et al.," n.d. Box 23: RSC, "What Should Be the Provision of a Model Medical Practice Act?" 1916. Box 25: RSC, "The Health of a Nation"; author unknown, prose poem about Dexter, Mich. Box 26: RSC, "The Medical Man in Politics"; Laurence Reid, "Senator: A Profile of the Gentleman from New York Who Talks on Movies and Health," *Reporter,* n.d.; scrapbooks: article from *Pittsburgh Post Gazette,* Apr. 15, 1929. Box 34: RSC, "A 'Physically Fit' Chart"; RSC, "Food Fads and the Baker's Bread"; RSC, "Are You Too Thin?"; *Minnesota Medicine,* Feb. 1923; "Fordham National Bank," *Business Survey,* Jan. 15, 1926. Box 35: scrapbooks: RSC's description of Washington, D.C., in 1898, from *New York Tribune,* June 18, 1938. Box 36: Randolph Teasdale, "The New York Physician Who Goes to the United States Senate," *Country Editor,* Aug. 1923; papers of Mrs. Royal Copeland (Frances), typescript of her unpublished book "Ladies of the Senate" (she had tried unsuccessfully to sell it as a serial to *Woman's Day, Good Housekeeping, Ladies' Home Journal,* and *Cosmopolitan*). Box 113G: James W. Ward, "Homeopathic Activities," *California State Homeopathic Society,* May 10, 1922. **Books:** Fontanarosa, *Alternative Medicine* (Oumeish Youssef Oumeish, MD, "The Philosophical, Cultural, and Historical Aspects of Complementary, Alternative, Unconventional, and Integrative Medicine in the Old World," p. 135); Marwil, *History of Ann Arbor;* Cocks, *Pictorial History of Ann Arbor;* Lockie and Geddes, *Complete Guide to Homeopathy;* Potter dissertation (p. 238 re Bond Bread, *New York Tribune,* Feb. 12, 1922; p. 293 re running for the presidency, "At first it was said half-jokingly"; and p. 349 re RSC's use of Senate stationery for personal business).

ELEVEN: "As the Wing of a Bird Fits the Air"

Information in this chapter was drawn from the following: Morris Fishbein, MD, "The Rise and Fall of Homeopathy," www.homeowatch.org/history/Fishbein.html; Stephen Barrett, MD, "Iridology," www.quackwatch.org.; Russell S. Worrall, OD, Jacob Nevyas, PhD, and Stephen Barrett, MD, "Eye-Related Quackery," www.quackwatch.org; www.redcross.org/; Food and Drug Administration, "The Story of the Laws Behind the Labels," *FDA Consumer,* June 1981, www.fda.gov (then click on to "FDA History"); www.breadworld.com; "World War II Combat Medic,"/The History of World War II Medicine; www.home.att.net/~Steinert/wwii/htm; Janet Mace Valenza, article on mineral water springs and wells, Texas State Historical Association; James Glanz, "Tiniest of Particles Pokes Big Hole in Physics Theory," *New York Times,* Feb. 9, 2001. **AMA Archives:** letter from Bureau of Investigation, "Dear Dr. Fishbein," Dec. 16, 1927; letter re RSC, "Dear Dr. Fishbein," Feb. 3, 1932; RSC letter to Fishbein, "Dear Sir," Dec. 13, 1927; "Announcing the Dr. Royal S. Copeland Hour," broadsheet and accompanying letter, Oct. 6, 1927; letter to AMA from D. J. Leithauser, MD, "Dr. Copeland an Authority on Medical Issues," Apr. 4, 1928; "Magic Materia Medica," condensed from *JAMA,* May 30, 1936; "Current Comment," *JAMA,* May 11, 1935, p. 1760; assorted documents on Pluto Water; selected letters re homeopathic queries, 1933 and 1934; "Health Specialists Graduate," *Los Angeles Ledger,* Jan. 12, 1929; "Chiropractors and Naturopaths: A Recurring Problem for the Virginia General Assembly," 1948; AMA Bureau of Legal Medicine and Legislature, "Memorandum Relative to Naturopathic Schools," Jan. 1944; "Professor Samuels and His Eye Water," in Cramp, *Nostrums and Quackery.* **RSC Collection/Bentley:** Box 15: assorted undated speeches. Box 17: "Farm Relief Speech of Hon. Royal S. Copeland," *Congressional Record,* Feb. 9, 1927. Box 20: assorted letters and documents about Dexter Poultry. Box 21: RSC, "What Is Homeopathy?" Box 25: Barbara Burke, "Senator Royal S. Copeland Calls Joint Meeting to Discuss Federal Cosmetic Bill," *Barbara Burke's Beauty Journal* 5, no. 1 (Jan. 1928); RSC speech, "Radioactive Waters," Apr. 29, 1939; "Consumers Charge Copeland Oversteps Law in Wrecking Tugwell Bill," Conference of Consumer Organizations, Mar. 1934; folder on RSC's writings on the economy; Garet Garrett article in *Saturday Evening Post,* Dec. 12, 1931. Box 26: speeches: "Remarks of Senator Royal S. Copeland in Relation to Conference Report on S.1077"; "The Tugwell Bill: An Analysis and Proposed Amendments," n.d. Box 34: "Tammany to Let Copeland Have Renomination," *New York Herald Tribune,* Apr. 14, 1927; RSC, assorted obituaries, 1938; "Copeland Ignores Demand He Quit" and other assorted news articles, 1933; "Ask Law to End Poison Menace in Beauty Aids," undated news article from unknown newspaper, ca. 1927. Box 35: "Radium Cure of Tumor a Triumph," *New York Herald,* Apr. 22, 1909. **Books:** Jacobs, ed., *Encyclopedia of Alternative Medicine;* Potter dissertation (p. 379 re Nujol; p. 401 re Stuart Chase and F. J. Schlink, *Your Money's Worth;* p. 494, re S.5 bill). Additional information from FDA Web site.

TWELVE: "A Very Great Advance"

Information in this chapter was drawn from the following: re clinical trials: U.S. Food and Drug Administration, www.fda.gov/fdac; re health: www.onhealth.com; www.nejm.org; www.marius.net/research. **AMA Archives:** *Digest of Official Actions;* re Copeland bill: Burrow, *AMA,* pp. 273–80; additional material from Campion, *The AMA and U.S. Health Policy*—see pp. 141–45 re osteopathy licenses (the author thanks Robert Tenuta for giving her a copy of this book); *Chiropractors and Naturopaths,* a brochure; "Memorandum Relative to Naturopathic Schools," Jan. 1944; AMA letter about naturopaths, osteopaths, and chiropractors, Feb. 19, 1942; "Legislation Pending in Congress Concerning Food, Drugs, Cosmetics and Therapeutic Devices," *JAMA,* Dec. 21, 1935; comments on the Copeland bill by William C. Woodward, MD, *JAMA,* May 30, 1936; Fishbein, *History of the American Medical Association* (this is one of the glorious reference books that were housed next to the table where I worked at the AMA Archives, which I was allowed to study only after much begging); selected entries from *The Guide to the AMA Historical Health Fraud and Alternative Medicine Collection.* **RSC Collection/**

Bentley: Box 5: RSC, "A New Party or a Coalition?: What a Defeated Candidate Learned," 1911. Box 20: assorted documents and letters re RSC's proposal for "Education for Character"; RSC telegram to RSC, Jr., June 13, 1938. Box 21: RSC, annual address to American Hospital Association, Sept. 14, 1932. Box 23: untitled RSC speech beginning "One who has had a scientific education . . ." Box 25: handwritten speech with the word "sympathetic" deleted, 1937. Box 26: scrapbooks; articles from *Albany Evening News,* July 15, 1937. Box 34: RSC and Bertie Backus, MS of "Education for Character"; RSC, "New Food, Drug, and Cosmetic Law"; "River-Harbor Improvements," *Beacon News* (Albany, NY), May 27, 1938; "Resume Fight to Earmark WPA Funds, *Syracuse Journal,* June 2, 1938; "Battlefield at Saratoga Becomes Park," *Troy Morning Record,* June 3, 1938; "WPA Men Afraid to Back Copeland"; assorted obituaries. Box 36: Frances S. Copeland, "The Good Guest" and "Ladies of the Senate," typescripts of articles. **Books:** Copeland, *Dr. Copeland's Home Medical Book;* Jacobs, ed., *Encyclopedia of Alternative Medicine* (aromatherapy, p. 205; "Edward Bach, M.D., devised the first precise system of soul healing . . . ," p. 55; dance therapy, p. 136; polarity therapy, p. 40; reflexology, p. 225; shiatsu, p. 262); additional information on dance therapy is from Royal Copeland's address to the AMA, "What Should Be the Provisions of a Model Medical Practice Act?," 1916; Grevitz, ed., *Other Healers* (re homeopathy as a subspecialty of internal medicine, p. 114); Potter dissertation (p. 475 re RSC and education plan; p. 51 re FDR on Copeland bill, from FDR memo of Feb. 16, 1937; p. 536 re RSC called a "stuffed stethoscope"; p. 537 re "nominee of Communists"; Shapiro and Shapiro, *Powerful Placebo* (p. 128); Starr, *Social Transformation* (overview of Social Security Act, pp. 268–69).

THIRTEEN: "Scientific Rule"

Information in this chapter was drawn from the following: author interviews, follow-up phone calls, and e-mail exchanges with Jennifer Jacobs and Michael Carlston, 2000–2004; author's notes and interviews from the Fifth Homeopathic Research Network Symposium, June 23–24, 2000; some additional information from the symposium's printed booklet. **Journal and magazine articles:** Michael Carlston, MD, "Kent and Swedenborg," *American Homeopath,* Summer 1995; Michael Carlston, MD, "The Mechanism of Homeopathy: All That Matters Is That It Works," *Alternative Therapies,* July 1995; Henry W. Eisfelder, MD, "Modern Medicine Rediscovers Homeopathy," *Journal of the AIH,* Nov. 1955; "The Evolution of US Drug Laws," *FDA Consumer,* June 1981; Alphonse Gay and Jean Boiron, "A Physical Demonstration of the Real Existence of the Homeopathic Remedy," *Journal of the AIH,* pp. 307–35 (orig. Éditions des Laboratoires P.H.P., Lyon, France, 1953); Marilyn Heins, MD, et al. (including Jennifer Jacobs, MD), "Productivity of Women Physicians," *JAMA,* Oct. 25, 1976; also "Comparison of the Productivity of Women and Men Physicians," *JAMA,* June 6, 1977; Jennifer Jacobs, MD, et al., "Treatment of Childhood Diarrhea with Homeopathic Medicine," *Pediatrics,* May 1994; Jennifer Jacobs, MD, letter to the editor, *New England Journal of Medicine,* Oct. 14, 1993; Jennifer Jacobs, MD, and Michel Labrecque, MD, and associates, letter to the editor, *Canadian Medical Association Journal,* Nov. 15, 1992; Leon Jaroff, "Homeopathic E-Mail," *Time,* May 15, 1999; Klaus Linde et al., "Are the Clinical Effects of Homeopathy Placebo Effects?" *The Lancet,* Sept. 20, 1997; Dawn Mackeen, "The Global Medicine Cabinet," *New York Times Magazine,* May 6, 2001; E. B. Nash, "Interrogations in Homeopathics," *Transactions of I.H.A.,* 1889 (re derivation of the word "complementary," p. 65), www.julianwinston.com/archives/periodicals/iha/php; David W. Ramey et al., "Homeopathy and Science: A Closer Look," www.colorado.edu/philosophy/VStenger/Medicine/homeopathy.html; Marjorie Rosen, "Controversial Founder of Quackwatch," *Biography,* Oct. 1998. W. Sampson and W. London, "Analysis of Homeopathic Treatment of Childhood Diarrhea," *Pediatrics,* Nov. 1995; Wallace Sampson, MD, position paper by the National Council Against Health Fraud, 1994; Karin Horgan Sullivan, "Alternative Therapies: Experts Say Homeopathy Does Work," United Press Syndicate, April 11, 1999, www.uexpress.com; Stuart Keith Sutton, "Sourdough, Homeopathy, and Evidence-Based Medicine," *The Lancet,* Jan. 20, 2001; Wanda G. Vockeroth, "Veterinary Medicine," *Canadian Veterinary Journal,* Sept. 1999. **Miscellaneous brochures:** advertisements and booklets collected by the author at the Fifth Scientific Symposium of the Homeopathic Research Network; Dennis Remington, MD, *A History of Meridian Stress Assessment,* BioMeridian—The Human Calibrations Company. **Newspaper articles:** Paul Lewis, obituary of Victor D. Herbert, MD, *New York Times,* Nov. 21, 2002; Kelly Scott, "Birth at Home," *St. Petersburg Times,* Sept. 6, 1997; Miriam Silver, article about Michael Carlston, *Press Democrat,* June 17, 2001; Laurie Tarkan, "Use of Antibiotics in Children Is Down, but Enough?" *New York Times,* July 23, 2002. **Web sites:** www.cityofhuntington.com (information about the city); www.telehomeopathy.net (information about Dr. F. H. Schmidt) (this Web site no longer exists); www.onebody.com ("Women's Health and Homeopathy: A Chat with Jennifer Jacobs, MD," Sept. 25, 2000) (this Web site no longer exists); www.quackwatch.org (Stephen Barrett, MD, "Electrodiagnostic Devices," and Stephen Barrett, MD, "Bee Pollen, Royal Jelly, and Propolis," 1999); www.ncschiropractic.com [Niagara Chiropractic Society]; www.chirobase.org (William T. Jarvis, PhD, "Why Chiropractic Is Controversial" and information on chiropractic schools); www.arthritis.com ([Arthritis Foundation], Judith Horstman, "Homeopathy"); www.nccam.nih.gov (*NCCAM Newsletter,* Fall 1991); homeoinfo.com_reference/web_sites/research/php (John R. Benneth, "Seven Kinds of Provings for Homeopathy"); www.hoopesvision.com ("History of Refractive Eye Surgery"); www.lasersurgeryforeyes.com ("History of Laser Eye Surgery"). **AMA Archives:** "About Controversy over Naturopathy," *U.S. News & World Report,* Nov. 11, 1976 (article clipped by AMA); Campion, *The AMA and United States Health Policy* (p. 419 re Council on Scientific Affairs; p. 195 re osteopathy; pp. 197–98 re decline of AMA's influence); *American Medical News,* re wellness, Sept. 24, 1982; *Digest of Official Actions; Guide to the AMA Historical Health Fraud and Alternative Medicine Collection;* AMA letter, "Dear Dr. Denison," Aug. 11, 1954; AMA letter, "Dear Dr. McCullough," Dec. 11, 1956; letter to AMA from Harris Coulter, legislative director, AIH, Aug. 14, 1979; "Memo to the Finance Committee, U.S. Senate, from Wyeth Post Baker, MD, re the US Homeopathic Pharmacopeia," May 13, 1965; "Public Is Warned on Useless Drugs," *New York Times,* Oct. 2, 1960; "Report 12 of the Council on Scientific Affairs," June 1997; Self-Medication files. **RSC Collection/Bentley:** Box 21: RSC, "The Proof of Homeopathy"; RSC, "Homeopathy in the 20th Century." Box 23: RSC, "The Teachings of Materia Medica." **Books:** Fontanarosa, *Alternative Medicine;* Garrett and Stone, *Catching Good Health* (interview with Jennifer Jacobs); Coulter, *Divided Legacy* (pp. 493–95 re homeopathic tests in 1950s; p. 515 re 1980 trial in Scotland); Jonas and Jacobs, *Healing with Homeopathy* (pp. 13, 17, 86); Coulter, *Homeopathic Science* (p. 4 re the Cincinnati Centennial Medical Exhibition); Schiff, *Memory of Water* (re Benveniste); Gevitz, ed., *Other Healers* (pp. 114–15 re Martin Kaufman, "Homeopathy in America"; pp. 157–91 re Walter I. Wardwell, "Chiropractors: Evolution to Acceptance"); Shapiro and Shapiro, *Powerful Placebo* (p. 47n re WHO and unorthodox therapies); *The Skeptic's Dictionary* (www.skepdic.com); Park, *Voodoo Science* (p. 56).

FOURTEEN: "Another Tool in the Bag"

Information in this chapter is drawn from the following: author interviews and e-mail and phone conversations with Jennifer Jacobs, MD, and Michael Carlston, MD; e-mail exchanges and/or telephone calls with Stephen Barrett, MD, Wallace Sampson, MD, and Frank Wilczek, PhD, in 2002 and 2003; in-person conversation with Murray Gell-Mann, PhD, June 29, 2003; author's notes from Homeopathic Research Network meetings in 2000 and 2002; court documents re *National Council Against Health Fraud, Inc. v. King Bio-Pharmaceuticals, Inc.,* California Supreme Court, Dec. 17, 2001. **Journal and magazine articles:** John Astin, PhD, et al., "A Review of the Incorporation of Complementary and Alternative Medicine by Mainstream Physicians," *Archives of Internal Medicine,* Nov. 23, 1998; B. Barzanski, PhD, et al., "Educational Progress in U.S. Medical Schools" (1999–2000, 2000–2001, 2001–2002), *JAMA,* Sept. 6, 2000, Sept. 5, 2001, Sept. 4, 2002; Carol Berkowitz, "Homeopathy: Keeping an Open Mind" (letter), *The Lancet,* Sept. 10, 1994; "OAM Sponsors Placebo and Nocebo Conference," *NCCAM Newsletter,* Jan. 1997; Michael Carlston, letter to the editor, *Pediatrics,* Jan. 1995; Edward H. Chapman, MD, letter to the editor, *Pediatrics,* May 1995; "International Bottled Water Association Position Paper on AMA Report," Mar. 14, 2000, www.bottledwater. org; E. H. Chapman et al., "Homeopathic Treatment of Mild Traumatic Brain Injury," *Journal of Head Trauma Rehabilitation,* 1999; John de Cuevas, "Mind/Brain/Behavior: The Pleasing Placebo," Jan. 20, 1995, www.focus.hms.harvard.edu/1995/Jan20_1995/ mind.html; Peter Fisher, "Progress of the Basics," editorial, *British Homeopathy Journal,* Oct. 1999; Phil Fontanarosa, MD, and George Lundberg, MD, "Alternative Medicine Meets Science," *JAMA,* Nov. 11, 1998; Megan A. Johnson, "Homeopathy: Another Tool in the Bag," *MS JAMA,* (medical student *JAMA*), Mar. 4, 1998; Ronald Koretz, "Is Alternative Medicine Alternative Science?" *Journal of Laboratory and Clinical Medicine,* June 2002; John Lacey, news release (re Kessler et al., "Study Indicates Alternative Medicine Here to Stay," *Annals of Internal Medicine,* Aug. 21, 2001), Harvard Medical School Office of Public Affairs, 2001; James A. Lalumandier, DDS, MPH, and Leone W. Ayers, MD, "Fluoride and Bacterial Content of Bottle Water vs. Tap Water," *Archives of Family Medicine,* Mar. 2000; Richard Layton, MD, et al., letters to the editor, and replies from Jennifer Jacobs, MD, *Pediatrics,* Dec. 1994; Thierry Montfort, "Medical Homeopathy in Action," *Resonance,* Mar.–Apr. 1995; Steven Novella, MD, "Homeopathy," *Connecticut Skeptic,* Summer 1996; Matt Nisbet, "Second World Skeptics Congress," *Skeptical Inquirer,* Nov.–Dec. 1998; Palmer et al., "Adverse Events Associated with Dietary Supplements: An Observational Study," *The Lancet,* Jan. 11, 2003; Robert L. Park, "An Upside-Down View of Health" (a review of *Healing with Homeopathy*), *Scientific Review of Alternative Medicine,* Fall–Winter 1999; Arnold S. Relman, MD, "A Trip to Stonesville," *The New Republic,* Dec. 14, 1998, as posted on www.quackwatch.org; "Report 12 of the Council on Scientific Affairs," AMA: 1997 (also report 4, Oct. 1, 1996), www.ama-assn.org/ama/pub/article/2036-2432.html; Linda Rosa, BSN, RN, et al., "A Close Look at Therapeutic Touch," *JAMA,* April 1, 1998; Wallace Sampson, MD, "The Braid of the Alternative Medicine Movement," *Scientific Review of Medicine,* Fall–

Winter 1998; Wallace Sampson, MD, and William London, "Analysis of Home Treatment of Childhood Diarrhea," *Pediatrics,* Nov. 1995; Isadora Stehlin, "Homeopathy: Real Medicine or Empty Promises?" *FDA Consumer,* Dec. 1996; Dana Ullman, "Implications of a Court Case," *Holistic Health Handbook,* 1978; Linda Villarosa, "Verdict Is Still Out on Some Alternative Therapies," *New York Times,* Apr. 13, 2002; Michael Weiser et al., "Homeopathic vs. Conventional Treatment of Vertigo: A Randomized, Double-Blind Controlled Clinical Study," *Archives of Otolaryngology—Head and Neck Surgery,* Aug. 1998. **Miscellaneous brochures:** David Tulbert, BSC, DC, "Hypothesis for the Structure and Action of Sub-Avagadro Homeopathic Dilutions," abstract in Homeopathic Research Network Fourth Scientific Symposium booklet, Sept. 1998. **Newspaper articles:** James Glanz, "Tiniest of Particles Pokes Big Hole in Physics Theory," *New York Times,* Feb. 9, 2001; "Alternative Medicine Panel Formed," Associated Press, July 13, 2001; Donald G. McNeil, Jr., "With Folk Medicine on the Rise, Health Group Is Monitoring" (re WHO), *New York Times,* May 17, 2002; Sheryl Gay Stolberg, "Alternative Care Gains a Foothold" (re quote by Dr. Daniel Moerman), *New York Times,* June 32, 2000. **Web sites:** www.consumerlab.com; www.fda.gov (warning letter from Public Health Service, FDA, to Bill Gray, MD, Apr. 2, 2003); www.hcahf.org/ (National Council Against Health Fraud, position paper on homeopathy, Feb. 1994; www.onebody.com ("Women's Health and Homeopathy: A Chat with Jennifer Jacobs, MD," Sept. 25, 2000); www.homeopathic.com/research (Dana Ullman, "A Unique Non-Melting Ice Crystal Found in Room-Temperature Water: Significant Implications for Medicine, Manufacturing, and the Environment," 1997); www.quackwatch.org (Stephen Barrett, MD, "Homeopathy: The Ultimate Fake"; Stephen Barrett, MD, "Be Wary of Alternative Health Methods"; Stephen Barrett, MD, "Some Notes on the Quantum Xrroid [QXCI] and William C. Nelson"; Stephen Barrett, MD, "Petition Regarding Homeopathic Drugs," Aug. 29, 1994; Rory Coker, PhD, "Distinguishing Science and Pseudoscience"; Patrick Curry, "Notes on James S. Gordon, MD," Feb. 28, 2002; "National Council Against Health Fraud's Statement on the White House Commission on CAM," Mar. 25, 2002); www.whccamp.hhs.gov/finalreport.html/ ("White House Commission on CAM Policy Final Report," Mar. 2002). **Books:** Fontanarosa, *Alternative Medicine* (Foreword, p. iii; Eisenberg et al., "Trends in Alternative Medicine Use in the United States, 1990–1997," p. 4; John A. Astin, "Why Patients Use Alternative Medicine: Results of a National Study," p. 16; Jacobs et al., "Patient Characteristics and Practice Patterns of Physicians Using Homeopathy," p. 422); Jonas and Jacobs, *Healing with Homeopathy* (pp. 102–7); Park, *Voodoo Science* (pp. 52–54). **Special document:** Here in its entirety is Dr. Stephen Barrett's "An Idea for Testing Homeopathy":

> A safety deposit box is obtained that can only be opened by insertion of keys by both a proponent and a skeptical researcher.
> A homeopathic pharmaceutical company provides ten coded sets of homeopathic and matching placebos.
> A copy of the code is placed in the safety deposit box.
> A set of code numbers is prepared by the skeptical researcher.
> The sets of remedies and placebos are delivered to the skeptical researcher in the presence of a proponent.
> While the proponent stays far enough from the remedies to be unable to read their labels, the skeptic recodes them, and records how they are changed.

The new code is placed in the safety deposit box. This procedure should guarantee that no one can tell which remedy sets are the active medications and which are placebos until the code is broken.

Select a condition whose severity is easily rated.

It has to be common enough to collect 150 cases for the study.

A skin condition such as psoriasis might be ideal.

Devise a rating scale.

Divide the 150 subjects into a group of 100 and one of 50.

The time period of the experiment should be set in advance.

All cases will be treated by allopathic physicians.

The larger group is also treated by a homeopathic physician in his standard manner. Half of the patients will receive homeopathic remedies and half will get placebos.

The smaller group receives no homeopathic treatment.

After each remedy (or placebo) has had time to act, the homeopath should judge from the response whether he believes he has administered the remedy or the placebo.

If homeopathic remedies are effective drugs, the patients who receive them should do better than those who receive placebos or do not receive any homeopathic treatment.

If homeopathic remedies are placebos (as critics charge), patients who receive the remedies and those who receive placebos should do equally well.

If the relationship with the homeopath has a beneficial effect, patients seeing the homeopath should do better than those who do not.

If homeopathic remedies are placebos, homeopaths should be unable to guess whether they have administered a placebo or not.

This protocol would permit the homeopath to individualize the treatment. If patients treated by homeopaths do better than those who are not, it may be possible to tell whether the effective part of the treatment was the remedy or the interaction with the homeopath.

FIFTEEN: "A Long-Felt Want"

Information in this chapter was drawn from the following: author interviews (in-person and telephone) and/or e-mail exchanges with Dean Crothers, MD; Murray Kopelow, MD (Oct. 29, 2002); Jennifer Jacobs, MD; and Wallace Sampson, MD. **Journal and magazine articles:** Elizabeth Barnett, MD, et al., "Challenge of Evaluating Homeopathic Treatment of Acute Otitis Media," *Pediatric Infectious Disease Journal,* Jan. 2000; James Brokow, PhD, et al., "The Teaching of Complementary and Alternative Medicine," *Journal of the Association of American Medical Colleges,* Sept. 2002; Michael Carlston, MD, et al., "Alternative Medicine Instruction in Medical Schools and Family Practice Residency Programs," *Family Medicine,* 1997; Victoria Stagg Elliot, "Behind the Scenes: How a Drug Becomes a Drug," *American Medical News,* Jan. 6, 2003; Jay Greene, "Complementary Curriculum," *American Medical News,* Jan. 17, 2000, and "Federation of State Medical Boards (FSMB) Developing Guidelines for Complementary Care," May 8, 2000; Jennifer Jacobs, MD, et al., "Homeopathic Treatment of Acute Childhood Diarrhea: Results from a Clinical Trial in Nepal," *Journal of Alternative and*

Complementary Medicine, April 2000; Jennifer Jacobs, MD, et al., "Homeopathic Treatment of Acute Otitis Media in Children: A Preliminary Randomized, Placebo-Controlled Trial," *Pediatric Infectious Disease Journal,* Feb. 2001; Leon Jaroff, "Something to Sneeze At," *Time,* Nov. 3, 2000; Wayne Jonas, MD; Ted J. Kaptchuk, OMD; Klaus Linde, MD, "A Critical Overview of Homeopathy," *Annals of Internal Medicine,* March 4, 2003; B. J. Kennedy, MD, "Origin and Evolution of Medical Oncology," *The Lancet,* Dec. 18, 1999; Wallace Sampson, MD, "Homeopathy Does Not Work," and Jennifer Jacobs, MD, "Homeopathy Should Be Integrated into Mainstream Medicine," Point/Counterpoint, *Alternative Therapies,* Sept. 1995; Stephanie Stapleton, "Medicine's Chasm: The Wide Gulf Between Conventional and Alternative Approaches," *American Medical News,* June 3, 2002; A. J. Vickers and C. Smith, "Oscillococcinum for Preventing and Treating Influenza and Influenza-like Syndrome," abstract from *Cochrane Review/The Cochrane Library,* no. 4, 2002; Pamela Wyngate, "Little White Pills Promise to Cure Ills," *Natural Foods Merchandiser,* Oct. 1999. **Newspaper articles:** Kenneth Chang, "A Tiny Force of Nature Is Stronger Than Thought" (re Casimir effect), *New York Times,* Feb. 9, 2001; Connie E. Dickey, Sgt. First Class, "Army Plays Big Role in Breast Cancer Research," *Army News Service,* Jan. 29, 1999; Claudia Dreifus, "Separating Remedies from Snake Oil," *New York Times,* Apr. 3, 2001; James Glanz, "Survey Finds Support Is Strong for Teaching Two Origin Theories" (re poll by People for the American Way), *New York Times,* Mar. 11, 2000; "Homeopathy: Concerns About Training and Certification," Personal Health column, *New York Newsday,* Feb. 6, 2001. **Web sites:** www.homeopathic.org (National Center for Homeopathy, "Homeopathy in the News," 2001); www.homeopathic.com/articles (Dana Ullman, "Homeopathy and Managed Care: Manageable or Unmanageable"; also in *Journal of Alternate and Complementary Medicine,* May 1, 1999); www.accme.org (information re accreditation); www.quackwatch.org (Stephen Barrett, MD, "Homeopathy: The Ultimate Fake"). **RSC Collection/Bentley:** Box 21: RSC, "Homeopathy"; RSC, "The Germ Theory of Disease." Box 23: RSC, "Autobiographical Sketch." **Books:** Goldstein, *Alternative Health Care* (p. 166 re licensing statistics); Carlston, ed., *Classical Homeopathy* (pp. 66, 67, 96, 97; also chap. 9, "Homeopathic Education and Certification," by Richard Pitt, p. 146; on p. 34, Carlston uses Eisenberg's 1997 statistics showing that "the use of homeopathy increased fivefold to 6.7 million adults—3.4% of the adult population" and that "self-treatment over professional care increased to more than 82%." He then states that "assuming that the popularity of homeopathy has continued to grow at the same pace, the number of adult Americans using homeopathy in 2001 would have risen to 12 to 13 million." Carlston goes on to say that "although these projections are impressive, a 1999 survey suggests they might significantly underestimate the popularity of homeopathy." The author has used the conservative figure of 15 million.); Lockie and Geddes, *Complete Guide to Homeopathy.*

EPILOGUE

Information in the Epilogue is drawn from the following: author interviews (in-person or telephone) and/or e-mail exchanges with Stephen Barrett, MD, and Eric Kandel, MD; Robert L. Park, "Alternate Medicine and the Laws of Physics," *Skeptical Inquirer,* Sept.–Oct. 1997; V. S. Rambihar, MD, letter to the editor, *The Lancet,* May 13, 2000; Stephen E. Straus, MD, testimony before House Appropriations Subcommittee on

Labor, Mar. 2, 2000; "Traditional Healing Practice Using Medicinal Herbs," *The Lancet,* Dec. 8, 1999; National Center for Homeopathy, "Homeopathy in Crisis Intervention," Sept. 27, 2002, www.homeopathic.org. **Books:** Coulter, *Divided Legacy* (p. 8); Kandel, Schwartz, and Jessell, eds., *Essentials of Neural Science and Behavior* (pp. 690–91); Jonas and Jacobs, *Healing with Homeopathy* (p. xvii); Shapiro and Shapiro, *Powerful Placebo.*

Selected Bibliography

Ballentine, Rudolph, MD. *Radical Healing.* New York: Harmony Books, 1999.

Boericke, William, MD. *A Compend of the Principles of Homeopathy.* Pomeroy, Wash.: Health Research, 1971 (copyrighted 1891 by Boericke & Runyon).

Bordin, Ruth. *Washtenaw County.* Northridge, Calif.: Windsor Publications, 1988 (courtesy of Bentley Historical Library, Ann Arbor, Michigan).

Burrow, James G. *AMA: Voice of American Medicine.* Baltimore: Johns Hopkins University Press, 1963.

Campion, Frank D. *The AMA and U.S. Health Policy Since 1940.* Chicago: Chicago Review Press, 1984.

Carlston, Michael, MD, ed. *Classical Homeopathy* (Series Editor: Marc S. Micozzi). New York: Churchill Livingstone, an imprint of Elsevier Science, 2003.

Cocks, J. Fraser, III, ed. *Pictorial History of Ann Arbor.* Ann Arbor: Michigan Historical Collections, Bentley Historical Library, University of Michigan, 1974.

Copeland, Royal S. *Dr. Copeland's Home Medical Book.* Philadelphia: John C. Winston Co., 1935.

Coulter, Harris L. *Divided Legacy: The Conflict Between Homeopathy and the American Medical Association.* Vol. 3, *Science and Ethics in American Medicine, 1800–1914.* Berkeley, Calif.: North Atlantic Books, 1982.

———. *Homeopathic Science and Modern Medicine: The Physics of Healing with Microdoses.* Berkeley, Calif.: North Atlantic Books, 1980.

Cozolino, Louis. *The Neuroscience of Psychotherapy: Building and Rebuilding the Human Mind.* New York: Norton, 2002.

Cramp, Arthur J. *Nostrums and Quackery.* 2nd ed. Vols. 1–3. Chicago: American Medical Association Press, 1912.

Cutler, Howard C., MD, and His Holiness the Dalai Lama. *The Art of Happiness: A Handbook for Living.* New York: Riverhead Books, 1998.

Davenport, Horace W. *Not Just Any Medical School: The Science, Practice, and Teaching of Medicine at the University of Michigan.* Ann Arbor: University of Michigan Press, new printing, 1999 (courtesy of the Bentley Historical Library).

Davidson, Jonathan R. T., MD, and Kathryn M. Conner, MD. *Herbs for the Mind: What Science Tells Us About Nature's Remedies for Depression, Stress, Memory Loss, and Insomnia.* New York: Guildford Publications, 2000.

DeSchepper, Luc. *Human Condition: Critical.* Santa Fe, N.M.: Full of Life Publishing, 1993.

Dossey, Larry, MD. *Reinventing Medicine: Beyond Mind-Body to a New Era of Healing.* San Francisco: HarperSan Francisco, 1999.

Fishbein, Morris, MD. *A History of the American Medical Association, 1847–1947.* Philadelphia: W. B. Saunders & Co., 1942.

Fontanarosa, Phil B., MD, ed. *Alternative Medicine: An Objective Assessment.* Chicago: American Medical Association, 2000.

Garrett, Raymond J., and TaRessa Stone. *Catching Good Health with Homeopathic Medicine.* Sebastopol, Calif.: CRCS Publications, 1990.

Garrison, Fielding H., MD. *An Introduction to the History of Medicine.* 3rd ed. Philadelphia and London: W. B. Saunders & Co., 1921.

Gevitz, Norman, ed. *Other Healers: Unorthodox Medicine in America.* Baltimore: Johns Hopkins University Press, [1958] 1990.

Goldstein, Michael S. *Alternative Health Care: Medicine, Miracle, or Mirage?* Philadelphia: Temple University Press, 1999.

Gordon, Richard. *The Alarming History of Medicine: Amusing Anecdotes from Hippocrates to Heart Transplants.* New York: St. Martin's Press, 1993.

Grun, Bernard. *The Timetables of History.* New York: Simon & Schuster, 1975.

Hafner, Arthur W., PhD, ed. *Guide to the American Medical Association Historical Health Fraud and Alternative Medicine Collection.* Chicago: American Medical Association, 1992.

Hahnemann, Samuel. *Organon of the Medical Art.* 6th ed. Edited and annotated by Wenda Brewster O'Reilly, PhD. Palo Alto, Calif.: Birdcage Books, 1996.

Haller, John S., Jr. *Kindly Medicine: Physio-Medicalism in America, 1836–1911.* Kent, Ohio, and London: Kent State University Press, 1997.

Hirshberg, Caryle, and Marc Ian Barash. *Remarkable Recovery.* New York: Riverhead Books, 1995.

Holbrook, Stuart. *The Story of American Railroads.* New York: Crown Publishers, 1947.

Jacobs, Jennifer, MD, ed. *The Encyclopedia of Alternative Medicine.* Boston: Carlton Books, 1997.

Jonas, Wayne B., MD, and Jennifer Jacobs, MD. *Healing with Homeopathy.* New York: Warner Books, 1996.

Kandel, Eric R., James H. Schwartz, and Thomas M. Jessell, eds. *Essentials of Neural Science and Behavior.* Norwalk, Conn.: Appleton & Lange, 1995.

Le Fanu, James, MD. *The Rise and Fall of Modern Medicine.* New York: Carroll & Graf, 2000.

Lockie, Andrew, MD, and Nicola Geddes, MD. *The Complete Guide to Homeopathy: The Principles and Practice of Treatment.* New York: DK Publishing, 1995.

Marwil, Jonathan L. *A History of Ann Arbor.* Ann Arbor: Ann Arbor Observer Company, 1987.

McAllister, Norma. *Judge Samuel William Dexter.* Dexter, Mich.: Thomson-Shore, 1989.

McCabe, Vinton. *Let Like Cure Like: The Definitive Guide to the Healing Power of Homeopathy.* New York: St. Martin's Press, 1997.

Nuland, Sherwin, MD. *Doctors: The Biography of Medicine.* 2nd ed. New York: Vintage Books, 1995.

Oz, Mehmet, MD, with Ron Arias and Lisa Oz. *Healing from the Heart: A Leading Heart Surgeon Explores the Power of Complementary Medicine.* New York: Dutton, 1998.

Park, Robert L. *Voodoo Science.* New York: Oxford University Press, 2000.

Plotkin, Mark J. *Medicine Quest.* New York: Viking, 2000.

Porter, Roy, ed. *Medicine: A History of Healing: Ancient Traditions to Modern Practice.* New York: Marlowe & Co., 1997.

Potter, Raymond. "Royal Samuel Copeland, 1868–1938: A Physician in Politics." PhD dissertation, Western Reserve University, 1967 (Ann Arbor: University Microfilms).

Sanders, James, and Ric Burns. *New York: An Illustrated History.* New York: Knopf, 1999.

Schaller, Warren E., and Charles R. Carroll. *Health, Quackery, and the Consumer.* Philadelphia and London: W. B. Saunders Co., 1976.

Schiff, Michel. *The Memory of Water: Homeopathy and the Battle of Ideas in the New Science.* San Francisco and London: Thorson, an imprint of HarperCollins, 1995.

Shapiro, Arthur K., and Elaine Shapiro. *The Powerful Placebo: From Ancient Priest to Modern Physics.* Baltimore: Johns Hopkins University Press, 1997.

Starr, Paul. *The Social Transformation of American Medicine: The Rise of a Sovereign Profession and the Making of a Vast Industry.* New York: Basic Books, 1982.

Ullman, Dana. *The Consumer's Guide to Homeopathy.* New York: Jeremy P. Tarcher/Putnam, 1995.

———. *Discovering Homeopathy: Medicine for the 21st Century.* Berkeley, Calif.: North Atlantic Books, 1991.

Vithoulkos, George. *The Science of Homeopathy.* New York: Grove Press, 1980.

Weil, Andrew, MD. *Natural Medicine.* Boston: Houghton Mifflin, 1990.

———. *Spontaneous Healing.* New York: Knopf, 1995.

Weiner, Michael, PhD. *The Complete Book of Homeopathy: A Comprehensive Manual of Natural Healing.* New York: MJF Books/Fine Communications, 1989.

Wilbur, C. Keith, MD. *Revolutionary Medicine, 1700–1800.* Old Saybrook, Conn.: Globe Pequot Press, [1980] 1997.

Winawer, Sidney J., MD, with Nick Taylor. *Healing Lessons.* New York and London: Routledge, 1999.

Acknowledgments

There really should be a fourth name in my dedication, but I know he would say, "Leave it be, it's fine as it is," so I have. But my husband, Christopher Lehmann-Haupt, went over every single word of my final draft and coaxed me into a clarity I thought was already on the page but wasn't quite yet. He is everywhere in this book, and I thank him with all my heart.

My daughter, Rachel Lehmann-Haupt, probably doesn't realize how important her reading of a very early chapter was to me. She pointed out an inconsistency in logic that I had somehow missed, and having this straightened out, I was set on a path that I hope I have never left. My son, Noah Lehmann-Haupt, was a title maven and would stop by my desk to see what latest one was Scotch-taped to my wall. He never stopped booing the one I clung to the longest, but when I found the present one, he was the first to cheer.

I feel very fortunate to be in the hands of Knopf. I thank my editor, Victoria Wilson, for her guidance and wisdom. Thanks, too, to her assistants, first Lydia Grunstra and then Zachary Wagman. I also thank Anthea Lingeman, Victoria Pearson, proofreaders Toni Rachiele and Laura Starrett, and, most especially, copyeditor Fred Wiemer.

I am very appreciative for the reality check provided by my agent, Lynn Nesbit. I also thank her assistants, Tina Simms and Elexis Loubriel. And I am always grateful to Bennett Ashley for his outstanding legal and people skills.

I thank Jennifer Jacobs, MD, and Michael Carlston, MD, for their willingness to be part of this book and for patiently answering my many questions over the years. I especially thank Jennifer Jacobs for reading and commenting on parts of the manuscript-in-progress.

I thank Stephen Barrett, MD, for his time, and for reading certain sections of the manuscript.

Ah, the Bentley Historical Library at the University of Michigan. What a place, as I've described at the beginning of the "Sources" section. Thanks to the staff: Kathy Marquis, the chief reference archivist who guided me for the first few years, and then Karen Jania, who took over as Reference Division Head in 2003; Malgosia Myc, a very patient and kind reference division Associate Head who helped me locate elusive prints; reference assistants Stephanie Alvarez and Leigh Jasmer; and the long list of graduate and undergraduate students who performed searches and photocopying—Jeff Bradley, Riva Pollard, Lisa Klopfer, Rosalie Ehrlich, Jennifer Yerty, Jennifer DeCapua, Trent Margrif, Amanda Aikman, Ben Heller, Sarah Keen, and Rebecca Bizonet. I would also like to thank Suzanne Chapman of the University of Michigan Art, Architecture, and Engineering Library and David Michener of the Matthaei Botanical Gardens.

For their time or help or cooperation or ideas or suggestions, I'd like to thank the following people (and in a few cases, groups, Web sites, or institutions): Phil Adair; Alan D. Aviles (general counsel, New York City Health and Hospitals Corporation); Barbara

Barrie; Ethan Basch, MD; Dan Belin; June Bingham Birge; Susie Bluestone; Vivian Boucherit; the late Karen Broderson; Kenneth R. Cobb (director, New York City Municipal Archives); Elizabeth Cooke; Dean Crothers, MD; Shelly Dattner (for long friendship and for her sensitive reading of a draft of the manuscript); Cindy DeVine (the secretary-receptionist at the Evergreen Clinic—thanks particularly for describing Jennifer Jacobs's office to me); Raefer Gabriel; Kate Ganz; Murray Gell-Mann; Robin Goland, MD; the late Ray Golden; Google; Dan Green; Jane Green; Blu Greenberg; Sarah Gund, pal extraordinaire; Wendy Harpham, MD (for sending articles, being my best survivor friend); Amy Hertz; Dalma Heyn; the Homeopathic Research Network; Stephen Hovytowner (Costume Institute of the Metropolitan Museum of Art); Hamilton Jordan; Eric R. Kandel, MD; Carol Kitman; Marvin Kitman; Betty K. Koed (assistant historian, U.S. Senate Historical Office); Misia Landau; Martin Leib, MD (for taking the time to read the opthalmological sections); Janet Levitan, MD; Jenifer Lingeman, MD; Loansome Document Services; Shahin Lockman, MD; Christopher Lukas; Susan Lukas; Richard Marek; Norma McAllistar; Kate McCarthy (NIH CAM newsletter); Jay Meltzer, MD; Mount Sinai School of Medicine (interlibrary loans); Annie Navasky; Victor Navasky; the New York City Department of Health; the New York Public Library, Mosholu Branch; Hugh Nissenson (for his sense of detail); Kore Nissenson; Marilyn Nissenson; Sherwin Nuland, MD; Emilie Osburn, MD; Alison Pavia; Paul Perkus (director, Municipal Research Center); Steven Pinker; Leslie Ann Price (Case Western Reserve University—for helping me try to locate Raymond Potter, though I was ultimately unable to do so, even with a general nationwide search service); Allen Podraza (director, AMA Archives); Letty Cottin Pogrebin; Putney School Library; Joyce Ravid; Mary Calder Rower; Raphael Rudnik; the late Faith Sale; Wallace Sampson, MD; Peggy Shapiro; Roger Shapiro, MD; Ruben Shapiro, MD; Selma Shapiro; Elaine Silver; Celia Soto; Brad Spotts; the late Jake Stump, MD; Robert Tenuta (AMA reference archivist); Betsy Tunis (National Library of Medicine); Nancy Van Blaricum (Dexter Historical Library); Pamela van Wagenen; Mildred Vogel; Vivian Wallace; Pennell Whitney; Dr. Frank Wilczek; Robert Williamson; Ada Zambetti.

Index

Page numbers in *italics* refer to illustrations.

corneas, 115; transplanting of, 116; ulcers of, 43, 45
Cornell Medical School, 109, 110
cortisone, 223
Cosmotarianism, 182
coughs, 8, 13, 20, 43–4, 152
"Courtship of Miles Standish, The" (Longfellow), 25
cowpox, 6–7, 67
Cramp, Arthur J., 176, 179, 182–3, 189
cramps, 6, 58, 131, 211
Crick, Francis, 238
Crothers, Dean, 235, 238, 260–1, 269, 270, 280
Cuprum, 128, 131
Cushing, Harvey, 209
Cutting Cafe, 72

Dairymen's League, 157
dance therapy, 222
Dartmouth Medical School, 16
Davis, John W., 181
DDD, 195
deadly nightshade, xiii, 8
Democratic Party, 45, 63, 149, 165, 166–7, 184
depression, 37, 49, 69, 72–3, 236
Depression, Great, 195
Detroit Free Press, 63–4, 161
Detroit Homeopathic College, 29
Dewey, John, 200
Dewey, W. A., 66, 76, 79, 112, 128, 155, 281
Dexter, Maine, 3
Dexter, Mich., 11–15, *12,* 25, 29, 41, 42, 70, 82, 95, 163–5, 167; churches of, 4, 164, 218; commerce and business in, 4, 5, 14, 164–5; early settlers, 3–5
Dexter, Samuel William, 3, 25
Dexter High School, 23, 24, 26, 29, 187
Dexter Leader, 14
Dexter Poultry Company, 191
Dexter Savings Bank, 14
diabetes, 99, 161, 175, 224
diarrhea, 131, 237–8, 251, 254, 269–70, 274–5
Dickens, Charles, 15, 229
diet, 50, 123, 159; vegetarian, 144, 182
digestive problems, 37, 39, 129, 131
digitalis, 21, 69, 70, 152, 155, 244

diphtheria, 66, 129, 234
disease, xv, 81; bacterial, 5, 27–8, 51, 123, 137; body type and personality relating to, 28; contagious, 51, 151–5, 158–9, 170; germ theory of, 5, 27–8, 51, 212; mortality rates and, 129, 158; prevention of, 123, 128–9, 158–9; viral, 5, 46, 141
DNA, 238, 241, 243, 250
Doctor Copeland's Home Medical Book (Copeland), 211–13, 214
Domagk, Gerhard, 201
Domestic Kits, 11, 16, 20
Domestic Physician (Hering), 16
Dover's Powder, 68
Downing, Augustus, 119–20
Dr. Charles' Flesh Food, 53
Dr. John Sappington Anti-fever Pills, 5, 7
Dr. Royal S. Copeland Hour, 189–90, 195–6, 200
Dr. Town's Epilepsy Treatment, 195
drug addiction, 157–8
drug companies, 27, 34, 101
drugs, *see* medicines
Dudley, Pemberton, 68
Duncan, Charles, 140–1
dynamite, 33
dysentery, 137, 152

ear problems, xiii, 6, 21, 211, 271–2
Eclecticism, 7, 10, 20, 23, 28, 31, 54, 67, 75, 122, 138
Eddy, Mary Baker, 24
Einstein, Albert, 137
Eisfelder, Henry W., 239–40
elections, U.S.: of 1920, 167; of 1922, 166–7; of 1924, 181; of 1928, 190; of 1932, 197
electricity, 29, 30, 44, 46, 164–5; lighting with, 29, 30, 73, *90, 94;* treatments with, 73, 138, 145
electrocardiograph, 68
Ellis Island, 156–7
Elmaleh, Rebecca, 281–3
emotional problems, 37, 38, 39, 131; *see also* depression
enemas, 50, 69, 146
Enzymol, 138
epilepsy, 62, 122
Equal Rights Amendment, 218

Volstead Act, 152
Von's Pink Pills, 195

Wagner, Robert F., 219
Washington, D.C., 167–70, 180
Washington *Evening Star,* 218
water, 44, 144, 145, 146, 213; bottled, 136,
    263; mineral, 34, 136, 174–6, 192, *193,*
    201; radioactive, 197–9
War of 1812, 25
Watson, James, 238
Watson, Thomas, 137
Wayne State University, 230
Weadock, Thomas, 45
weakness, 6, 10, 155
Webster, Daniel, 25
weight loss, 145–6, 159, 169, *169*
Weil, Andrew, 264
Wesley, John, 42
What Is Homeopathy?, vii, 110–11
White, George Starr, 137–8
whooping cough, 129
Wilczek, Frank, 256
wild hops, 7, 13, 38, 48

Wiley, Harvey, 84, 135–6
Wilhelmina, Queen of Holland, 160–1
Wilson, Woodrow, 190
Wise, Stephen S., 200
women's suffrage, 169
Woodward, William, 209
World Health Organization (WHO),
    237, 249, 254, 268, 273
World War I, 134, 141, 143, 148, 190, 222
World War II, 222, 223, 225
Wright, A. E., 113–14
Wurtz, John G., 126, 127

x-rays, 46, 77, 79–80, 161

yarrow, 5, 126
"Your Health" column, 160–1, 162, 167,
    169, 181, 183, 189, 219
Your Money's Worth, 192

Zendajas, 195
zinc, 6

A Note on the Type

This book was set in Adobe Garamond. Designed for the Adobe Corporation by Robert Slimbach, the fonts are based on types first cut by Claude Garamond (c. 1480–1561). Garamond was a pupil of Geoffroy Tory and is believed to have followed the Venetian models, although he introduced a number of important differences, and it is to him that we owe the letter we now know as "old style." He gave to his letters a certain elegance and feeling of movement that won their creator an immediate reputation and the patronage of Francis I of France.

Composed by North Market Street Graphics
Lancaster, Pennsylvania
Printed and bound by Berryville Graphics,
Berryville, Virginia
Designed by Anthea Lingeman

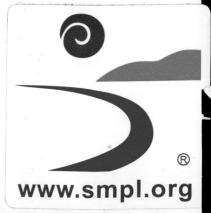